The International Behavioural and Social Sciences Library

SOCIAL ORIGINS
OF DEPRESSION

TAVISTOCK

The International Behavioural and Social Sciences Library

MIND & MEDICINE
In 6 Volumes

SOCIAL ORIGINS
OF DEPRESSION

A Study of Psychiatric Disorder in Women

GEORGE W BROWN AND
TIRRIL HARRIS

First published in 1978 by
Tavistock Publications Limited

Routledge
2 Park Square, Milton Park, Abingdon, Oxfordshire OX14 4RN
711 Third Avenue, New York, NY 10017

Routledge is an imprint of the Taylor & Francis Group

First issued in paperback 2011

British Library Cataloguing in Publication Data
A CIP catalogue record for this book
is available from the British Library

Social Origins of Depression
ISBN 978-0-415-26458-7 (hbk)
ISBN 978-0-415-51092-9 (pbk)
Mind & Medicine: 6 Volumes
ISBN 978-0-415-26512-6
The International Behavioural and Social Sciences Library
112 Volumes
ISBN 978-0-415-25670-4

Social Origins of Depression

A study of psychiatric disorder
in women

George W. Brown
and Tirril Harris

TAVISTOCK PUBLICATIONS

First published in Great Britain in 1978
by Tavistock Publications Limited
2 Park Square, Milton Park, Abingdon, Oxon, OX14 4RN

Phototypeset in V.I.P. Palatino

ISBN 0 422 76320 1

Study me then, you who shall lovers bee
At the next world, that is, at the next Spring;
   For I am every dead thing,
   In whom love wrought new Alchimie.
     For his art did expresse
A quintessence even from nothingnesse,
From dull privations, and leane emptinesse.
He ruin'd mee, and I am re-begot
Of absence, darknesse, death; things which are not.

JOHN DONNE
A Nocturnall Upon S. Lucies Day

Contents

V. Interpretation and conclusions

VI. Appendices

Acknowledgments

We report the results of a large-scale social enquiry – large in the sense of the questions asked, the time taken, and those who have been involved. We have been singularly fortunate in those who have worked with us and look back on the research with a great deal of pleasure. It is also a simple statement of fact that the research would not have been possible without the help of many people and in these acknowledgments we hope to convey not only our gratitude but the inevitable collaborative nature of such a research programme. Our pleasure in acknowledging this help is only clouded by the knowledge that we are bound in some way to fall short of recording the full extent of our debt.

The work has depended on the support of the Medical Research Council for most of its length. The Social Science Research Council gave us important support for the first community survey in Camberwell in 1969/71 and the survey in the Outer Hebrides in 1975. They also awarded one of us a Fellowship to enable full-time work on the material for a year. We also owe a great debt to the Foundations Fund for Research in Psychiatry, New Haven, who at an early stage of the work, at short notice, rescued us from financial difficulties.

From the start we have had close ties with psychiatric colleagues at the Institute of Psychiatry and have greatly valued their interest and support and their general tolerance of our not infrequent criticisms. Jim Birley who worked on earlier research with schizophrenia gave us encouragement and support when it was much needed at the beginning. John Cooper and John Copeland (who were then both working on the UK/US Diagnostic Project) encouraged us to go ahead with using for the first time the Present State Examination (PSE) in the general population survey. In this they were pioneers and we wish to acknowledge our debt for their intellectual and practical help. John Copeland collaborated closely during the first two years and did much of the clinical interviewing with the psychiatric patients and, with Michael Kelleher, also interviewed women in their homes in the first survey of Camberwell. Julian Leff, Sheila Mann, and John Wing of the Medical Research Council's Social Psychiatry Research Unit collaborated with us in the second Camberwell survey. Robert Kendell generously allowed us to examine in more detail some of the data he had collected for his important study of types of depression. The work has also depended on the good will of psychiatrists such as Douglas Bennett and Tony Isaacs, who work in Camberwell and who gave us permission to contact their patients and were always willing to give us help and advice. We are also particularly indebted to Una Macleod who encouraged us to extend the work to the Outer Hebrides and who joined us as a collaborator in our first survey in North Uist.

Then there are those colleagues with whom we have collaborated more closely and to whom we are, of course, particularly indebted.

Freda Sklair played an invaluable role in the developmental work in the first years of the programme and with Jennie Frankland did a great deal of the initial interviewing of patients. Much rested on their energy and enthusiasm. Freda Sklair and Sue Ulrich also helped with the interviewing in the first Camberwell survey. During the analysis of this material Julian Peto, although not a member of the team, devoted a good deal of time to helping us solve some difficult mathematical problems: Appendix 4 was written by him and we are grateful, not least, for the insights he gave us into such work. In 1971 Maire Ní Bhrolcháin joined us and made important contributions to the basic analysis. Some of her work on issues involving depressive symptomatology will be published separately, but her spirited determination during discussions of these with us was a major spur to the development of the theory in this book, and for this we are much indebted. In the second Camberwell survey we were helped by Janet Cabot, Sue Davidson, Marie Moyer, and Sue Pollock. Sue Davidson and Sue Pollock also helped in the North Uist survey and Sue Davidson played an important role – giving not only her assistance with the analysis but her patient support during the drafting of the book. In North Uist we also collaborated with Ray Prudo who contributed a great deal to the analysis of the psychiatric material and gave us the support necessary to use the psychiatric interview in a quite new setting. (Since then he has extended the full survey done in Camberwell to the island of Lewis – but this is not reported in this book.) We would also like to thank Elaine Murphy for her helpful advice about the psychiatric ratings. Sandra Cook has given us invaluable help in the final months of the analysis with the computer and rescued us from many difficulties. We have also been part of a wider group, the Social Research Unit of Bedford College, and have gained much from our colleagues and students. We are particularly indebted to Margot Jefferys who has supported us through various crises and been an unfailing source of encouragement; to David Tuckett for his painstaking criticisms of an earlier draft, and to Ray Fitzpatrick for his helpful comments. The Unit itself is part of the wider international research fraternity and many visitors from abroad have been a source of encouragement to us, particularly David Mechanic from the United States, Heinz Katschnig from Vienna, and Robert Finlay-Jones from Australia, whose comments on the early stages of the book were much appreciated. We must record a particular debt of gratitude to Pamela Bath, Christine Robson, Maureen Evans, and Sherry Seidel whose patience during the typing of the manuscript did much to keep us going. And special thanks must be given to Seija Sandberg and Nigel Harris who have had to live with the book through its various stages of development.

Finally, of course, we owe a debt of gratitude to the women themselves who have spoken to us with such openness and tolerance. Although we think, by and large, they were pleased to help us, we are sure that at times a number would have preferred not to have gone over painful memories. Some clearly were willing to do so because they thought our research might be useful and we hope we have to some degree justified this trust. Although they all knew we were to publish our findings, we, of course, have taken every step to disguise accounts of our interviews. All names are false and we have always changed enough of the basic circumstances to make it very difficult for anyone to recognize themselves. For their help we are most grateful.

Part I
Introduction

1 Sociology and the aetiology of depression

It is common for social investigators to justify their work in terms of the extent and importance of the problem they have tackled. Although their assertions are for the most part politely accepted, in time, as claims accumulate scepticism is inevitable. We are therefore diffident about beginning by asserting the particular significance – in scope and severity – of the condition we have chosen to study, clinical depression. But since we do believe that it is common – at least in urban centres – and that it is peculiarly unpleasant we feel obliged to confront the understandable scepticism that now tends to be evoked by yet another indictment of our way of life. There is good reason to believe that depression is not just another problem but a central link between many kinds of problem – those that may lead to depression and that may follow from it. It is not only, for instance, closely linked to poor housing; it is also highly correlated with a whole range of serious physical disorders. Our claim for the significance of the condition is, therefore, based on its pivotal position in the explanation of what is wrong with our society. For, as we will argue later, while we see sadness, unhappiness, and grief as inevitable in all societies we do not believe that this is true of clinical depression.

It was in order to establish clearly that depression did hold this pivotal position that we chose to study it. There is a long history of sociological concern with the aetiological role of psychosocial factors in medical conditions. C. Wright Mills in *The Sociological Imagination* argued that the relation of 'personal troubles' to 'public issues of social structure' was *the* central feature of all classical work in social science. Sociology has been concerned not only with the workings of social systems as a whole, but with the impact they have on individuals caught up in them. One thing sociology seeks from its collaboration with medicine is new ways of looking at such effects – how far is psychiatric or physical disorder the result of living in a particular form of domestic, economic, and political society? This interest can, of course, be seen in Durkheim's *Suicide* published in 1897 and in Marx's concern not only with an understanding of capitalist society but with its influence on the health and well-being of the individual.

In seeking to relate 'personal troubles' to 'public issues of social structure' there has been a difference of emphasis. There is a long and highly complex series of links between economic, cultural, and political systems and their eventual impact on particular individuals. We have concentrated on demonstrating that there *is* a link between clinical depression and a woman's daily experiences, in the belief that once this is done we will be in a stronger position to sort out the intricate links with wider structures. Other writers have shown, understandably, a greater initial concern with these wider links – say the relation between social mobility, ethnic background, and disorder (Dohrenwend and Dohrenwend, 1969). But it is a matter of emphasis – our work, we believe, already indicates something about these wider ramifications.

Given that we start with a woman's immediate experiences, where should a sociologist look for social 'facts' capable of influencing psychiatric and physical disorder? Cigarette smoking is without doubt linked to lung cancer, yet there is an important social component that increases a person's chance of smoking – that is of contacting the aetiological agent. A schoolchild, for example, may take to cigarette smoking not because it is enjoyed but because of the value it is given by his friends. One way to proceed, therefore, is to study the process by which such factors influence chances of contact with a pathological agent. The model of disease underlying this approach suggests that social factors influence alcohol consumption, cigarette smoking, and sexual behaviour but thereafter play no role in the aetiology of cirrhosis, cancer, or venereal disease – these are brought about by essentially mechanical means. A person's *awareness* of the environment plays no causal part once contact between agent and host is made. Enthusiastic gardening may reduce a man's risk of coronary disease; but it will do this whatever his feelings – whether he loves, hates, or is indifferent to the activity (Morris *et al.*, 1973). It is only important that he should do it.

This is not the only way to proceed. Consider a study by Meyer and Haggerty (1962) of sore throats in the children of fifteen middle-class families. Throat cultures were made every two or three weeks over the course of a year and at times of any obvious throat infection. By means of regular three-weekly interviews and diaries kept by the mother, events that disrupted family or personal life were recorded. Three measures of 'disorder' were then used: illness associated with streptococci, a new streptococcal culture *without* overt illness, as well as non-streptococcal respiratory infections. All three were about four times more likely to be preceded by than followed by a distressing event, such as witnessing a bad road accident or a father losing his job. They were also more likely in the context of 'chronic family stress'. Since events were recorded independently of any knowledge of the acquisition of streptococci *without* illness, the result is unlikely to be due to bias and there is thus a case to be made that emotional and physical factors combined in some way to produce illness. It is not just that social factors in some way brought the child in contact with streptococci, but that they lowered his resistance to them once contact was made.

We are not in this study concerned with the way social factors lead to increased risk of contact with a physical agent but with the possibility of a more direct involvement of the social environment in disorder. With such an approach it is not even essential for there to be a physical agent such as streptococci. Physical and psychiatric disorder may be produced by cognitive and emotional response alone (although there must, of course, always be a bodily basis to the disorder itself). Sociologists, we believe, have most to contribute in this second approach to aetiology: they can investigate whether something such as enforced rehousing can raise the chance of developing psychiatric disorder, irrespective of the physical changes involved. They will be concerned not just with the fact that as the result of rehousing a housewife walks further to the shops or sees fewer friends *but with how she perceives and reacts emotionally to these changes.*

Sociologists are not alone in taking this perspective and no one has found it easy to translate into effective research. It may therefore be useful to begin by discussing aetiological research in psychiatry in general terms. At the risk of drawing too sharp a distinction we will refer to the intensive or clinical, and the survey or epidemiological approaches. Since we will argue that the two should be brought much more closely together, we begin by emphasizing their differences. The clinical or intensive approach concentrates on the individual. Detailed knowledge of the person and his disorder allows the investigator to make sense of the meaning that the symptoms have for him. This is its strength. The snag is that this very detail makes it difficult to move beyond the individual case. The statistical survey has the reverse problem. Comparability tends to be maintained at the expense of ignoring much of the complexity of the individual. Sociology has traditionally been concerned both with the outside world (for example, with rates of migration) and with inner experiences (what the migrant makes of his new country). It has, therefore, straddled somewhat uneasily both intensive and survey approaches, although throughout its history there have been strong pressures from within the discipline for it to move one way or the other.

The clinical approach

Freud serves as an example of the strengths of an intensive approach. He was concerned with biographical detail. Consider the way he dealt with the question of aetiology in his *Introductory Lectures on Psychoanalysis*. (He is discussing a woman who had developed a delusion of jealousy about her husband after receiving an anonymous letter.)

'There are delusions of the most varied content: why in our case is the content of the delusion jealousy in particular? In what kind of people do delusions, and especially delusions of jealousy, come about? We should like to hear what the psychiatrist has to say about this; but at this point he leaves us in the lurch. He enters into only a single one of our inquiries. He will investigate the woman's family history and will *perhaps* give us this reply: "Delusions come about in people in whose families similar and other psychical disorders have repeatedly occurred." In other words, if this woman developed a delusion she was predisposed to it by hereditary transmission. No doubt that is something but is it all we want to know? Was this the only thing that contributed to the causation of the illness? Must we be content to suppose that it is a matter of indifference or caprice or is inexplicable where a delusion of jealousy arises rather than any other sort? And ought we to understand the assertion of the predominance of the hereditary influence in a negative sense as well – that no matter what experiences this woman's mind encountered she was destined some time or other to produce a delusion? . . . But can psychoanalysis do more here? Yes, it actually can. I hope to be able to show you that, even in a case so hard of access as this, it can discover something which makes a first understanding possible. And to begin with I would draw your attention to the inconspicuous detail that the patient herself positively provoked the anonymous letter, which now gave support to her delusion, by informing the scheming housemaid on the previous day that it would cause her the greatest unhappiness if her husband had a love affair with a young girl. In this way she first put the notion of sending the anonymous letter into the housemaid's head. Thus the delusion acquires a certain independence of the letter; it had been present already in the patient as a fear – or was it as a wish? Let us now add to this the small further indications yielded by only two analytical sessions . . . She herself was intensely in love with a young man, with the same son-in-law who had persuaded her to come to me as a patient. She herself knew nothing, or perhaps only a very little, of this love; in the family relationship that existed between them it was easy for this passionate liking to disguise itself as innocent affection. After all our experiences elsewhere, it is not hard for us to feel our way into the mental life of this upright wife and worthy mother, of the age of fifty-three. Being in love like this, a monstrous and impossible thing, could not become conscious; but it remained in existence and, even though it was unconscious, it exercised a severe pressure. Something had to become of it, some relief had to be looked for; and the easiest mitigation was offered, no doubt, by the mechanism of displacement which plays a part so regularly in the generating of delusional jealousy. If not only were she, the old woman, in love with a young man, but if also her old husband were having a love affair with a young girl, then her conscience would be relieved of the weight of her unfaithfulness. The phantasy of her husband's unfaithfulness thus acted as a cooling compress on her burning wound.'

(Freud, 1971: 251–53)

Although this is only one case, a 'first understanding' is possible and the interpretation of the delusion carries a good deal of conviction. And yet the questions he raises have never been systematically answered. We do not know what kinds of people have such delusions; nor do we know whether delusions arise in a particular person at some time irrespective of their experience. Nor, indeed, can we have any confidence about the causal link he asserts between conflict and delusion. To answer these questions we would have to know how often married women in general fall in love with close relatives (or were involved in some comparable 'impossible and monstrous thing') and how often delusions followed. These frequencies could show whether women with delusions of jealousy were more likely to have experienced such a conflict than those without them. *This cannot be done without studying a good number of instances of what is to be explained*. And with this we are brought to the central problem of aetiological research. If we are to deal with more than one instance, it is necessary to settle what is to count as an 'impossible and monstrous thing'. If this is not done before we begin to *test* our ideas, it is easy to fit fact to theory or at least to be seen to do so: to see 'monstrous things' when we know there is neurosis and not to see them when there is no neurosis. If psychoanalysis had been able to make this one step, it would have moved itself some way away from accusations of pseudo-science. But the step is not easy and has not been taken. That it has not is understandable; it would be too easy to lose the very thing that is important about an intensive approach, a sense of the uniqueness of experience for the individual. But, for whatever reason, psychoanalysis has never seriously put its mind to the task. The same could be said for much else in psychiatry; but we will stay with psychoanalysis as it illustrates all the problems of bringing together intensive and survey approaches. Freud was continually faced with the impact of the environment. Indeed, early in his work he viewed seduction and assault in childhood to be a crucial aetiological factor in sexual neurosis. A major change in his thinking occurred when he came to see the majority of these events as fantasies. At this stage his interest appears to have turned almost exclusively to matters of internal workings of the mind; he no longer appeared to be much concerned with actual experience:

> 'I believe these *primal phantasies*, as I should like to call them, and no doubt a few others as well, are a phylogenetic endowment. In them the individual reaches beyond his own experience into primaeval experience at points where his own experience has been too rudimentary. It seems to me quite possible that all the things that are told to us today in analysis as phantasy – the seduction of children, the inflaming of sexual excitement by observing parental intercourse, the threat of castration (or rather castration itself) – were once real occurrences in the primaeval times of the human family, and that children in their phantasies are simply filling in the gaps in individual truth with prehistoric truth.'
>
> (Freud, 1974: 418)

The point has often been made that the ability of the approach to explain any set of findings in terms of such general formulations gives psychoanalysis the hallmark of pseudo-science – nothing is seriously tested (e.g. Cioffi, 1970). While we believe this to be essentially correct, such criticism tends to place too little weight on the importance of the insights obtained by Freud and his followers – and the possibility, when viewed historically, that their achievements would have been impossible without some way of lightening the onerous duty of continually seeking the refutation of ideas. However, be this as it may, psychoanalysis has for the most part followed Freud's style of work and failed to subject aetiological ideas to serious test. It has continued to hold a highly ambivalent attitude to the real world – both in terms of *what* actually happened and its *timing*. There are certainly great difficulties in translating occurrences in the world into effects on the mind, but to remain largely concerned with internal mental processes must mean giving up a precious chance of subjecting aetiological ideas to empirical test.

A psychoanalyst is likely to object that it *is* the internal workings of the mind that are important, though perhaps set off by external events. Even if this is so, it is possible that internal processes can be approximately parallelled by happenings in the world. We use the term 'approximate' in the sense that generalizations may be possible when the data for a number of individuals is viewed statistically; and this may be quite enough to provide a causal framework or model to which clinical interpretations can be linked. While much could be said in defence of psychoanalysis and linked clinical work (e.g. Cosin, Freeman and Freeman, 1971), there seems no escape from the bald conclusion that case studies cannot provide a means of selecting between alternative ideas about aetiology, and the orthodoxies that have grown up about such work have veiled this issue with dogmatism. At some stage theories have to be subjected to test. If ideas about aetiology are to be tested we must have some way of moving from such therapy-based interpretations of the individual. To be more specific: we must deal with the meaningfulness of experience for the individual without leaving ourselves open to the accusation that we have simply imposed our interpretations *post hoc*.

The survey or epidemiological approach

Epidemiological surveys usually consider the distribution of a disorder within a definite population and relate it to factors such as age, sex, social class, and place of residence. Durkheim, for instance, related rates of suicide to institutional and general features of societies as a whole – marriage, family life, widowhood, and religion. He sought in them signs of social malaise arising from industrialization and the decay of traditional society. His well-known concepts of 'egoism' and 'anomie' fitted into his general theme of the weakening of social bonds. Durkheim's *Suicide* remains a superb example, despite shortcomings, of the power of the survey method to move from correlations (that depression is more common among women who are widowed) to statements about causality (that widowhood can bring about depression). Unfortunately this does not mean that the survey has no deficiencies. Curiously, one of its greatest failures is where, at first acquaintance, it might appear to be strongest: in measurement – the placing of like with like. In discussing Freud's patient with delusions of jealousy we indicated that a central problem was to be able to settle, in a systematic way, which happenings were, for instance, the 'impossible and monstrous things' capable of provoking such conflict. Nothing need be said of the likely shortcomings of official statistics (say of suicide) so often used in survey research. But as an alternative source of material, research workers have almost entirely relied on administrating to large numbers of people some form of the standardized questionnaire, with its dispiriting pretensions to measure almost anything by means of a few, often fixed-choice, questions:

> 'Continuing refinements of the structured questionnaire with efforts to eliminate interviewer bias can lead us up a blind alley – when carried to an extreme we will conclude that the best interviewer is a tape recorder containing the questions and the best recorder of replies a second tape recorder. A questionnaire addressed to the subject of the research which becomes very highly refined and standardised in its administration so as to allay our anxieties about interviewer bias may very well throw away the most valuable characteristic of the interviewer, his humanity.'
>
> (Gruenberg, 1963: 590–91)

Although used in almost all large-scale sociological enquiries, there must be the gravest doubt about the ability of such questionnaires to collect accurate and unbiased accounts of anything complex or of emotional depth. They are of little use in tackling the task of measurement highlighted by Freud's case example. It is not too dramatic to assert that much that has been done in the social sciences must be under question, because such questionnaires cannot be trusted to have placed like with like. This will become clear in later chapters.

Failure has not been, however, just a matter of inaccurate and biased measurement. Even when entirely accurate, much that has been measured has been only a most distant indicator of what might be at work in bringing about the disorder. Suchman some years ago in discussing stress and cardiovascular disease made the point that in social research:

> 'nothing is as sterile as demographic group comparisons. Rates analysed in relation to such categories as sex, age, race, marital status, occupation and geographical region are an essential part of the social book-keeping of modern society. In and of themselves, however, these rates offer little by way of explanation. If one's purpose is to explain the relation between demographic factors and coronary heart disease, one cannot help but get lost in a morass of inconclusive correlations . . . Where does the fault lie? The answer is probably to be found in the essential meaninglessness of gross demographic population categories when viewed as "causal" var-

iables indicative of social processes. These may be convenient, easily studied labels for subdividing populations, but they are not dynamic social ideas and cannot, except in a very limited superficial sense, represent the kind of social phenomena that may cause disease or anything else.' (Suchman, 1967: 110)

Brenner (1971, 1975), in an analysis of fluctuations in death rates for heart disease and alcohol-related disorders such as cirrhosis, shows an average two to three-year delay between peaks of unemployment in the United States and the death rate peaks for these disorders. He favours a link between rates of unemployment and the raised death rates. But as Eyer (1977) has pointed out, since the business cycle itself is about four years long on average, it is possible to see the peak of death from heart disease and death from cirrhosis coinciding with the boom of the cycle. And this, of course, is a very different emphasis. Eyer argues against any kind of delayed effect and for a direct response to the consequences of social stresses inherent in an economic boom. But this could not be tested and it is a typical impasse reached by much survey-type research. In Suchman's terms, because gross variables are used, we have no way of knowing how a boom impinged on the individual – did those who died tend to work longer hours, see less of their families, drink more, feel under conflict, show signs of strain, and so on? And how did others who experienced similar changes react? Did they also react adversely – though in other ways? But it is important not to over-state the point. Brenner's analysis does have an element of the dynamic social ideas called for by Suchman. It is not that 'demographic type' measures are of no use, it is that they are not enough. What is required is their *combination* with concepts and measures dealing directly and in detail with the immediate (not necessarily contemporaneous) experience of the individual.

Edward Shils sees the same problem from a somewhat different viewpoint. In a discussion of the history of sociology he notes:

'The unity which transcends specialisation in sociology rests on this common devotion to a relatively small number of "key words". That unity is very expensively purchased. The key words and the ideas which they evoke have become inexpungibly enmeshed in the sociological tradition, so much so that they can never be merely an honorific decoration. They have become constitutive of sociological analysis. But the fact remains that they weigh like an Alp on the sociological mind. Theory is recognized as such by the presence of those alpine key words in all their misty and simple grandeur. This is not good enough. Sociology needs a much more differentiated set of categories, a much more differentiated set of names for distinguishable things. It must name many more things and name them in agreed and recognizable ways. The "slippage" between "concepts" and "indicators" must be reduced by increasing and refining the variety of "concepts".'   (Shils, 1970: 819)

We need to translate concepts such as 'alienation' and 'anomie' into measures that reflect, albeit often indirectly, recognizable experiences of the individual.

So far we have concentrated on some of the weaknesses of the survey. Its ability to test ideas about aetiology is beyond dispute. Its basic design can be used to compare individuals who have developed disorder with those who have not, in order to isolate 'factors' of causal importance. It does not have to rely on an experimental design to do this, although the underlying logic of its approach is the same as that found in experimental work (see Campbell and Stanley, 1966; Susser, 1973; Rosenberg, 1968). Since the extent to which a survey can reap these benefits is largely dependent on the calibre of its measures we will turn to a less well recognized strength – the way it facilitates the generation of new ideas. Unlike the case of intensive research, this feature of the survey tends to be overlooked. Particularly important is the way new ideas can emerge as part of the *ongoing* job of testing aetiological propositions. Also valuable is the impetus it can give us to leave ideas rather than to stay with them, often the crucial step in creative work. Once developed, ideas (such as Freud's views about the role of fears of castration in neurosis) tend to be held tenaciously; without the unremitting pressure of dissenting data it is surprisingly difficult to give them up. Gruber illustrates this in his fascinating analysis of Darwin's *Notebooks*: how patently inconsistent ideas were entertained for many years, apparently obvious ideas not taken up, and obvious deductions not made. The apparently brilliant insight was so often anticipated that its eventual formulation appeared all but inevitable:

'If scientific thought moved more swiftly, perhaps we could single out a characteristic type of sequence of great creative import, such as "first theorize, then observe" – or the reverse. But in a long process, carried out by a living person, many different sorts of act occur repeatedly in different sequences, and, since each act may itself be prolonged and interrupted by other acts, important acts sometimes occur in parallel with each other, extended over the same period of time'   (Gruber, 1974: 123)

In survey research there can be the same lengthy cross-fertilization of data and ideas. New variables are introduced, usually one or two at a time, into existing data. Are widows living with children less likely to commit suicide than those living alone? And in the light of the answer new questions arise to be tested. What about widows who have never had children or those with children living nearby? Since possible tabulations of possible factors probably run into millions, it is never a matter of learning what is there: there has to be selection – hopefully guided by theory – of what is looked at. Worrying about data that so often appears to go round in circles can take years. One of the destructive results of the new computer technology is that it can brutally cut short this interweaving of evidential and theoretical activity.

An interesting point made by Gruber's analysis of Darwin's *Notebooks* is that significant advances do not necessarily, or even usually, come from an entirely new idea as such. (Given the amount of speculation in psychiatry about causality it is probably difficult in any case to have an entirely new idea!) As important as a new idea is the combination of existing ideas in a novel way. The survey approach with its tradition of looking at a number of factors simultaneously in relation to the dependent variable (e.g. suicide) seems particularly well-suited to suggest such insights:

> 'It is a serious error to suppose that the main features of a complex idea are adequately characterised by the more elementary ideas which make it up. If that were the case, the discovery of a new component idea and its introduction into a theoretical structure would always be the most prominent kind of event in the growth of the complex structure.
> In fact, however, very profound changes in the nature of a complex idea may depend mainly on the rearrangement of its components to form a new structure.'   (Gruber, 1974: 156)

We have discussed in very general terms some of the strengths and weaknesses of the survey; it has great potential but, with some notable exceptions, its promise has not been fulfilled. At this point it may be useful to discuss more fully particular epidemiological studies of psychiatric disorder. We have chosen two of the best and in our comments we intend in no way to detract from their importance or depreciate their achievements.

Two epidemiological studies of psychiatric disorder

The Midtown survey found that 23 per cent of a sample of 1,660 inhabitants close to the centre of New York were psychiatrically *impaired*. In the first report, *Mental Health in the Metropolis*, a series of demographic variables including age, sex, marital status, parental and own socio-economic status, rural-urban origins, and religious affiliation were related to the prevalence of psychiatric disorder (Srole *et al.*, 1962). A second volume related psychiatric disorder to factors that are part of the biographical experience of the individual (Langner and Michael, 1963). Past influences were: parental physical and mental health, childhood health, a broken home, parental quarrelling and disagreement, childhood economic deprivation, and the way the person perceived parental character; and in the present they were: work worries, socio-economic worries, the adequacy of interpersonal affiliations, and marital and interpersonal worries. This information was collected by standard questions and is of somewhat dubious worth; the reporting of parental character and even parental health, for instance, may clearly have been influenced by the psychiatric state of the respondent, the very phenomenon under study. But, leaving this to one side, the findings in the second volume are intriguing because they show that, although biographical factors relate quite highly to psychiatric disturbance, they do not explain its association with a lower social-class background.

The various biographical factors were used in a combined stress score, which showed a consistent association with psychiatric impairment: the mere *numbers* were important rather than any particular combination (Srole *et al.*, 1962: 377). Events in the life history seem to 'pile up' bringing with them increasing impairment, rather than there being one factor that by itself automatically spells mental disorder for those who experience it. However, these biographical factors were only very modestly associated with parental socio-economic status. Lower-class persons did report somewhat more 'adult' stresses, but no more from childhood (Srole *et al.*, 1962: 151). The surprising conclusion is that those in the low-status groups show greater psychiatric impairment *even when the number of stress factors experienced is controlled*. Therefore, even if the measures are accepted without question, they fail to explain the association between social class and psychiatric disorder. Although there was a sizeable association between social-class background and disorder, there was no understanding of the reason for the correlation. In terms of our previous discussion the link between social structure and the individual remained completely open.

The second survey, of a Canadian maritime population, involved a good deal of ethnographic field-work, and yet the links made between the individual and the wider social structure are on the whole no more convincing (Leighton, 1959; Hughes *et al.*, 1960; Leighton *et al.*, 1963). In spite of the descriptive material collected in the ethnographic surveys, much of the third volume containing results consists of speculations about demographic associations. About sex differences in psychiatric disturbance they comment:

'Certainly an outstanding characteristic among all the welter of changes in modern times is alteration of the sentiments of and toward women and in the roles open to and expected of them. There are similar changes for men, but they are not on the whole of the same magnitude. One may also note that men are affected by the changing position of women because they are husbands, brothers, sons and fathers of the women who are touched by their problems. This latter no doubt takes its toll, but it is not the same thing as being in the direct line of fire.' (Leighton et al., 1963: 366)

Altered attitudes to women were not measured and it is, in any case, difficult in such general comments to sense much hint of the dynamic social ideas called for by Suchman. Nonetheless this survey is a good deal more sophisticated than most and it does go some way to test its core notion that the social disintegration of a community or village is related to its rate of psychiatric disorder. (Indicators of social disintegration were economic inadequacy, cultural confusion, widespread secularization, few and weak group associations, few and weak leaders, few patterns of recreation, high frequency of crime and delinquency, high frequency of broken homes, high frequency of interpersonal hostility, and a weak and fragmented network of communications (Leighton et al., 1963: 26)).

For a crucial test two communities were picked out (by local informants) as outstandingly high on integration and three as outstandingly disintegrated. Results were in the expected direction although one of the two integrated communities was close in its rate of disorder to the less integrated areas (see Leighton et al., 1963: figure 19, 331).

The authors are fully aware that the most parsimonious interpretation of these results is that the differences are due to long-term selective processes. The disintegrated villages had been economically depressed for a long period: it is likely that more 'disintegrated personalities' failed to move elsewhere. However, it is unlikely to be the sole explanation. Alexander Leighton (1965) in a separate paper has described one of the disintegrated and depressed villages, which after 1950 gradually reached a state of comparative independence and self-sufficiency. At the turn of the century it suffered a major loss of economic support, and, although some inhabitants moved, enough remained to perpetuate the community. At the time of the first survey there was severe poverty, and the families showed a high rate of broken marriage, parental quarrelling, and child neglect. In spite of the smallness of the village there was a surprising degree of isolation between families. After the initial survey social conditions began to improve, including employment opportunities. Correlated with the changes there was an overall reduction in psychiatric disorder so that by the second survey, fifteen years later, the community's rate was the same as that of the county as a whole. While material on the *same* individuals is not reported, it seems likely that there had been a real change in the amount of psychiatric disorder, suggesting that in spite of the possibility that the more healthy had moved away, environmental factors are important in actually producing or alleviating psychiatric disorders.

Overall reaction to the study, given the years of effort that went into it, is a sense of disappointment. Measurement of psychiatric disorder leaves much to be desired, social factors are poorly specified, and the disintegrated communities so profoundly underprivileged that the generality of any finding must be in doubt. But most of all there is disappointment that studies based on interviews with respondents (and intensive ethnographic field-work) should give so little sense of how the disorders are grounded in their day-to-day lives. Both this and the Manhattan study fail to close the gap between 'social structure' and individual disorder. Of particular interest, therefore, are studies – so far rare – that combine some of the features of survey and more intensive, case-like, research.

We have already mentioned Meyer and Haggerty's study. This was in a number of ways a landmark: while the size of the effect was modest, it demonstrated that the onset of a particular illness could be linked to the day-to-day lives of those studied. One consequence of such an approach is to force both investigator and reader into serious concern with causal issues. The issues that demand to be settled are both more obvious than in larger enquiries and apparently more tractable. Did the event really come before the sore throat? Perhaps it was the effects the crisis had on the change in daily routines (meal-times, etc.) rather than the emotional effects of the event as such for the child? Meyer and Haggerty's study can answer some of these questions and not others. It still lacks much of the convincing detail of the more clinical type enquiry; and it fails to relate the details of daily life that it did collect to wider societal phenomena such as social class. However, the impetus to explore further is there. What is needed is work on larger population groups and the development of theory about what is going on within the immediate social milieu of the person, investigating whether this links, and in what way, to broader social processes.

This sums up our review so far. Social research has by and large so far failed to link in a persuasive and testable way broad social categories (social class and sex), intervening processes (e.g. sex roles), proximal causes (e.g. major crises such as loss of a confidant) and disorder (e.g. depression). However, a number of studies begin to show how this might be done.[1]

Should we study illness or illnesses?

So far we have tended to concentrate on the methodological weaknesses of aetiological research. In a recent authorative review Cassel allocates greater blame to theoretical shortcomings:

> 'Despite increased efforts, however, attempts to document the role of social factors in the genesis of disease have led to conflicting, contradictory, and often confusing results. There is today no unanimity of opinion that social factors are important in disease etiology, or, if they are, which social processes are deleterious, how many such processes there are, and what the intervening links between such processes and disturbed physiologic states may be. In part this unsatisfactory state of affairs is a function of the methodologic difficulties inherent in such studies, particularly the difficulties of measuring in any precise form such relatively intangible processes. To a larger extent, and underlying these methodologic difficulties are, I believe, inadequacies in our theoretical or conceptual framework.'   (Cassel, 1974: 471)

While Cassel is perhaps a shade too pessimistic about what has been achieved, his argument is persuasive and it leads aetiological research in a rather different direction to our own.

He argues that we have been led astray by the role micro-organisms play in certain diseases. Following the classical model of tuberculosis and the tubercle bacillus, particular social stressors have been seen in research so far as leading to *particular* diseases. He argues instead that social stressors raise susceptibility to disease in general and we should, therefore, begin to study disease as a whole. There is evidence for this view. For instance a Swedish study looking at risk factors for heart disease, found, as expected, that factors such as raised serum cholesterol, smoking, and alcohol consumption were associated with a higher risk of death from ischemic heart disease, but they also found that these same factors increased risk of *any* early death (Tibblin, Keys and Werkö, 1971). Syme notes that although New York and California have higher coronary rates than North Dakota and Nebraska, the proportionate mortality from coronary heart disease in these states is about equal. North Dakota and Nebraska have low death rates from coronary heart disease, but their all-cause death rate is also low. He suggests that the problem is not to explain why New York and California have a higher *coronary* rate than North Dakota and Nebraska, but why New York and California have a higher *death rate* as a whole than North Dakota and Nebraska (Syme, 1967: 176). In spite of this kind of evidence we disagree with Cassel's emphasis. First, such a general effect, even if it exists, is not without important exceptions. We will show for instance that *different* kinds of life-event influence the onset of schizophrenia and depressive disorders. We also make clear that this could not have been demonstrated if 'depression' and 'schizophrenia' had been lumped together in some general category of 'psychiatric disorder'. Much the same may well occur for physical disorders (e.g. Cobb and Rose, 1973). At present disorders seem best combined only after it is established that they have aetiological factors in common.

Our second objection can be illustrated by Cassel's own examples. He notes that a 'remarkably similar set of circumstances characterize people who develop tuberculosis and schizophrenia, alcoholics, victims of multiple accidents, and suicides'. Common to all of these people is a 'marginal status in society'. Leaving aside the question of evidence for this statement (which is poor) the concept of 'marginal status in society' is remarkably general and so vague that it could encompass both a link between, say, social isolation and suicide, and one between overcrowding and schizophrenia. Isolation and overcrowding are probably both characteristics of 'marginal status in society', but can hardly be said to represent a common social stressor. Before this could be claimed more specific causal links would need to be established – a point already made in general and in relation to the Midtown and Nova Scotia studies. The present point is that there must be a danger that only the broadest and vaguest social measures are likely to show associations across a wide range of disorder.

So far this discussion may be met largely by agreement from our colleagues in the social sciences. But our critique of Cassel leads to a position where we may well differ from most. We have concentrated largely on one psychiatric condition (depression) and in order to do this we have taken the existing framework of psychiatric diagnostic classification seriously.

Brewster Smith, a relatively moderate critic, argues that in using diagnostic categories we are captives of a metaphorical clinical terminology that, for good reasons, became current in a social context different from the one we now face, and that it

'leads us to a continued preoccupation with symptoms and syndromes, to a strategic commitment to the search for disease entities, to the appraisal of human effectiveness in terms of the sum of a person's symptom-like liabilities with inadequate attention to the concurrent sum of his strengths . . . The health-and-disease model also biases us toward a pre-emptive concern with the individual organism, so to speak in vitro, and, by extension, with intrapsychic processes. It predisposes us to neglect the context of structured social relations in which effectiveness or ineffectiveness is displayed, which contributes to their genesis, and which must be dealt with by programmes of intervention that aim at increasing the balance of effectiveness.'   (Smith, 1974: 124)

The argument, as far as it goes, is convincing: concern with symptoms and syndromes has been associated with a gross neglect of the role of the current environment and a person's possible strengths in combatting it. Psychiatrists come to their work after a long training in physical medicine and most are concerned to find a physical basis for the major psychiatric disorders. Diagnostic practices have been caught up in this basic concern. But it does not follow that this is an inevitable consequence of concern with diagnosis: all that it is necessary to rectify the situation *is not to allow it to happen*. Classification (a major job of diagnosis) can be used in support of *any* explanation of psychiatric phenomena.[2] This can be seen in the continued use of diagnostic terms by some of psychiatry's foremost critics. R. D. Laing, in spite of his acerbic strictures, still uses the term schizophrenia – albeit with ill-grace. He does so, because like everyone else, he needs to communicate. Clinical work as well as research is impossible without a means of reducing the variety of psychiatric phenomena to a provisional order. This can only be done by classification. And once this is accepted, it would be foolish, in setting up a diagnostic system, to neglect the impressively detailed descriptive work by psychiatrists over the last century.

However, concern with diagnosis has created considerable confusion in psychiatry; not least in understanding the role of social factors in aetiology. Brian Cooper (1976) in a valuable review of the history of the concept of reactivity in psychiatry notes how:

'The 19th-Century preoccupation with specific disease-entities strongly influenced psychiatric thinking about aetiology. It was argued that, before a mental disease could be classed as exogenous, a necessary and sufficient external cause must be demonstrable in every case; if the external factors exercised a merely quantitative, or contributory effect, then the prime cause must be internal, and the disease an endogenous one. This line of argument inevitably weighted the scales in favour of an endogenous hypothesis, since the predisposing internal factors did not have to be demonstrated, whereas any supposed external factors did: in all cases of doubt, the onus of proof rested with the environmental hypothesis.'

While medical thinking has changed a good deal, traces of this kind of argument can still be found. However, use of diagnostic terms does not need to imply any view about aetiology. For example, the use of a diagnostic classification that discusses 'psychotic' and 'neurotic' *symptom patterns* in depression need not and should not initially imply anything about the presence of precipitating events, even though psychiatrists have traditionally assumed there is a link. Any such assumption is bound to lead to circularity in aetiological research. If one of the criteria for classifying someone as 'psychotically' rather than 'neurotically' depressed is the absence of a precipitating event, then it is bound to follow that research based on this criterion will pinpoint a connection between events and neurotic rather than psychotic depression. It is important to prune from the existing diagnostic categories *any* variables which are to be considered of possible aetiological importance (Blumenthal, 1971; Ní Bhrolcháin, 1977). Another common pitfall is the notorious unreliability of the diagnostic categories, which has been documented in a series of studies and recently highlighted by the study of British and American psychiatrists: it emerged that a large proportion of patients diagnosed as schizophrenic by American psychiatrists were diagnosed by British psychiatrists as suffering from depression (Cooper et al., 1972). Once again the answer to this is not to allow it to happen, but to strive for strict standards of reliability in establishing the boundaries of any category. There can be no doubt that this can be done – certainly in a research setting. If such pitfalls are avoided, the use of the conventional classification in aetiological research can be seen more optimistically as a process of refining and distilling the experience of a century of psychiatric experience. This has seemed preferable to attempting an independent contribution from outside psychiatry: one which would, even if successful, only with difficulty be integrated into the tradition and practice of those dealing with psychiatric disorder.

We therefore turn next to a discussion of the nature of the condition we have sought to explain – depression.[3]

2 Depression

It was with the considerations of the last chapter in mind that we set out to study a particular condition rather than psychiatric disorder in general and in doing so to take seriously existing psychiatric classifications of depression. We felt that, if we could guard against the obvious pitfalls we have discussed, any disadvantages would be far outweighed by the advantages of working within a tradition where our work would have meaning, and, just as important, be subject to informed criticism.

First of all we had to face the problem of 'illness behaviour' (cf. Mechanic, 1968; Tuckett, 1976). Very far from all instances of psychiatric and physical disorders receive treatment. There is also every likelihood that the reasons why some do not receive treatment are related to factors of aetiological significance (e.g. Mechanic and Newton, 1965). For instance, while caring for her young children may increase risk of various disorders it may at the same time inhibit a woman from seeking medical help. For this reason we determined to study untreated instances of depression which we expected to pick up in a random sample of the community, as well as women who were depressed and receiving different forms of medical care. It was thus not possible to rely solely on the definitions of depression of the various doctors and clinics; it became imperative to develop standards that we could use for depressed women who were not in treatment.

Another feature of the research, which perhaps needs some explanation, is its concentration on women. This stemmed not only from the decision to look at untreated depression but also from the decision to take as a comparision group a random sample of people without depression from the same community from which the patient group was drawn. In order to avoid bias, the sample not only had to be random but we also needed as many people as possible to agree to co-operate in what we knew would be a lengthy interview. The interviewer had to collect a great deal of social material as well as establish whether or not the women were suffering from a psychiatric disorder. Such an interviewing programme is expensive and one way to reduce its cost was to study women only, as they probably suffer from depression more often than men. Women usually form about two thirds of all depressed patients treated by psychiatrists (Silverman, 1968: 73; Wing and Hailey, 1972) and community surveys, at least in urban areas, have arrived at much the same conclusion regarding untreated depressive conditions, although it is less securely established (e.g. Warheit, Holzer and Schwab, 1973). If such findings were to be trusted, we would need to approach only half as many women as men to obtain the same number with depressive disorders. It also seemed likely that women, who are more often at home during the day, would be more willing to agree to see us for several hours, the time we needed to collect our material. The decision proved to be justified in the sense that we did find that depression was relatively common among women in Camberwell and that most of the women we approached were willing to talk to us at length about their lives and appeared to enjoy doing so.

Clinical depression versus depressed mood

With this general outline of the research it is now necessary to describe what we sought to explain: what does it mean to say that a woman is suffering from clinical depression? Psychiatrists all agree that it involves far more than a depressed mood. (It is of interest that the women we saw were far more likely to use terms such as 'nerves' about themselves than 'depression'.) Just how much more than a depressed mood is clinical depression? Aaron Beck has described its central core in terms of the self seeming worthless, the outer world meaningless, and the future hopeless, and many psychiatrists would probably agree with this. Most of us will have experienced these feelings if only briefly. We will also have a passing familiarity with many of the emotional and bodily phenomena associated with Beck's triad: the ease with which one can be reduced to tears by relatively trivial matters, a general and persistent feeling of sadness, the loss of interest in things and people normally dear and exciting, the restlessness and sense of being unable to settle into any task or decide upon small issues, the ease with which one feels tired and wearied. We may also have felt so self-disparaging and in such despair as to have entertained, even if not seriously, thoughts of suicide. But this very familiarity makes it all the more difficult to describe clinical depression. Is it, for example, merely a matter of intensity and duration of such easily recognized experiences? Or does it have a different quality? Is it, in other words, a question of different degrees of the same type of phenomena or of different types of phenomena that separates clinical depression from a disturbance of mood?

The answer is that there is no general agreement. In practice psychiatrists have given the name depression to a wide variety of clusters of symptoms. Although someone defined as clinically depressed would usually be expected to experience some of the changes of mood we have just outlined (crying, sadness, loss of interest, restlessness, and tiredness) accompanied in varying ways by other cognitive, somatic, and behavioural symptoms (feelings of guilt, sleep and appetite disturbance, social withdrawal, irritability, and so on) not even a depressed mood is considered as a necessary feature of the diagnosis. Patients who complain of loss of energy and interest, without feelings of sadness, guilt or futility, but with some of the other behavioural and somatic accompaniments are considered by many psychiatrists to be 'masked depressions' (for example, Watts, 1966; Sargant and Dally, 1962).

The variety of possible forms of clinical depression has been acknowledged by the subcategories described in the manual of the *International Classification of Diseases* (8th Revision). Its description of 'manic-depressive psychosis' suggests a disease that is more probably genetically transmitted, more likely to respond to a particular range of drugs (especially lithium) and more likely to alternate episodes of dysphoric mood with episodes of elation and frantic activity. The description of 'endogenous depression' suggests a depression that arises autonomously and is likely to have a larger number of somatic accompaniments than 'neurotic depression', which is considered more likely to be a response to certain environmental circumstances and to involve various behavioural features associated with nervousness. 'Reactive depressive psychosis' suggests a depression with the extreme features of the other psychotic depressions, such as 'endogenous depression', yet arising in response to circumstances. These different categories have, however, been assembled in an unsystematic way; and as can be seen, their defining characteristics subsume a number of dimensions that are neither exclusive nor exhaustive.

These subcategories of the *International Classification of Diseases* can also be criticized for confusing the business of classification with the search for causes and consequences in just the way we have already discussed in Chapter 1. Aetiological assumptions are included in the definitions rather than examined independently. If an apparent precipitating event is allowed to influence clinical classification, it becomes difficult, if not impossible, to establish whether, say, 'reactive depressive' conditions described in clinical terms are in fact more often brought about by environmental factors than other forms of depression. To assume this in the classification itself rules out the possibility of testing the assumption properly. In spite of these shortcomings, one distinction, that between 'neurotic' and 'psychotic' depression, deserves discussion. (The terms 'reactive' and 'endogenous' have been used at times to make much the same distinction.) A common debating point in psychiatry is whether they are separate entities or whether they represent two extremes of a continuum of symptoms with most cases of depression tending to fall somewhere in the middle. The issue in its formal aspects is similar to the focus of our present discussion, the distinction between clinical depression and an ordinary depressed mood. Are psychotic and neurotic depressive conditions qualitatively different? Or is there a dimension of symptoms along which a patient is more or less psychotic, less or more neurotic? Similarly is there a sharp qualitative distinction between a clinical depression and a badly depressed mood, or is it as impossible to specify when one becomes the other as it is to pinpoint the moment at which water becomes ice? A qualitative difference would make the conditions relatively easy to distinguish; if there is a continuum there is bound to be an element of arbitrariness in selecting a point at which they can be said to divide.

While the separation of clinical depression and depressed mood has received relatively little attention, that between psychotic and neurotic depression has been subjected to a great deal of research (e.g. Kendell, 1968; Kiloh and Garside, 1963). The distinction has proved to be important in our work and we will deal with it later in more detail. While there has been continued dispute about whether qualitatively different conditions are involved, hallucinations, delusions, agitation, retardation, weight loss, early morning waking, feeling worse in the morning (diurnal variation), and constipation seem generally to be judged as indicators of psychotic depression. Indicators for neurotic depression have been feeling worse in the evening, crying a great deal, being a worrying type of person, finding it hard to make decisions, as well as a variety of non-symptom features such as being younger, which we have already argued should be kept distinct in the development of the clinical classification itself.

Factors influencing psychiatric opinion about diagnosis

This lightning tour through some existing diagnostic categories of depression, illustrating the complex task of distinguishing whether a person is clinically depressed or just distressed or low, may have done more to confuse than to clarify. But there are still further complexities. While the *International Classification of Diseases* gives us some clue to the possible boundaries of clinical depression, many things influence diagnostic practice and, although it is impossible to document their precise influence, they merit some consideration. One is technical: the *perceived* effectiveness of currently available treatments. (Treatment does not necessarily have to be effective to influence clinical practice.) Therapeutic refinement can lead to diagnostic refinement. The fact that electroconvulsive therapy (ECT) seems to have some favourable influence on those depressions considered psychotic but not those considered neurotic is a powerful argument for the division, vague as it is, between the two types of depression. Similarly, the notion of 'masked depression' was originally developed because some patients with conditions resembling anxiety states responded well to anti-depressant drugs.

A further factor influencing diagnostic practice has probably been the increasing use of anti-depressant drugs by psychiatrists and general practitioners. Many who prescribe benzodiazepines or trycyclic drugs to tense and weepy women probably experience no philosophical struggle in deciding whether or not they are 'psychiatrically disturbed' but their activities might well be changing current opinion. One way of reacting to this is conservative: to argue that it is necessary to distinguish between a 'true' clinical depression (meaning the sort of depression that used to be given treatment before the new drugs became widely available) and a pseudo-clinical depression which is only 'clinical' in the sense that something can be done about it in a clinic. But it should be stressed that such a 'true' concept would have been developed in the first place as a result of a similar social process – the classifying of cases for whom clinicians were trying to do something. It would be absurd to suggest that pioneers such as Kraepelin, Freud, and their successors worked in a world in which they met the entire range of clinical conditions of possible relevance to psychiatry. Indeed, a third influence on the boundary drawn by psychiatrists around depressive conditions is just the social factors that determine the range of patients seen by them in their day-to-day practice and at what point in the course of their illness they see them (i.e. nosocomial influences – see Svendsen, 1952). There is every likelihood that psychiatrists tend to see only conditions that have reached a particular stage of development and rarely encounter the early phases – something that again will influence diagnostic practice. Who seeks treatment is influenced by public attitudes to 'mental illness', by the views of general practitioners about what is worthy of referral to a specialist, and, in addition, by political and economic factors that determine the development and distribution of psychiatric services. The expansion of out-patient psychiatric facilities means that the average psychiatrist today sees a different mix of patients from one practising twenty-five years ago. The present widespread use of psychotropic drugs by general pracitioners also means that the situation is still changing. As they gain greater confidence in using such drugs, general practitioners are likely to refer fewer patients with 'straightforward' affective disorders and relatively more with affective conditions who have also troublesome long-term 'personality' and 'neurotic' difficulties. Ingham and Miller (1976) have recently published a discussion of this filtering process and emphasized the need to study persons at every stage of the referral procedure. We have attempted to do this by considering in-patients, out-patients, patients attending general practitioners, and an unselected sample of women in the general population.

As far as those that attend are concerned, most psychiatrists appear reluctant to define anyone who has presented himself for treatment as *not* really in need of it; that is they are usually unwilling to define a clinic attender as not clinically disturbed. Psychiatrists certainly do at times have doubts about the appropriateness of treating some of those referred to them; but such doubts do not often seem to be publicly expressed. (One possible explanation for the briefness of much psychiatric out-patient treatment and the high proportion of patients who attend clinics no more than once or twice is that psychiatrists indirectly convey their feelings of doubt and impotence to their patients.) Because of this situation, there has been little opportunity for psychiatrists to establish clearly the lower limit of the boundaries of the concept of clinical depression: the division between normal variations in mood and the clinical state has been more the territory of general practitioners. And here the tasks of the medical practitioner and of the research worker make different demands: a general practitioner can proceed in a situation of considerable ambiguity, perhaps not deciding the clinical status of a patient's complaint until after matters have been made clear by spontaneous recovery, or an increase in severity to a point where there is no doubt that some sort of therapeutic attention is needed. If a general practitioner does hesitate to treat a widow's grief, there is little risk in his hesitation; he can ask to see her again and make up his mind later. By contrast, when a research worker is unable to classify he jeopardizes his whole undertaking. For example, if a random sample of women in the general population, designed to act as a comparison group for a group of clinically depressed patients, contains a high proportion of women with apparently similar conditions, it becomes crucial to ask how many of these should be excluded from what is supposed to be a non-depressed comparison group. If the worker cannot employ a criterion that is consistent with the characteristics of the patient group, he will be hindered in his search for factors that vary between the two groups. It is the demand for comparability that forces the research worker to do something to resolve the problem.

A recent series of studies by a group of American psychiatrists in St Louis, interviewing people shortly after the loss of their spouse, is one of the few pieces of work that has made an attempt to confront this problem.[1] They conclude that

> 'grief is grief, and is not a model for psychotic depression . . . Thus while the normal depression of widowhood serves as an excellent model for the depression resulting from a clear-cut loss, it is also different from clinical affective illness, and should be considered separately in studies of affective disorders in psychiatric patients.'
> (Clayton, Desmarais and Winokur 1968)

This conclusion if taken strictly logically, implies that no depression following a clear-cut loss should be called a case of affective illness, which, as we have seen, would not accord with modern clinical practice, where both reactive and non-reactive depressions are treated as illnesses. Furthermore, their actual figures are consistent with a radically different interpretation. Only three symptoms (depressed mood, sleep disturbance, and crying) were experienced by more than half the group of bereaved subjects and they argued plausibly that these seemed to correspond to grief. Following the criteria of Feighner and his colleagues (1972) they considered a clinical depressive disorder in addition required at least four of the following eight symptoms: (i) loss of appetite or weight loss, (ii) sleep difficulties including hypersomnia, (iii) fatigue, (iv) agitation or retardation, (v) loss of interest, (vi) difficulty in concentration, (vii) feelings of guilt, and (viii) thought of suicide or wishing to be dead. In the light of current psychiatric practice these are reasonable criteria and, as will be seen in the next chapter, they are strikingly similar to the ones our psychiatric colleagues and we were developing at about the same time to define depression (1969–71). In fact, the St Louis study found that as many as 35 per cent of their widows 'manifested enough symptoms at one month (after the bereavement) to be either definitely or probably depressed'. Thirteen months after bereavement 16 per cent still fitted this category. It seems that within the first three months, widowhood had produced in a third of the women symptoms similar to clinical depression.

In distinguishing grief from depression Clayton and her colleagues have made a useful step. We would agree with them that the reactions they describe are for the most part probably not 'psychotic'. But it is not possible to follow them when they suggest that these conditions are of no relevance to the understanding of affective illness or depression where there has been no preceding clear-cut loss. For a start, without close enquiry who can be sure that there has not been some less dramatic loss? For as Freud said, the object lost in melancholia need not necessarily have died but simply have been lost as an object of love – and very often, as we will see in later chapters, there occur, before the onset of all types of depression, losses when this term is allowed to have a wider meaning than that of bereavement. Furthermore, no reason is given why the third or so of women with severe symptoms should not be viewed as clinically depressed. Not to do so is simply to let prior assumptions about aetiology intrude into one's efforts at classification. This is a startling example of the logical shortcoming discussed earlier: the confusion of aetiological considerations with classification. And it is precisely because we wished to avoid this confusion that, starting with similar standards to the eight symptoms outlined by Feighner and his colleagues, we came to a different conclusion: that women with *major* symptoms after loss were clinically depressed and that this classification could serve to advance psychiatric knowledge.

An example of a case of depression

In order to illustrate the similarities between our standards and those of the St Louis group and to give more substance to these rather general remarks, we will describe one of the women we came across in our random sample of women in Camberwell whom we decided was clinically depressed during the year of study. She is, we believe, typical. The example will not only serve as a useful background when we come to describe our procedure for establishing the presence of clear psychiatric disorder in the general community, but will also show the importance of attention to matters of the timing of onset and fluctuation of symptoms. We give with the clinical account details of social incidents of possible aetiological significance, but in deciding whether a woman was a 'case' these were entirely omitted from consideration: the decision was based on the symptom picture alone.

Mrs Trent, with three children under seven, was married to a van driver. She lived on the ground floor of a typical two-storey Camberwell house in two rooms and a kitchen. Twelve months before our interview she reported feeling 'quite herself'. This did not mean she was completely symptom-free; she used to experience pains in the head, eye-aches, and occasional dizziness. She also used to avoid going in lifts and kept away from crowds and certain animals because they made her feel nervous and uncomfortable. She did not report enough anxiety about any of these for them to be considered phobias. Eight months before interview her third child was born and her husband lost his job. Although she had known that the firm had not been satisfied with some of his work, she said that this came as a surprise, but she did not worry very much, and indeed he found another job within three weeks. Within a fortnight, however, he was called to head office and given the sack without any explanation. It was during the next few weeks that she started to worry about his getting another job. The only explanation that she could see for his losing his job the second time was that the firm's reference for him was a poor one and had only arrived after he had started work. About seven weeks later, and five and a half months before interview, her worries had progressed to a point where she had become very tense, feeling tight and tensed up in her back and legs and unable to relax in general; she felt depressed and miserable and had difficulty getting off to sleep. She was getting migraines which she had not had for some time and she felt lacking in energy. She began to be irritable, although she said she usually 'bottled up feelings like that'. These changes interfered with her ability to concentrate not only on her children and her housework, but also on reading the newspaper. Her appetite deteriorated quite noticeably. We judged this to be the point of onset. During the next two months these changes became more marked. She felt very exhausted, irritable, and miserable, and would often cry during the day. She had some sleeping pills which she took at nights but she often woke up during the night, sometimes with nightmares, and only rarely because of her baby who was sleeping through the night at this stage. Her relationship with her husband deteriorated. She lost all interest in sex, they had rows about money, and she 'thought the marriage was finished'. Three times she packed her bags and walked down the road, but each time she came back because of the children. She became self-depreciatory, feeling she could not cope with anything. She lost interest in her appearance and in the house: some days she would only just manage to keep the baby looking decent. It sometimes seemed so hard to keep her mind out of a muddle about what she had to do that she seriously thought of ending it all. Her appetite waned further and she took to going to bed during the day for hours at a stretch. This phase lasted for about six weeks, after which she gradually began to feel more energy and interest in the home and children. She began to sleep better at night, though she was still occasionally taking sleeping pills at the time of interview. She began to realize that far from 'just sticking it out for the sake of the children', it was only that 'things had got on top of us' in the marriage. Her improvement took a definite turn for the better three weeks before interview. She was no longer feeling so exhausted that she would spend time in bed during the day. Her concentration improved a little – she could now listen to the radio and if she saw the television she would keep her mind on it without her thoughts drifting off. Her interest in sex had returned in the last month, and she said that her sexual relationship with her husband was better than it had ever been before, since she had always been a bit cold. She still felt her concentration was worse than usual – and she was still tending to brood on things, and she felt tense and irritable with the children, her sleep and appetite were still not back to normal, but she was quite convinced she was on the road to recovery

Throughout the time of her depression, a period of about five and a half months, she had not talked to her doctor of her psychological symptoms, although she had consulted him about the migraines. The sleeping pills had been prescribed, she said, in connection with these. She seemed to take it for granted that after her initial visit to discuss the migraines it would have been wrong to bother him with these other complaints which she related quite clearly to her financial and marital worries.

Our approach to diagnosis

The situation at the beginning of our research was thus that we were trying to look at aetiological factors for a condition whose existence was best established by a complex judgement which took account not only of the number and type of a variety of symptoms, but also of their intensity, duration, and fluctuation – all of which are illustrated by Mrs Trent. Among psychiatrists there was a general agreement that the more a depressed mood was accompanied by interference with bodily functioning or with social activities the more likely it was to be 'clinical' depression, but no one had quantified this. It was relatively easy to know that someone like Mrs Trent, who felt that life was without hope, who thought seriously of ending it all, who cried a lot, and who had a negative self-image, would be more likely to be considered clinically depressed if she had, like her, also given up some of her normal pursuits, if it had interfered with her housework or child care, or if she had lost her appetite, had trouble sleeping, lost her energy, or had been exhausted or badly constipated. But there were no clear guidelines which laid down precisely that a woman was or was not clinically depressed – a woman who, say, felt constantly sad when alone, and being a retired widow, spent most of the day in bed letting her house get untidy but who cheered up and would go out if someone contacted her. Was it a sign of 'clinical' disturbance to wait for social contact to rescue her from her misery and anxiety instead of going out to seek it herself? On the other hand, was it not 'normal' to feel lonely and sad if one saw few people and had no compelling reason to get out of bed in the morning? And if it was normal, was it a 'clinical' disturbance?

We have explained our decision to throw in our lot with the best in the clinical tradition and we accepted that at present, at least, there was no other way of validating a measure of clinical depression than by using *clinical judgments* about what should be counted as a 'case'. We have noted already that psychiatric standards concerning diagnosis are bound to be influenced by a range of wider social factors. In this potential flux our aim was to deal with phenonema about which there would be general agreement among psychiatrists and on the basis of these delimit clusters of symptoms that most would have little hesitation in calling clinical depression. We had no shadow of doubt that our measure would be provisional – that it would change at least in some degree as better methods of measurement were developed and as theory about what we were studying accumulated. It would be a start. But this procedure only needs apology if that of science does:

> 'The ad hoc method of dealing with problems of clarity or precision as the need arises might be called "dialysis", in order to distinguish it from analysis: from the idea that language analysis as such may solve problems or create an armoury for future use. Dialysis cannot solve problems. It cannot do so any more than definition or explication or language analysis can: problems can only be solved with the help of new ideas. But our problem may sometimes demand that we make new distinctions – ad hoc, for the purpose in hand.'
> (Popper, 1976: 31)

Since our first major objective was to understand the causes of depression among women treated by psychiatrists, we based our *patient* study on women judged by the research psychiatrists collaborating with us to be suffering from primary depression uncomplicated by obvious physical factors. They made their judgments after completing a full clinical interview based on the PSE, or Present State Examination. This is a standardized clinical-type interview which at this time had been extensively tested on in-patient populations (see Wing, Cooper and Satorius, 1974). In addition to the patient series we needed a comparison group, which served two purposes. First, to tell us about the rate of life-events and difficulties among women living in the same community but without psychiatric disorder; and second, to allow us to study depression among women in the general community who might not have sought medical help. These two tasks were, of course, complementary; in order to obtain the comparative material we had to exclude women with psychiatric disorder. Therefore when we came to extend the work to the random sample of women living in Camberwell, all were given a shortened version of the PSE. For these women we added a further stage after the use of the PSE, where we made an overall judgement as to whether or not a woman was suffering from a definite psychiatric disorder. We called such women *cases*. Mrs Trent is a typical example. The symptoms covered by the shortened PSE schedule have the advantage of corresponding closely to those considered relevant in any diagnostic interview and their ordering follows a principle of grouping under the headings of recognizable clinical syndromes such as nervous tension, free-floating anxiety, muscular tension, phobic anxiety, depressed mood, hallucinations and delusions, obsessional symptoms, expansive mood and ideation, sleep disturbance, and many more. There is a glossary of definitions of symptoms which, together with a suggested list of questions and probes concerning them, acts as a guide to both interviewing and rating. As well as deciding whether a woman was suffering from a definite disorder (i. e. a case) we made ratings of severity and diagnosis and also established the date of any onset in the year before interview. We will now discuss these tasks in turn, beginning with the use of the PSE to collect information about symptoms.

(a)   *Psychiatric symptoms*

Although there is a manual explaining in detail the use of the PSE, it is essential that this is supplemented by training in interviewing and in rating. Both our teams were fortunate enough to be trained by psychiatrists at the Institute of Psychiatry.

If in response to standard questions (or to something said spontaneously) the interviewer believes that a symptom may be present, it is up to him or her to question until there is enough information to make a decision about its presence or severity. At this stage a particular point would be made to ask a woman tending to 'over-report' symptoms to give more details. For example, two women might reply 'yes' to the question on anergia: 'Do you seem to be slowed down in your movements; or to have little energy recently?' and both might report that this had affected them quite a bit. But upon further probes it might emerge that the first woman had only noticed it really when coming up the four flights of stairs to her flat, and this only in the last two days while she was recovering from influenza, whereas the second one had felt it continuously during the whole month, had had no physical illness, and had had to spend more time in bed, or resting, and had given up doing various things. The second woman would be given a positive rating for anergia, but not the first. (Mrs Trent, of course, would be rated as positive.)

Every interviewer has to cover a standard number of questions, and criteria are laid down to help decide when to go on to ask supplementary questions or probes. We cannot stress enough the value of these in sifting the central data about symptoms from the surrounding remarks which vary so much with a respondent's reporting style. One of the reasons we ruled out the use of a straightforward pencil-and-paper questionnaire to do the job of collecting material about symptoms was that, for our purpose at least, self-rating questionnaires would be likely to contain important biases. Our experience with middle-class women, for instance, suggested that they were particularly conscientious in reporting minor examples of tension, anxiety, and the like when compared with their working-class counterparts. Also it is hard, if not impossible, to build into questionnaires like the Hamilton Rating Scale, the Zung Scale, and the Beck Depression Inventory a means of establishing the date of onset of the disorder, which was essential if we were to examine the role of social factors in onset. Ratings for the PSE are made as far as possible on the basis of clinical information alone (intensity, frequency, and duration of symptoms) though social data are taken into account when rating a few special items. In conjunction with psychiatric colleagues we undertook studies of inter-rater reliability for the shortened schedule, which showed that non-medical interviewers could reach high standards of reliability that were comparable with those of medically trained interviewers (Cooper et al., 1977; Wing et al., 1977).

(b)   *The rating of caseness and borderline caseness.*

Our second task was to establish which women in the general population were suffering from psychiatric disorder, particularly depression. Women considered to have a definite psychiatric disorder at any time in the twelve months before interview were classified as *cases*, and women who had psychiatric symptoms that were not considered frequent or severe enough for them to be rated as cases were classified *borderline cases*. (For our measure of prevalence of psychiatric disorder in the general community we used presence in the three months and not the whole year before interview.) Almost all the women who were cases were suffering from a depressive disorder but we dealt with all psychiatric conditions in this same way. While the judgment itself was made on the basis of clinical criteria the principle that guided the development of the standards for caseness was that a psychiatrist would not be surprised to see a woman defined as a *case* in an out-patient clinic and, if she were to attend, he would be likely to see the woman as benefitting from some form of psychiatric treatment. Our clinical criteria attempted to translate this underlying conception into a usable measure of disorder. It is clear from our own work and that of others that psychiatric symptoms are common in the general population. Taylor and Chave (1964) for example, in a survey of a New Town, found that a third of adults reported 'sub-clinical' neurotic symptoms. We have attempted in the rating of *caseness* to differentiate, within this broad spectrum of disorder, women with symptoms of sufficient severity to merit psychiatric attention according to psychiatric standards generally accepted in this country. In addition, there were the borderline cases and also women with psychiatric symptoms that were not severe enough to be classed even among the borderline cases.

Central to the whole rating procedure was the development of anchoring examples of cases and borderline cases. In order to be rated as a case, it was necessary for a woman not only to have a central disturbance of mood but also other symptoms recognized by psychiatrists to be part of either a depressive or an anxiety syndrome – for example, sleep disturbance, loss of concentration, loss of appetite and weight, being slowed down in movement, and having diurnal variation in mood. This, of course, is illustrated by Mrs Trent. A woman whose symptoms were considered short of caseness, and whom we allotted to the borderline case group, was Mrs Allen.

She was a forty-one-year old woman with two children. Six months before interview she began to get tension headaches which she seemed to have all the time. Eventually she went to the doctor who prescribed librium. The headaches lasted about two months; and during this time she also felt more nervous tension, felt that she could not relax, that her mind was always busy, often brooding about the past. She would cry two or three times a week if she was on her own in the evenings. She could not really be bothered with food, but she did not lose any weight, and her sleep was not disturbed. She felt more irritable and more tired than usual; everything seemed an effort, but she managed to carry on with her housework and other tasks. At the time of interview these symptoms were considerably improved.

But not all women suffering from psychiatric symptoms were considered to be borderline cases. Mrs Stacey was a married woman in her thirties with three small children. She seemed mildly depressed and said her mood 'went up and down', but reported no worries. She had some symptoms which were probably psychosomatic, such as back-ache, indigestion, and blotches on her skin. She also reported feeling tired recently for no obvious reason. She did not show any symptoms of anxiety, but she was very shy, and was rated as showing a patholog-ical lack of self-confidence, although she did not actively avoid other people. She had some troubles getting to sleep, but not for more than one hour, and she did not report any irritability. About three years before she did have a definite psychiatric episode at the time of an abortion. We did not consider her symptoms sufficient to rate her as a borderline case.

Further examples are given in Appendix 1.

(c)   *Onset and course of the disorder*

Detailed descriptions of the range of fluctuations during the course of depressive disorders do not form part of existing diagnostic instru-ments, which follow the rather static description of depression in psychiatric text-books. Rating scales to measure onset and course of depressive disorders had, therefore, to be specially developed. They involved an additional set of questions covering the twelve-month period focussed on the timing of onset and changes in the course of the disorder.

The dating of onset itself is, of course, crucial in aetiological research: onset can only be influenced by something occurring before it. A considerable effort was made to date onset accurately – if at all possible to within a period of one week. We will discuss our method of interviewing in a later chapter. In our earlier schizophrenic study we obtained almost complete agreement on the date of onset between patient and relative when seen separately by different interviewers (Brown and Birley, 1968; Birley and Brown, 1970). However patients had been specially selected because of a recent and acute onset of symptoms. In the depression study patient and relative were again seen separately for the first fifty interviews. Agreement was somewhat lower than in the schizophrenic study. Nevertheless forty-three (86 per cent) of the fifty patients and relatives clearly described the same onset; six out of the remaining seven cases were due to 'private onsets' reported by the patient alone, the relative describing a later exacer-bation. In thirty-four (79 per cent) of the forty-three cases where patient and relative reported the same onset they dated it within three weeks of each other.

We also wished to describe the course of the disorder after onset. In order to do this we developed the concept of *change-point* when increase or decrease in the number of symptoms led to a noticeable change in a woman's psychiatric state. Interviewers were allowed to use no more than three change-points to describe major clinical changes in the year, the first being at onset. In addition they always described the point of interview (or 'admission' in the case of patients). Patients were only included if they had had an onset in the year; all had to have been free from an obvious depressive disorder for some time previously – other than a few mild symptoms. However, any woman in the Camberwell survey could be included as a case irrespective of whether she had had an onset in the year. (As will be seen only about half the cases had experienced an onset in the year covered by our interview; the rest had been disturbed more or less continuously for more than a year and were called *chronic* in contrast to *onset* cases.)

The establishment of change-points enabled us to examine whether major changes in psychiatric state after the original onset were also related to social factors preceding the change.

Change-points, by definition, occurred at a particular point in time and were dated, if possible, to a one-week period. Only under exceptional and clearly defined circumstances could change-points occur within four weeks of each other. While *any* change for worse or better could in principle be included, in almost every instance sudden changes involved worsening of the condition – and this, in practice, is with what we will deal when we discuss change-points.

The end-point of a change, or a time when the rate of increase in symptoms became much slower or where a period of stability of the symptom-picture emerged, we called the levelling-off point. Between a levelling-off point and the next change-point (or admission to in-patient or out-patient status if there was only one change-point) we described the course of symptoms according to whether they fluctuated week by week, day by day, whether they were stable, or indeed if there was even some improvement. This all required a meticulous attention to dating which we will describe when we discuss our methods of interviewing.

In Mrs Trent's case there was really only one change-point, at the time of onset five and a half months before interview, which levelled off after two months. The symptoms were stable for about six weeks after that and then began to fall off, at first gradually and then more markedly. Two more examples from our patient series will further illustrate our approach.

For the first patient the change-point represented an increase both in the number of symptoms and in the severity of the existing ones. Mrs Davies was in her late forties, married, with one teenage son living at home. She had had one previous episode of depression soon after the birth of her son. Although she had tended to experience palpitations and to show obsessional traits such as checking over and over again whether she had turned off the taps, she had been well until three and a half months before admission when she became more tired than usual, and had to force herself to do things. As she put it 'my arms and legs felt too heavy – there was no go in me'. Things began to get more and more on top of her, every little task seemed too big; she felt miserable and anxious and became much more irritable than usual. She would worry about her husband and her son, often wishing she had not married, and felt guilty that she ill-treated them. She also had bouts of crying. During this period, which lasted about three months, she had frequent colds and nosebleeds.

About two and a half weeks before admission she caught influenza and four days later she became very disturbed although her temperature was no longer high. She heard voices; she thought she was going to die, that the vicar had come to say a prayer for her, and that her husband was taking her to the mortuary rather than to hospital. She thought her lodger, who was a family friend, was going to leave despite his constant denials. She wanted but was unable to cry. She complained of 'thoughts in her head which she could not shift' and was preoccupied with worry over what would happen to her husband and son if she was ill. Her loss of energy now was even more severe; she stayed in bed most of the time leaving most of the household jobs undone. She had lost interest in everything; when visitors came she just lay in bed; she hardly ate anything 'just two or three mouthfuls' and had already lost weight. She took a long time to get off to sleep, and would wake every hour or only sleep until the early morning. Her irritability increased so that now she would sometimes yell out, and her husband had trouble quietening her down. This very marked change in overall severity was rapid, the levelling-off point was within one week of the change-point, in contrast to the more gradual levelling-off of the onset itself.

In our second example there were once again an onset and a further change-point. While the change after onset represented a much milder worsening than with Mrs Davies, it was still enough to count as a change-point rather than a fluctuation in the level of symptoms. Mrs Gray was thirty-nine with two adolescent children and married to a business man. She did some work at home for a local factory. At the beginning of the year she was well, though she had always shown obsessional traits of personality such as coming down in the night to check that the gas was off. About sixteen weeks before interview she became depressed, crying on and off throughout the day. She became tired and irritable, shouting at the children, and her interest in sex declined. She found it something of an effort to keep up with the household chores. She usually felt worse in the mornings. The only place she felt all right was in bed during the day. But at night she sometimes woke up suddenly with the feeling that something awful was going to happen and worried about who would look after the children if it did. She developed 'muzzy' headaches and her legs became aching and heavy and she worried that she might have leukemia, but medical tests showed there was no cause for alarm. This dispelled that particular worry but the other symptoms remained without showing much change.

About three weeks before interview she suddenly got worse, crying much more than before. She could not go on a bus or into a shop. If she did she 'felt something come over her'; she would feel shaky inside, her mouth would dry up and she had to run home. She began to feel that she could not swallow, her appetite waned, and she lost weight. Normally a very sociable person, she now could not be bothered to talk to anyone, and could not bring herself to go out. She had feelings of being unreal, feeling numb, and like a machine when walking, almost unable to feel herself moving her limbs. Household chores became even more of a burden, though she forced herself to do them perfunctorily; she gave up the 'home work' from the factory. She felt she could not think straight, nor make up her mind even about little things like going on holiday. She also had great difficulty getting off to sleep at nights. The general practitioner whom she now consulted for her depression suggested she go to the Maudsley hospital; at first she refused, but some days later her sister and brother-in-law came over in the evening and managed to persuade her to take his advice. Even her husband, who earlier had thought she should 'snap out of it', was now in favour of her seeking psychiatric help.

This change-point levelled off after ten days, whereas after onset she had tended to get gradually worse over about a month before going to the general practitioner about her headaches and her legs. The levelling-off point for onset was rated as occurring after four weeks. From this point until the change-point her symptoms had been fairly steady and were rated on the fluctuation measure as 'nil or little fluctuation'.

(d)   *Severity*

It is clear from the descriptions we have given of Mrs Gray and Mrs Davies that their symptoms differed in severity at different points in time. To take account of this we developed a simple five-fold scale of 'overall severity' ranging from 1 (marked) to 5 (mild) which we found could be used with a reasonably high inter-rater reliability.[2] Thus Mrs

Davies, whom we have just described, started at the lowest point (5) and then just before admission became very much worse, reaching a rating of marked (1). This degree of change was unusual – the average movement being less than two scale points. Mrs Gray, for example, was 'moderate' (3) at onset and (2) by the change-point, illustrating a less marked worsening compared with Mrs Davies. Mrs Trent, who did not seek psychiatric care, was rated (3) at onset and had no other change-point. At time of interview, when she had greatly improved, she was rated 'mild' (5). This scale of overall severity took account of the total symptom picture including symptoms of, for example, anxiety, suicide attempts, and bizarre behaviour which might not be considered by some a central part of the depression. While this decision might be considered controversial, we did also have separate severity scales for more restricted items such as appetite change, depressed mood, overactivity, and interference with daily routine. (A list of our clinical measures and further examples of overall severity appear in Appendix 2.) We shall return to the problem of measuring severity later in chapter 13.

(e) *Diagnosis*

Within the sample of depressed *patients* we also wished to make distinctions in terms of the neurotic-psychotic sub-categories of depression discussed earlier. Patients with any manic features were excluded from this part of the study. Once again this distinction relied ultimately for its validity on clinical judgment. We chose the terms 'psychotic' and 'neurotic' deliberately because they do not imply anything in terms of aetiology unlike the counterpart terms 'endogenous' and 'reactive'. However, our category of psychotic was a broad one – out of the 111 psychiatric patients finally used in our statistical analysis of the psychotic-neurotic distinction, sixty-two were classed 'psychotic' and forty-nine 'neurotic', by a research psychiatrist from the Institute of Psychiatry.[3] Our psychotic category undoubtedly corresponds quite closely to the way the term 'endogenous' is used by the many psychiatrists who focus on the somatic symptoms of retardation, weight and appetite loss, early morning waking and diurnal variation of mood, which they see as setting these depressions apart from the 'reactive' or 'justifiable' ones (Pollitt, 1965). We will deal in more detail with the psychotic/neurotic distinction in a later chapter; but at this point it is perhaps worth noting that Mrs Davies with her hallucinations, delusions, marked withdrawal, and waking early in the morning presented us with an obvious 'psychotic' picture, and Mrs Gray was equally obviously 'neurotically' depressed with her agoraphobia and inability to swallow. Two points should be noted. A 'neurotic' picture is more easily characterized by lack of psychotic features than by features of its own, although those in the neurotic group were a little more likely to be more active and more anxious. Second, 'typical' symptoms of either group can occur in the other: for example, Mrs Gray did feel worse in the mornings but was diagnosed neurotic. The judgment was always an overall one based on the total picture.

Finally, we had to make other diagnostic classifications. The PSE collected information about the entire range of psychiatric symptoms and it was to be expected that not all the cases in the community would be cases of depression. Depressions therefore had to be distinguished from other disorders. In practice, however, all the cases in Camberwell were some form of affective disturbance, and the only other diagnoses encountered were thus some form of anxiety.

The relationship between anxiety and depression is often a close one and this differentiation was made at the *syndromal level* rather than at the level of individual symptoms. A rating, for instance, of depressive disorder is quite compatible with the presence of anxiety symptoms. What is important is the constellation of the symptoms and the course they have taken. For instance, a depressive disorder might well have such symptoms as difficulty in getting off to sleep, worrying, tension, restlessness, and change in appetite, and all these could on occasion be part of an anxiety state. We developed yet another system of classification of our community cases which allowed us to take into account this dimension of anxiety symptoms. Where either anxiety or depression dominated the clinical picture and other disorders were absent, the simple diagnosis of 'anxiety' or 'depression' was used, but where there were symptoms relating to both, the problem of deciding which was the major one had to be faced. Examination of the disorder as a whole throughout its course, as well as its state at interview, usually made the distinction possible.[4] In those individuals where one clinical syndrome was superimposed on another (e.g. phobic anxiety with onset of depression in the year of interview) women were considered to have two separate syndromes which were rated independently.

In this mixed group we used our categories of case and borderline case separately for each of the two syndromes. It was thus possible to describe a woman as a case of depression and a case of anxiety, where her anxiety symptoms were so marked that even in the absence of her depressive ones she would have been diagnosed as suffering from some form of phobia or anxiety state; for example, if she had frequent panic attacks on going out and was confined to the home as a result. Where a woman had some depressive symptomatology and also some anxiety symptoms which on their own were not severe enough for her to be judged a *case* of anxiety, we described her as case depression and borderline case anxiety. In theory we could have described a woman with definite agoraphobia and mild depressive symptoms as a case of anxiety with borderline case depression. In practice we did not find anyone who fitted this category.

To sum up our measurement of psychiatric disorder, in our community sample we distinguished three major groups of women: with definite psychiatric disorder (cases), less disturbance (borderline cases), minimal or no symptoms ('normals'). For patients and cases in the general population we established the date of onset and major changes in condition in the year of study in order to relate these to various social factors of possible aetiological significance. The overall severity of symptoms at the various change-points was also rated. Finally, for patients we distinguished 'psychotic' and 'neurotic' depressive conditions; and for patients, cases and borderline-cases, whether the women had primarily depressive, anxiety, or mixed conditions. Further examples of these various categories of cases can be found in Appendix 1 and some of the other ratings in Appendix 2.

Illness and abnormality?

There remains a final issue already touched upon in chapter 1. What are the implications of working with such ratings and categories? Do we, for example, see the patients and women rated as 'cases' in Camberwell as ill? In the first place, we do not believe that the question has to be answered for research to proceed. Research requires only that psychiatric phenomena can be reliably classified and applied to various groups with strict comparability. Such a response may seem evasive, but it is not easy to give a clear answer to this question without first clarifying the issues surrounding it.

There have been four main grounds on which objections have been made to the application of the term 'illness' to psychiatric symptoms:

(i) There is a difference between physical illness and mental illness. The former is more objective because it involves physiological symptomatology and aetiology; mental illness is a matter of subjective opinion and value-judgment made about deviations from normal behaviour (Szasz, 1961; Goffman, 1972). In its hardest form this critique maintains that mental illness is simply an infringement of social rules by ordinary people (Scheff, 1966).

(ii) Mental illness is more vaguely defined than physical illness, involving definitions that are more subject to social values (Szasz, 1962).

(iii) The ascription of the term 'illness' removes the responsibility of the sufferer for his action, and this responsibility is just what is required if the patient is to take control of his life-style in order to recover. Thomas Szasz, whose basic commitment is to private one-to-one psychotherapy, believes that the patient's sense of control is sapped if he is forced into a sick role by being defined as ill.

(iv) The term illness implies that the locus of remedies should be a clinic which attends to individuals rather than the reform of the wider society, which is what is required for the prevention of mental illness.

These approaches to the topic are subject to a number of errors. Many of them stem from a failure to move beyond the dualistic conceptual framework of the mind-body distinction, which results in the exaggeration of the differences between what are portrayed as two different types of phenomenon, the mental and the physical.

(a) Physical illness also depends upon judgment, and upon a preconception of what is 'normal' or usual in any context; for example the standards of health of the young and the elderly are not the same (Sedgwick, 1973; Lewis, 1953; Ausubel, 1961).

(b) Physical illness can also involve variations in opinion, and be vaguely defined (Bloor, 1976).

(c) Empirically few people would confuse depressive symptoms with social rule-breaking. Social science critics often seem to work with an undifferentiated concept of mental illness that does not square with the complexities of reality; in practice it means that they use examples of bizarre forms of behaviour derived from lay notions of madness rather than examples of the duller realities of affective disorder. They therefore fail to come to terms with one of the most cogent reasons for preserving the term illness for mental disorders, namely that they cause the sufferers considerable distress. Further, we find the 'rule-breaking' approach inadequate insofar as many of the depressed women in our community survey were patently not the victims of labelling either by social or medical agencies or by their own social circle, although their symptoms were almost indistinguishable from those of women in treatment.

(d) The arguments of the third criticism are correct in drawing attention to the consequences of being labelled ill in our society: the 'sick' are, by and large, not held to be responsible. (For the classic discussion of this see Talcott Parsons, 1951.) But they exaggerate the extent to which this implies that patients are treated as 'ineffective' (in Brewster Smith's terms) in controlling their condition. Moreover, the distinction claimed between physical and mental illness is again invalid. No doctor would deny the responsibility of a diabetic patient for the course of his condition if he rejected advice about his diet. Imparting an attitude of responsibility for the course of a condition through giving insight into its dynamics is as much part of good physical medicine as of the psychotherapy extolled by Szasz.

Criticism (iii) derives from a critique of certain treatment settings where mental patients are 'dehumanized' by the attitudes shown towards them. One of the attitudes involved is indeed the belief that such patients are not ordinary responsible agents. Paradoxically, however, this can be itself humane if it is not combined with indifference or arrogance. For many who agree with the concept of illness for mental conditions see it as a way of avoiding the use of stigmatizing and punishing labels; these believe that it is unfair to class a depressed woman who steals a scarf from a shop on the spur of the moment along with someone who plans and carries out a burglary. They argue that the concept of illness, by removing her moral responsibility, can be used to make a fundamental distinction between the two.

There is a slight confusion in all these arguments about the boundaries of the concept of moral responsibility, as if it were *totally* excluded from areas where the concept of illness applied. As we have just seen this is not the case in the practice of physical medicine, where responsibility is merely seen as reduced not removed by the intervention of some other agent (for example a virus).

A final point can be made here: recognition of the ethical and social issues raised by these critics in no way logically invalidates the study of the aetiology of psychiatric phenomena.

(e) With regard to the fourth criticism, the use of an 'illness' perspective has not necessarily involved individualistic repair rather than social reform. Indeed, historically the control of infectious disease was largely due to improved diet and water supply and was made possible by the search for discrete aetiological agents (McKeown, 1971). There is no necessary incompatibility between individual treatment and social prevention – although in practice the balance of resources is usually tipped too far in favour of the former. The way to right this imbalance is not to deny the relevance of medical intervention but to demand a fairer distribution of resources. Our research with its emphasis on social causes of illness depends on the same logic of approach.

One response to the confused debate is to try to deal with the matter empirically; does what we know of depression square with a disease model? As outlined by John Wing, the criteria for this model are that:

(1) a limited syndrome can be reliably recognized; (2) plausible guesses can be made about aetiology, pathophysiology, and underlying processes of normal functioning; (3) the most effective use of pharmacological and social treatments will depend on a proper diagnosis of the disease; and finally (4) the diagnosis implies a prognosis that can be fairly accurately made in statistical terms if the social conditions under which the individual is living are known (Wing, 1973: 161). We believe that the relevance of these criteria to depression cannot be ruled out.

We did find it feasible to identify a limited syndrome, by relying on detailing specific symptoms many of which were not hitherto publicly recognized, and not by making judgments about rule-breaking behaviour. The women we saw did not find it easy to 'snap out of it', to change the course of the condition, that is, once it was under way; it did seem as if their responsibility was in some way diminished, and that prescription of physical treatments was sometimes helpful to them. We therefore decided not to take a crusading stand against the use of the term illness. We were concerned with understanding the genesis and control of a condition, and the research could quite well proceed without any final label being appended to that condition. We saw the humanitarian interests of much of the anti-mental illness lobby as a well-intentioned check on the excesses of psychiatry, but we felt that these interests would not necessarily be furthered by the rejection of the concept of 'illness' but by confronting more directly the implications of using it; for example by asking why mental patients were not encouraged to become more 'effective' in Brewster Smith's terms, that is to see themselves as having some responsibility for the course of their condition. But whatever the opinion of the reader about the label, in the end its use (or its abandonment) in no way changes the substance or the implications of our results.

This also applies to the parallel question whether those classified by diagnostic categories are in some way abnormal. An unwillingness to stigmatize a patient as abnormal often leads to the rejection of current diagnostic labels in favour of novel, often vague descriptions, such as distress. Logically, however, the use of diagnostic classifications to describe clusters of symptoms does not imply any belief either about the abnormality or the illness of the person with those symptoms. Though we use the word 'normal' at various stages to describe women who were not, in our terms suffering from a psychiatric condition, this is intended as a shorthand (perhaps a misleading one) and not a manifesto of our own stand. In some circumstances we believe it is as normal to develop depression as it is to develop a blister when a hand has been burnt by a hot stove, although it is unusual to have a burnt hand in a random selection of hands. We are only willing to see clinical depression in general as abnormal in this sense of 'unusual'. And, of course, the unusualness is significant because of the associated distress and handicap. Here we will let the matter rest. Whatever answer is reached, no-one doubts the suffering involved in what we have classed as depression. Whether illness or not, whether abnormal or not, there is something to understand and perhaps in time to control.

3 Research design

So far we have dealt with depression in general terms: we now consider our own investigation. Our approach developed from the hypothesis that clinical depression is an understandable response to adversity, and it was this we wished to investigate. We could imagine practically anyone developing depression given a certain set of environmental circumstances. We do not view all psychiatric disorder in these terms and would certainly see it as an inappropriate perspective for schizophrenia. We therefore looked at clinical depression in terms of rates of disorder in a population and sought to explain differences through the everyday lives of particular individuals. It was only by trying to link rates of disorder between social class groups, and similar broad social categories, to detailed knowledge about the lives of particular individuals that we felt at all confident about reaching an understanding of the processes underlying differences in rates. It was in this way that we attempted to bring the survey and clinical traditions closer together. We began by developing a causal model of depression based on the day-to-day experience of each woman. While we did not entirely ignore the woman's past, we concentrated on her recent experience because we considered it had been unwarrantedly neglected elsewhere (perhaps as a result of psychoanalytic influences) and because it was obviously easier to collect accurate information about the present. Only when this model had been established did we attempt to use it to arrive at some understanding of rates of depression in the general population.

In setting up the model we first described, as accurately as possible, crises and ongoing difficulties in the period before each onset of depression, at the same time doing all we could to deal with the methodological problems inherent in such research – for example, insuring that these events and difficulties had occurred *before* onset of depression.

The first two components of our model were therefore clear – the 'dependent' variable, the onset of depression and the 'independent' variable, factors capable of producing depressive disorder. We call the latter *provoking agents* and include life-events occurring at a particular point in time (e.g. losing a job) and ongoing difficulties that may or may not have begun with a discrete incident (e.g. a husband's unemployment or a son's alcoholism). This was not enough however. Even if we established that life-events and depression were causally related, the question would arise as to why only some women with an event develop depression. We saw in the opening chapter that social scientists have usually simply speculated about what might lie behind such an association; others have often been tempted to use ideas about basic constitutional and genetic variation to explain differences in response. Our answer was to consider whether social factors – both past and present – *also* performed this role. In principle, there seemed no reason why influences should be restricted merely to provoking onset; they might well also leave a person vulnerable to the effects of a current provoking agent. This had been largely ignored, although Cassel (1974) has recently discussed the possible existence of such factors in both physical and psychiatric disorder and reviews a few studies that hint at their presence. These are the second main set of aetiological factors in our model.

Three points should be noted. First, that while we emphasize the negative aspect by calling these *vulnerability factors*, they can equally be called protective factors. The fact that lack of work outside the home increases risk of developing depression once a major loss has occurred (say of a husband) can be seen as employment serving to protect or as unemployment serving to make vulnerable. Second, vulnerability factors are only capable of increasing risk of depression *in the presence of* a provoking agent. Alone they have no effect at all. In practice, however, this clear-cut distinction depends a little on definition. To take again the example of employment. We have in mind unemployment as an ongoing situation causing vulnerability. Therefore if a sudden loss of a job produced depression it would be clearly best seen as a provoking agent and not as a vulnerability factor. It is quite possible for something such as unemployment to have more than one aspect of causal importance; when unemployment acts as a provoking agent it may do so in terms of a sudden loss, and when it acts as a vulnerability factor, it does so in terms of its correlation with isolation and boredom. While this kind of 'overlap' does not occur often in our model it is important to recognize that it is possible.

Finally, vulnerability factors should be seen initially as part of the particular life-circumstances of the individual. They may, of course, also form part of some general characteristic of society as a whole – Durkheim's concepts of egoism and anomie come to mind – but this is a distinct issue. If vulnerability factors are associated with general social categories, such as social class, there is a presumption that common experiences underlie the association. This is one reason for studying them. But this must be demonstrated, not assumed. We have managed to go a certain way towards this broader objective.

There is yet another set of factors in our model which influence depression but, unlike provoking agents and vulnerability factors, do not increase the risk of developing it. We call these *symptom-formation* factors as they influence only the form and severity of depression. A number of experiences discussed in the psychiatric literature as increasing risk of depression are probably better seen as symptom-formation factors. Again, however, the distinction is a conceptual one. It may at times be possible for different aspects of the same experience (say loss of mother in childhood) to act both as a vulnerability and as a symptom-formation factor. However, when this occurs we believe that distinct aspects of the underlying experience are involved. In the present instance it might be the fact of loss of the mother that increases *risk* of depression and whether or not the loss was by death or other means, say adoption, that influences the *form* of any depression. The model is concerned to establish that different aspects are involved; it is the job of theory to say why it should be so.

At its simplest our causal model is therefore:

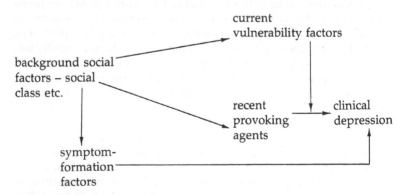

Whilst theoretical concerns were not absent during the building of the model, they did take second place to methodological issues. But, as we became more confident about the causal links of the model, they began to take up more of our time. A model, however well established, can only tell us a limited amount. In the earlier parts of this book, therefore, we will concentrate on the causal model itself while endeavouring to rule out possible artefacts that threaten its validity. We will be concerned essentially with which factors lead to yet other factors.[1] As we proceed we will turn more to theoretical considerations. Here our answers are bound to be less certain than those concerning the model itself. But without such theory research cannot proceed – it is largely by working to reduce the tension between model and theoretical ideas that progress is made.

Research design

If we are to argue that something is of causal importance in depression, it is necessary to show that it is more common before onset of depression than in a comparison group who did not develop depression. A number of studies have looked at the role of life-events in depression,[2] but hardly any have met the minimal demands of an acceptable research design – a comparison group selected at random from the general population. Almost all have used medical or other psychiatric patients. Such groups are quite inadequate to serve as comparison groups because there is now evidence that life-events can play an aetiological role in physical conditions and other types of psychiatric disorder (see Brown *et al.*, 1973a).

Two groups of women form the core of our enquiry – 114 psychiatric in-and out-patients living in Camberwell and two separate random samples, totalling 458 women living in the same community. In order to reduce problems of different cultural influences West Indian women were excluded and any women who had not lived in the United Kingdom or Eire for at least fifteen years. The basic design is simple: in order to establish whether events and difficulties occurred more commonly before onset of depression these two groups of women are compared. Insofar as differences emerge (and various methodological objections are met) provoking agents can be claimed to exist. It is, of course, necessary to make sure that the patient and comparison groups are comparable in terms of factors, such as social class, known to relate in the general population to the rate of the provoking agents. It is also essential to exclude women suffering from psychiatric disorder. Quite a large proportion of the random sample of 458 women in Camberwell were suffering from definite psychiatric disorder, only four had received psychiatric care during the year and almost half were not being treated by a general practitioner. We have already referred to these women as 'cases' and they were excluded from the comparison group, reducing the sample of women used for comparison from 458 to 382. The inclusion of such women could only serve to reduce misleadingly any difference between the comparison group and the patient series. But this is not the end of the matter. Since many of these excluded women were depressed they were not just a potential source of bias but an essential part of our overall design, for they enabled us to make a second and quite independent check on anything found in the patient series. One in twelve women in Camberwell had developed a definite depressive disorder in the year before we saw them and this was quite sufficient for us to examine factors involved in onset, using the other women in Camberwell as a comparison. This comparison provided, however, for more than a simple replication. It is highly likely that social factors of aetiological importance in depression also influence *who* receives psychiatric care. For example, if having young children increases risk of depression, it may also, once a woman is depressed, hinder her from seeking and receiving psychiatric treatment. To the extent that such 'illness behaviour' influences those receiving care, conclusions about aetiology based only on a patient series will be hazardous. We might, in the present example, erroneously conclude that having young children plays no role in depression. The community cases enable us, therefore, to study aetiological processes among a group of women uninfluenced by such selective factors, and second, to examine whether there were social factors influencing both the risk of depression and the receiving of medical attention.

Third, the community survey also told us about *chronic* cases – that is about women who had suffered from a psychiatric disorder for more than a year before our interview. (A further one in twelve women had done so.) We could therefore make a direct estimate of both *prevalence* of psychiatric disorder in Camberwell (based on all women with psychiatric disorder) and *incidence* (based on women developing a disorder in the year.) Therefore in addition to their usefulness in developing a causal model, these measures could be related to social categories such as 'social class'. It was important to base such comparisons on the community 'cases' and not the patients because of the strong possibility that these very factors influenced selection into treatment.

In order to fill out our knowledge of possible selective processes linked to treatment we also looked at a small group of thirty-four women receiving treatment from their general practitioners for a clear depressive episode. This group was additional to the women in our random community sample receiving care from their local doctors.

While these additional groups of women are of considerable importance, the 114 patients receiving psychiatric treatment were a vital part of the research. They provided a ready source of women from Camberwell suffering from recognizable depressive disorders with a range of severity and symptoms impossible to obtain in such numbers in a general population survey without prohibitive expense. They were particularly important for the investigation of symptom-formation factors where a wide range of clinical phenomena is required. Most of the major findings of this study have therefore been checked on more than one group of women.

Except for the use of discriminant function analysis in chapter 14 dealing with depressive symptomatology, we have kept to simple statistical methods: in most instances Chi-square has been used to test statistical significance and gamma the degree of association.

We will now say a little more in turn about the groups of women that we studied.

Patients

The main patient group had recently contacted a psychiatrist either as in-patients (73) or out-patients (41). All were between eighteen and sixty-five and resident in Camberwell. In-patients were selected from admissions to the Maudsley, Bethlem, and St Francis hospitals. Records of hospital admissions were regularly screened to identify possible subjects and a research psychiatrist interviewed them with the systematic clinical interview already outlined in chapter 2. For out-patients a number of psychiatrists were regularly telephoned after their out-patients clinics to ask for names of any patient presenting with a depressive disorder that had apparently begun in the previous year. Case records were checked and, if included, a clinical picture obtained by the same systematic clinical interview – this time carried out by a trained lay interviewer. The material for out-patients was discussed in detail with a psychiatrist collaborating in the research. All patients in the study had been given a diagnosis of primary depression uncomplicated by any underlying condition such as alcoholism or organic psychosis. Patients were included if there had been an important change in their condition in the twelve months before admission (in-patients) or first out-patient contact (out-patients).

A systematic clinical interview was always carried out by one of two sociologists irrespective of whether the patient was seen by the research psychiatrist. In addition a good deal of social data was collected. For the first fifty patients the other interviewer saw a close relative, collecting information on events, difficulties, and other social data as well as details about psychiatric onset. Total interviewing time with patient and relative averaged six hours. All interviews were tape-recorded and rating always made without knowledge of information collected by the other interviewer.

Thirty-five male patients were also seen.

Comparison groups

Two surveys of women living in Camberwell were carried out – the first in 1969/71 of 220 and the second in 1974/75 of 238 women, giving in all a sample of 458 women. The women, like patients, were aged between eighteen and sixty-five and drawn from households selected at random from local authority records of households. The records used had been drawn up for local taxation purposes. The rateable unit in 7 per cent of instances was found, in fact, to contain more than one household (defined by communal eating arrangements). When this happened we chose a household at random. In 15 per cent of the selected households there was more than one woman aged between eighteen and sixty-five (the target population) and in these instances a woman was selected at random. There are therefore likely to be small biases in our selection – women in multiple household addresses and in larger than average households will be slightly under-represented.[3]

Three interviewers were used in the first Camberwell survey and four in the second. All received several months training. The interviews were the same as the interviews given to patients, the year before the day of interview being covered. A somewhat shortened version of the same psychiatric interview (the PSE) was used and date of any onset in the twelve months before interview established for anyone considered to have experienced a psychiatric disorder in the year. A relative was not interviewed.

In both surveys we collaborated with psychiatric colleagues at the Institute of Psychiatry. In the first survey we arranged for a psychiatrist to return to see any woman we considered to be possibly a case and also to visit a sample of women we considered a borderline case or 'normal'. In the second series we arranged for a psychiatrist to see any woman we considered a case or borderline case and a sample of 'normal' women. In both instances they gave the same shortened version of the PSE. In most instances the woman was seen within a few weeks of the first interview. In no instance did we include a woman as a case if this was not finally agreed by a psychiatrist either on the basis of his own interview or (in a few instances) from listening to our tape-recording of the interview.

Some of the findings of the first series were published in 1975 but in the present report of the research the total series will be used. Any significant differences between the results for the two samples will be noted.

We have already mentioned the small special samples of women seen by their local doctor. We regularly approached two sets of general practitioners to ask them for the names of any women whom they had just seen who had clearly had a recent onset of depression. We saw all women they mentioned and in this way interviewed thirty-four women whom we considered to be suffering from a definite recent onset of clinical depression (i.e. all were cases). They were given the interview we have already described for patients.

Now we have dealt with the various groups of women, it is possible to summarize the various time periods involved.

Time periods

In following the accounts of the patient and general population series four points in time must be kept in mind:

1 Date of research interview = I
2 Date of admission (for in-patients) and out-patient attendance (for out-patients): in both instances we refer to 'admission' = A
3 Beginning of the twelve month period covered for everyone – B
4 Furthest point covered by detailed interviewing about life-events and difficulties = F

For the general population in most instances we simply covered:

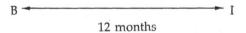

12 months

But if there had been an onset of caseness within three months of B a thirteen week period was always covered before onset. This could therefore extend the period of detailed interviewing to a maximum of fifteen months:

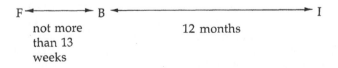

For patients, while we covered a twelve month period before interview (I), this interview always came within a few weeks of 'admission'

(A). Again if onset occurred within three months of B, we covered a thirteen week period before onset:

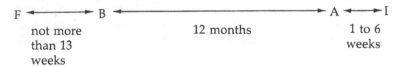

F	B	A	I
not more than 13 weeks	12 months	1 to 6 weeks	

We managed to keep the period A – I to a matter of a few weeks by regular checking with the hospitals for new 'admissions'.

All the women we have discussed so far lived in Camberwell and we should say a little of this Inner London borough.

Camberwell

From Camberwell Green, the centre of Camberwell, the dome of St Pauls can be seen less than three miles away. The growth of Camberwell followed the great expansion of Victorian London. The original villages of Peckham, Camberwell, and Dulwich were old, and the expansion that engulfed them and turned the district into a suburb began between 1800 and 1850 with a rise from 20,000 to 55,000 people and then with a rapid acceleration to reach a population of 260,000 in 1910. By 1969 it had a population of 170,000. During the decade 1871–81 the population increased by more than 75,000 people (Dyos, 1961). Today the area has great social and architectural variety: residents we saw ranged from a few with titles to families living in conditions akin to those of Dickens' London. While there is a clear geographical basis to these social distinctions, as in many parts of London, different types of housing can be found in close proximity. In an analysis of the 1961 census material by the Centre for Urban Studies 45 per cent of Camberwell was grouped as 'stable working class', 28 per cent as 'almost suburban', 23 per cent as 'local authority housing', and 5 per cent as 'poor'. In our first survey in 1970 just under a third of the women were living in local authority housing, a half in private tenancy, and about a fifth were 'owner occupiers'. In spite of this heterogeneity Camberwell is a working-class area in the sense that in 1961 69 per cent of the economically active males were manual workers compared with 54 per cent for London as a whole (and only 33 per cent for Chelsea – albeit an exceptional borough). Like other Inner London boroughs Camberwell has, since the end of the 1939–45 War, suffered a marked reduction in population and in local industry. The most obvious change has been the large scale housing development carried out by the local authority. Many acres of Victorian housing have been cleared and replaced by high-rise flats. Much rebuilding was going on during the period covered by our surveys: we saw one woman who had just had to move from the house in which she was born and had lived for fifty years, another who had had fire engines in her road three times in the previous weeks to cope with fires started by local youths in the demolition debris surrounding her house, and a local small shopkeeper worried at the loss of customers as the houses about her disappeared. Current opinion sees much enforced rehousing as misguided and, as we write, *The Times* notes the comment of a local councillor, on the completion of the largest of these estates, that nothing like it should ever happen again. But the changes should not be exaggerated – much of old Camberwell remains.

We chose Camberwell because of the contacts we had with the Inst: tiute of Psychiatry and the Maudsley Hospital situated not far from Camberwell Green. John Wing and his colleagues (1972) have described the development of its psychiatric services in some detail. The most conspicuous event was the building of the Maudsley Hospital by the London County Council, which was opened in 1915 and which became a postgraduate psychiatric medical school in 1924. Patients could be admitted voluntarily and could also be treated as out-patients. Most admissions, however, took place in one of the large outlying mental hospitals. Wing has described the psychiatric provision in Camberwell in 1964 as one of a rather traditional London service modified by the presence of an undergraduate (King's College) and a postgraduate (Maudsley) teaching hospital. The Maudsley out-patient department is substantial and covers a large proportion of the care in the area as well as providing a service for the rest of London. Its emergency clinic provides a twenty-four hour service. There is also an acute clinic at King's College Hospital, the general hospital opposite the Maudsley. While there were further developments during the period of our study, the important point is that the services are generous compared with elsewhere in London. In Camberwell there were 5,822 out-patient attendances per 100,000 population which is about two and half times the national rate (Wing and Hailey, 1972: 96). Attendances were rising during the five years before our first survey although there is some hint that the rate of increase had reached a peak by 1970.[4]

Throughout the interviewing of the two community samples care was taken to minimize the number of women who declined to be interviewed. This quite often meant that as many as ten visits were made to a household until either someone was found to be in or in some instances until we had managed to contact the particular woman we had selected from that household.

The percentage of refusals was 17 per cent which, given the nature and length of the interview, compares favourably with other surveys.

Finally we saw a small group of women living 500 miles to the North. While nearly all our work has been based on Camberwell, we have recently begun to extend our research to other communities, and we will report some preliminary findings from North Uist, the first of a series of Scottish islands we are studying.

Women in the Outer Hebrides

A random sample of 154 women aged between eighteen and sixty-five living in North Uist in the Outer Hebrides were seen in 1975 in order to establish whether they were suffering from any psychiatric disorder. Since this sample represented 40 per cent of eligible women and only 5 per cent of the women refused to be seen, a reasonably accurate estimate of the prevalence of disorder on the island was probably obtained.

Although the majority of the women used Gaelic as their first language, all spoke good English and the five interviewers (three of whom had had experience of interviewing in the earlier Camberwell series) were not aware of any particular difficulties in communication; nor did they experience difficulty in applying the same standards for rating the severity of individual symptoms or overall psychiatric state. The only general practitioner on the island collaborated fully in the work and the research would have been impossible without his help.[5]

The 'dependent' variable – depression

We have dealt with the concept of depression in chapter 2 and in this chapter we have detailed the various groups of depressed women that we studied. It may therefore be useful at this point to describe these women in terms of some of the main psychiatric measures we will be using.

The Present State Examination in its published form asks about symptoms in the last month. While we questioned in this way, we *also* modified the instrument to cover the twelve months before interview (or in the case of patients before 'admission'). We did this in order to obtain details of any onset of psychiatric disorder in this period. Therefore, at the end of each section of questions (e.g. on 'tension' or 'anxiety'), we asked whether the woman had experienced the symptoms at any time in the year. In addition we established the dates of any onset or change-point in the year.[6] In what follows we therefore present results for the general population in three ways:

(a) prevalence of caseness or borderline caseness in the three months before interview;
(b) prevalence of caseness or borderline caseness at any time in the twelve months;
(c) the proportion of women developing psychiatric disorder, i.e. incidence, at any time in the year. In practice these (*onset* cases) all had a predominant depressive component.

The first measure, the three month prevalence, is the key measure used to describe the amount of psychiatric disorder in Camberwell. The third is the measure used to test for factors influencing onset of depression.

We found that as many as 17 per cent of the 458 women we saw in Camberwell were psychiatrically disturbed at some time in the year – that is were 'cases' (15 per cent in the three months). Most of these were suffering from depression, but there was a small group of other cases such as anxiety states, phobic states, or hypomania. A further 19 per cent were considered borderline cases in the year (18 per cent in the three months).

The following list gives a breakdown in terms of caseness and borderline caseness, chronicity and diagnostic category during the year.

Cases – 17 per cent of sample

Onset cases –
    total 37: 8%
Case depression – 25
Case depression: borderline anxiety – 9
Case depression: case anxiety – 2
Case tension: borderline depression – 1
Case anxiety – 0

Chronic cases –
    total 39: 9%
Case depression – 14
Case depression: borderline anxiety – 14
Case depression: case anxiety – 4
Case anxiety – 5
Case other – 2

Borderline cases – 19 per cent of sample

Onset borderlines –
    total 31: 7%
Depression alone – 25
Depression: anxiety – 5
Anxiety alone – 1

Borderline cases – 19 per cent of sample

Chronic borderlines –   Depression alone – 26
total 56: 12%   Depression: anxiety – 14
                               Anxiety alone – 16

Remaining 'normals' – 64 per cent of sample – Total 295

When we come to present our results we shall often talk of a group of normal women whom we will compare with cases and patients. In practice this group contains both borderline cases and all the 'remaining normals'.

A comparison of the various treatment groups reveals, as might be expected, a gradation in our ratings of overall severity. Taking the top two points of the severity scale 96 per cent of in-patients, 44 per cent of out-patients, 17 per cent of those attending general practitioners, and 11 per cent of community cases were severely disturbed – that is rated 1 or 2 on the five-point scale of overall severity. One problem arising in this comparison is that, although those receiving treatment were probably seen somewhere near the 'peak' of their disorder, cases in the general population were seen at some random point in their disorder. Furthermore there may well be certain rating biases associated with the fact that the latter group were not interviewed in the context of receiving care. We have therefore taken the 'peak' level of disorder recorded during the year for cases.

Having established that the community cases are on the whole less severe than the psychiatric patients, it is interesting to examine whether they differed substantially in the quality of their depression. One method was to assess the women in terms of the criteria elaborated by Feighner and his colleagues and discussed in the last chapter.

This required the simultaneous presence of five of a list of symptoms; the presence of four was an indication of probable disorder. Of the women whom we considered cases during the one month before interview, 70 per cent were either definite or probable depressions according to the Feighner criteria, at the peak of their episode. Of those classified as cases during the three months before interview, but not at one month, again 70 per cent were Feighner positive. It is quite possible to see this as a minimal estimate of the seriousness of our cases since we were unable to use one of the items on their list of symptoms: agitation and retardation in Feighner's sense can only strictly speaking be assessed at the time of interview and not rated on the basis of written descriptions of the related, but slightly differing, scores for restlessness and anergia on the PSE schedule. At the time our interviewers and psychiatric colleagues saw the women they were not instructed in the use of Feighner's criteria and so did not make the appropriate ratings. Our cases were therefore required to reach a score of four or five out of seven rather than eight items; a restriction which would be expected to reduce the number who were positive. Of those who had only been cases earlier in the year, i.e. more than three months before interview, results were less clear-cut, but this was almost certainly related to difficulty in judging co-existence of symptoms at such a distance in time.[7]

Another way of deciding whether general population cases differed in their depression from psychiatric patients was to look at their sub-scores on the PSE. A detailed analysis of some or our cases has been made by John Wing, who collaborated with us in our second random sample. He compared them with depressed in- and out-patients (not our own patient sample, but drawn from the same hospital) (Wing, Nixon, Mann, and Leff, 1977). Symptoms which were similarly distributed in all three groups were depressed mood, muscular tension, worrying, irritability, and early waking. Symptoms that differed markedly between the groups, being rare in the community cases and quite frequent among in-patients were hallucinations and delusions, pathological guilt, slowness, and underactivity. Intermediate between the two were symptoms such as inefficient thinking, suicidal ideas, agitation, subjective anergia, and self-depreciation, which were not uncommon among the general population cases, but more common among psychiatric patients. The relative lack of pathological guilt among the community cases is reminiscent of Clayton's finding among her recently bereaved sample. It was largely this absence of guilt which led her to define her subjects as 'not depressed'. Viewed as a whole these results suggested that although the cases in the general population did differ from psychiatric patients viewed as a single category it was with in-patients that the differences were marked. If compared with out-patients, the cases fell well within the same range both in terms of severity and in terms of types of symptom; for example, more than half the out-patients were given ratings on the bottom three points of the overall severity scale. These findings provided some sort of confirmation, not only of our ratings of caseness but also of the decision to investigate social factors conjointly in treated and untreated cases: it seemed that we were succeeding in classifying like with like.

With this overall account of our design we turn to the measurement of the first of our provoking agents – life-events.

Part II
The Provoking Agents

4 Measurement of life-events

There is a large and apparently causal link between life-events and depression. At least half the depressed women we studied had a recent life-event of aetiological importance. However before this is discussed it is essential to deal with some of the methodological issues surrounding the establishment of causality in non-experimental research. It is not just a matter of statistics and technical issues – although these can be involved. Methodological considerations start from the fact that it will usually be possible to reach alternative conclusions about the same set of results: methodology concerns anything that enables the researcher to rule out explanations that compete with the one favoured. Returning to the investigation of life-events and sore throats in children, perhaps it was not emotional upset but change in routine brought about by the crisis that led to the raised rate of illness? This is an explanation that still assumes that there is a causal link. More fundamentally the whole idea of a causal link might be rejected; it might be suggested, for instance, that the regular fortnightly questioning conveyed to parents what the study was about and some parents, in order to be helpful, made an effort to think of a crisis to 'give' to the investigators once they knew their child had a sore throat. And that this and not a causal link explains the association between life-events and sore throats. Investigators have to do what they can to anticipate such objections. The first, for instance, might be met by excluding from the analysis events likely to have led to changes in a child's routine (e.g. admission of mother to hospital) and demonstrating that the association still held with the remaining events (e.g. the child witnessing a bad road accident). In response to the second, more fundamental, objection it can be pointed out that the association holds not only for overt illness but for the acquisition of strep throats without overt illness. Since parents could not have been aware of such changes in their child the main results become more plausible. These are typical methodological arguments and illustrate how the issues can usually be appreciated without special statistical or mathematical knowledge. One further point should be borne in mind. It is unnecessary to demonstrate that a methodological objection is correct, only that it is a reasonable possibility. It was only possible, not obviously true, that the parents of children with sore throats had made an effort to remember events to 'give' the investigator. The objection is plausible enough to deserve some response.

In this chapter we start with methodological problems surrounding the definition and measurement of life-events, using for illustration some early work with schizophrenia.

Life-events and distress

Lindemann's classic paper on reaction to bereavement and David Mechanic's well-known *Students Under Stress* dealing with university examinations, like most work on life-events, concern distressing circumstances. However there is no need for research to restrict itself in this way. Barbara and Bruce Dohrenwend (1974a), while seeing life-events as disrupting – or threatening to disrupt – usual activities, do *not* view them as necessarily involving negative experience, and a wide range of incidents can therefore be studied – finishing school, starting a job, leaving parents, marriage, birth of a child, death, divorce, promotion, and move of a house. But this at once raises the question of where we stop. Hans Selye, who published the first of his influential papers based on animal experiments in 1936, has argued that stress is a natural by-product of human activities. In similar vein Lawrence Hinkle writes:

'The ordinary activities of daily life – the ingestion of food, or the failure to ingest food; muscular activity, or the absence of muscular activity; breathing, or not breathing; sleeping, or not sleeping – all affect the dynamic steady state. Their effects are not qualitatively different from those of the "stressors" that are used in the laboratory. It has been aptly said "to be alive is to be under stress".'
(1973: 43)

Since the reasoning behind this kind of broad definition is the notion that stress-is-a-part-of-our-smallest-activities, one response to the question of where we stop is to reject this view of stress. Mason (1975) argues that too little attention has been given to the fact that laboratory experiments with animals using physical stressors such as exercise, heat, and cold are usually *also* emotionally disturbing. Responses of the pituitary-adrenal cortical system first studied by Selye may be largely due to psychological responses to the experimental situation on the animal's part. If much of biological stress research can be seen in these terms, there is not the same case for considering change as such as stressful irrespective of its meaning for the subject.

But although this simplifies the issue it still leaves us with the dilemma of what should be included as a life-event. Even if we reject the idea that 'to be alive is to be under stress' there is still a need to settle where to place the threshold for disruption or disturbance. The Dohrenwends, who quote Hinkle's passage, are clearly worried by its implications and note that although they 'do not doubt the truth of this generalisation, it nevertheless is a highly abstract truth' (1974: 4). They deal with the question by returning to the notion of distress, concluding that life-events differ in stressfulness and it is necessary to distinguish the more from the less stressful. Fortunately our early work with schizophrenic patients provided an answer which gives a flexible solution. We first became interested in life-events in 1959 when talking to the relatives of schizophrenic patients about what had led to admission. One wife told us how her husband's doctor had insisted that he stay at home until he could be admitted to hospital for a minor hernia operation. (In fourteen years he had never before had time off work.) A fortnight later to her amazement he took off his clothes and rushed into the nearby church, shouting about a plot to get him. As we continued we found other incidents closely antedating onset of schizophrenic symptoms. In the next interview a wife told us how her son had come home from school to say, to everyone's surprise, that it had been settled that he was to go to sea as a trainee merchant naval officer almost at once, a year earlier than they had thought. Within two days of his leaving, her husband developed schizophrenic symptoms. In the next but one interview a couple, who had been planning for over a year to move into a new home, took a week off work, 'planning everything like a military operation'. All went well at first; symptoms developed suddenly on the seventh day of these preparations, on the night of the move itself, when the patient woke his wife with a flood of strange talk about someone stealing their gas stove.

Our first reaction was to be puzzled by the variety of the incidents. Some were unexpected but others had been eagerly sought; some were major catastrophes but others involved no more than a change in routine; some involved nothing by way of a change or disruption of routine and others even the occurrence of something much desired. No definition in the literature appeared to fit (see Mechanic, 1968: 301). Most definitions emphasize the need for a novel pattern of problem-solving or threat to an important life-goal. We could not readily square the heterogeneity of our incidents with such formulations. Although we were in no position to say what was important, it was clear that the move planned 'like a military operation' did not demand novel patterns of problem solving (the couple had done it before and could scarcely have been better prepared) not did it involve any threat to important life-goals (they had eagerly sought it).

While at this point we did not wish to commit ourselves to a rigid definition, our interviews did suggest that schizophrenia might be precipitated by marked emotions of *any* kind – by joy and excitement as well as by distress and fear. This would be enough to explain our puzzlement about the bewildering variety of events. Tomkins (1962 and 1963) has discussed eight innate affects and the wide range of stimuli that produce them – interest or excitement, enjoyment or joy, surprise or startle, distress or anguish, fear or terror, shame or humiliation, contempt or disgust, anger or rage. We therefore came to see life-events in terms of the emotions they might arouse irrespective of the quality of the emotion involved; and as some psychologists have argued, it is the *appraisal* of the environment that leads to emotion and to 'stress' (e.g. Arnold, 1961; Lazarus, 1966). We will also need to keep in mind that it is likely to be the meaning of events that is significant rather than change as such.

Measurement of life-events in the schizophrenic study

In the schizophrenic study itself we therefore started with the somewhat vague belief that marked emotion could be enough to precipitate florid symptoms. At this point we made a critical decision that has had major methodological ramifications throughout our research programme. We decided to define or measure events in terms of the likelihood of their having produced strong emotion rather than by the emotion they actually produced. The implications of this decision will only gradually emerge, but it is clear that it had the considerable advantage of allowing us to avoid the onerous task of establishing the emotional arousal consequent on previous events.

We therefore drew up a comprehensive list of events which could be dated to a particular point in time and which we believed would for most people be likely to be followed by strong negative or positive emotion. These were the basic units of study. It did not matter that a particular event was not in fact followed by emotional arousal. We largely restricted ourselves to events involving the respondent (henceforth called the subject) and his 'close ties'; that is members of his or her household or a close relative (i.e. spouse or cohabitee, parent, sibling, child, or fiance), but at times particularly dramatic incidents involving more distant relatives or even strangers were included as long as the subject had been present (e.g. witnessing a serious road accident). In the depression study we also included confidants as close ties. A confidant was an especially close friend, defined as one to whom the subject felt able to confide any problems or worries with complete trust.

The list contained thirty-eight types of event falling into the following eight groups:

(i) changes in a role for the subject such as changing a job and losing or gaining an opposite-sex friend for the unmarried;[1]

(ii) changes in a role for close relatives or household members, such as a husband staying off work because of a strike;

(iii) major changes in health, including admissions to hospital and developing an illness expected to be serious; and

(iv) similar changes in close relatives or household members;

(v) residence changes and any marked change in amount of contact with close relatives and household members;

(vi) forecasts of change, such as being told about being rehoused;

(vii) valued goal fulfillments or disappointments, such as being offered a house to rent at a reasonable price;

(viii) other dramatic events involving (a) the subject, e.g. witnessing a serious accident or being stopped by the police when driving, or (b) a close relative or household member, e.g. learning that a brother had been arrested.

In every instance the events can be seen as involving *change* in an activity, role, person, or idea.[2]

Two illustrations will be enough to give a general idea of our standards; a more general sense can be got from Appendix 3 which gives examples of most types of event.

(1) For major changes in health we included events occurring to those with whom the subject lived as well as close relatives. All admissions to hospital for the subject were included, but only those that were urgent or lasting one week for other persons. Illnesses not followed by admission were counted only if in our judgment they involved a possible threat to life or were alarming enough for serious implications to be suspected. Accidents were covered by similar criteria. There was one exception: we included any new contact with a psychiatric service by a close relative. Deaths of anyone at home and close relatives were included but otherwise only when the respondent had been present or involved in the immediate aftermath (such events were rare).[3]

(2) Marked changes in social contact included anyone leaving home after a stay of at least three months, someone coming for as long as three months, and the start of a relationship with someone of the opposite sex (if it seemed likely to continue for some time) or its ending (if it had lasted for at least eight weeks). Close relatives were included where frequency of contact had been reduced by at least two-thirds and where the usual rate of contact (including telephone calls) had been at least once a month.[4] In order to meet these criteria a total break was usually involved – the person most often moving some distance from London.

In addition to the list of events which, with the necessary probes, was used as an interview schedule, we developed a reference book of several hundred pages which included extensive instructions along the lines of the preceding paragraphs for each of the thirty-eight classes of event. These guided the interviewer and enabled a decision to be made about what to include. It was insufficient, for example, simply to ask about accidents. It was necessary to settle before the main study began whether to include, say, an accident to a woman's husband which required out-patient treatment but about which she knew nothing until he came home. But the definitions had a more fundamental purpose than accuracy of measurement. We were concerned that in the actual study any decisions left open might be influenced by knowledge about whether the event had antedated a schizophrenic attack. This is the first of a number of specific methodological issues, which we will discuss, based on the logic we have already outlined: is there anything about the way data were collected that would enable a would-be critic to conclude that a putative causal link could be the result of an artefact? That, for example, more events occurred before onset of schizophrenia because the interviewer had lowered his threshold for inclusion of an incident as an 'event' when he knew the person to be schizophrenic. The definition of accidents therefore served a methodological purpose. A case could be made for both including and excluding the accident to the woman's husband. (We in fact excluded it.) The important point was to settle the matter *before* we began our main research and then apply a common set of standards to everyone.

We spent a good deal of time developing these standards and in the main research we did not often come across events about which we had not already made a ruling. However, the approach did mean that at times apparently significant events were excluded. One schizophrenic patient, for instance, broke down within days of learning that her son had sat an examination that would play a part in determining his chances of going to a grammar school. She had been educated until she was nineteen but had failed every examination. Although she had married a man with an unskilled job, she sent their children to a small private school – something extremely rare in London. The event's likely symbolic importance is obvious. It was not included as it had not been explicitly settled that such examinations would be included before beginning the main study.

This example also illustrates a more general point. It does not matter if 'rules' developed for methodological purposes lead at times to such 'errors' as long as it is still possible to argue that there has been no exaggeration of the size of the causal effect. In the present instance, the exclusion of the child's examination could only serve to reduce the size of any association between life-events and onset of schizophrenia. We believe this holds for all our methodological procedures. We have aimed not so much for complete accuracy as for an ability to decide about the role of social factors in the aetiology of psychiatric disorders. But we were not unmindful of the need for accuracy and, before continuing with methodological problems of life-event research, we will discuss this aspect of our measures, in both the schizophrenia and the depression studies.

Reliability and accuracy of our life-event measures

Accuracy is a basic (if somewhat pedestrian) matter of sound methods of data collection. It is related to methodological issues in the sense that without a fair degree of accuracy they are likely to prove irrelevant.

There has been a fair amount of controversy about the possibility of collecting and accurately dating events and onset of psychiatric disorder. Since only events occurring before onset can play an aetiological role, we, in fact, made a considerable effort to date events precisely. The period of study (three months for schizophrenia and twelve months for depression) was divided into weeks and events allocated to one of these. Where dating was not immediately clear, an attempt to relate events to 'anchor dates' such as public holidays, a birthday, or a firm's outing often helped, and if nothing like this appeared to be relevant, already established dates (such as moving house) were used as a check. Whenever possible we checked from another source the date of any event that was in doubt; hospitals, general practitioners, housing departments, and police were all at times approached – always with the subject's permission. Where there was still doubt about the dating of an event, a range of uncertainty was plotted and its midpoint taken in the analysis.

We found that respondents, particularly in the study of depression, often found it easier to describe *onset* when there was some anchor point to which to relate their account; indeed when the respondent did not give a suitable incident we usually did our best to provide one by referring to a Bank Holiday, Bonfire Night, an important public event, and the like. Not infrequently an actual crisis or life-change was mentioned quite spontaneously. The respondent was always encouraged to relate onset to other things and if there was a nearby event we usually asked a direct question about their proximity (but nothing about cause and effect). We were aware that there might be a tendency for the respondent or interviewer to place event and onset nearer than they should be. We can only state that we did our best to avoid this. Indeed the interviewers were encouraged to ask 'leading questions' of the sort 'Are you sure the change you mentioned came *after* your mother's accident? Could it have come before?' In general we believe that the chance of such bias will be lessened if the event and onset are asked about in detail and the justification for the dating of each scrutinized as much as possible during the interview itself.

In 1970 Hudgens and his colleagues in St Louis published a paper in the *British Journal of Psychiatry* concluding that a causal link had not been convincingly demonstrated between life-events and psychiatric disorder. A major point of the argument was that they found in their own study only a 57 per cent agreement between accounts of patients and additional respondents about events occurring in the previous twelve months.

There are two issues. The simplest is the reliability of a measure in the sense of whether two raters can agree – say about whether a particular incident should be included as an event. The second is the more complex question of validity: is the measure doing what it claims to do? There are many different forms. The most obvious is whether two separate respondents report the occurrence of a particular event. These two issues are related in that a measure with low reliability cannot be shown to be valid. A husband and wife may both mention the same incident when seen by separate interviewers. But, if one of the interviewers fails to record the incident as an 'event', measurement will be unreliable and since the couple will, in effect, be recorded as disagreeing, this will contribute to its invalidity.

The reliability of our basic life-event measures was in fact very high (with correlations of at least .90 between raters). However, similar high levels of reliability can usually be achieved on such rating tasks if sufficient time is spent in developmental work and training (e.g. Brown and Rutter, 1966; Rutter and Brown, 1966). The issue of validity reflected in the amount of agreement between patient and relative about events when seen separately by different interviewers is more open – and in any case more fundamental. Low validity is compatible with a highly reliable measure. Fortunately agreement between patient and relative was high. In the schizophrenic study there was an 81 per cent agreement between the two about the occurrence of the *same* event and practically no disagreement about time of onset of the disorder. (It should be borne in mind, however, that the schizophrenic patients were specially selected because of a recent and acute onset of symptoms. Patients were accepted only if we considered that onset could be dated to within a period of seven days.) For the first fifty patients in the depressive study an additional respondent who knew the patient was seen. As in the schizophrenic study interviewers never discussed material until all the ratings had been made. Agreement was the same as for the schizophrenic study although a year and not three months was covered: agreement was 79 per cent about events reported by the patient *or* relative in the period before onset (of the total events 11 per cent were reported by the patient alone and 10 per cent by the relative alone). There was no difference in the amount of agreement shown by household and non-household respondents, or by whether the patient reported the other respondent as a confidant or not. Nor did severity of the patient's condition make much difference. Agreement about the dating of onset was also good – results have already been given in chapter 2 (p. 35).

The difference between the St Louis and London studies merits some comment. For high levels of agreement to be obtained it is essential for interviewers to have a list of specific questions about possible events with the backing of very clear definitions of what is to be included. Without both of these, the reporting or recording of events will almost certainly be biased and it is difficult to make a meaningful comparison between the accounts of patient and relative. Hudgens and his colleagues 'recorded all events which the patient considered important whether we did or not' (1967). But this means that differences between patient and relative were bound to occur about what they considered to have been worrying or distressful; such an approach makes certain that some of the disagreement between patient and relative will be about the *importance* of the event rather than its occurrence. For example, the St Louis group report a number of disagreements between patient and relative about the 'death of a spouse, relative or friend'. But since the disagreements all involved the death of someone who was a 'distant relative' or who was a 'friend', it is probable that either the patient or relative considered the death not 'important enough' to mention.

There are other reasons to expect differences between the two approaches. In the St Louis study we are told that subjects and their relatives were questioned about the occurrence and absence of events in a standardized list of areas such as legal trouble, trouble in school or job, or sickness in relative, friend, or spouse. It is not clear, however, how far the interviewer used a detailed check list of different types of illness, examples of different types of legal trouble, financial difficulty, and so on. We found it necessary not only to ask such fairly specific questions, but also at times to give indications of the sort of thing we had in mind. For instance, they give an example of disagreement about a 'marital separation' and state that 'the husband did not call this separation'. Our approach is quite different. As already outlined, a specific question would first be asked along the lines 'Have you and your wife been separated for any length of time over the past twelve months?'. The length of any 'separation' would then be established and only then a decision made about whether it had lasted long enough to count as an 'event' in terms of the rules that had already been established. The respondent was not left to decide on what was an 'event'. Nor were his first responses to questions necessarily accepted. Interviewers were encouraged to do a certain amount of further questioning to help ensure that all possibilities and all relevant persons had been covered. For example, we found it was not enough to make a general statement at the beginning of the interview about the relatives in whom we were interested; as the interview progressed respondents were often reminded of the relatives we were interested to hear about ('What about your sister?' etc.). The interviewer was also always on the look-out for any hint of the occurrence of an event and added further questions as appeared necessary. In other words we relied a great deal on the skill, judgment, and sensitivity of the interviewer, although, at the same time, there was a good deal of control over her activity.

We conclude that there is no reason why recent life-events cannot be collected with a good deal of accuracy – certainly enough for scientific purposes. Before we return to methodological issues surrounding life-event research we will present briefly some of the results of the research on schizophrenia.

Schizophrenia and life-events

In 1960 a pilot study showed that life-events were particularly common in the three weeks immediately before the onset of a schizophrenic attack. In the main study this was confirmed: 60 per cent of the schizophrenic patients had had at least one event in the three-week period before onset, compared with an average of only 23 per cent in the three preceding three-week periods. A very wide range of events were involved. The higher rate was restricted to the three weeks immediately before onset. A survey in the general population showed that 20 per cent of 325 men and women had had at least one event in each of the four three-week periods before interview, confirming that the effect appeared to be restricted to the three weeks before onset.[5]

The concept of 'independent' events

An obvious objection to any claim that these findings represent a causal link is that many of the events in the schizophrenic group could have been brought about by the insidious onset of the illness itself – that, for instance, the patient's odd manner for some time before onset had led to a broken love affair. If this were so, there would be no need to see the events in the three weeks before onset as playing a causal role although they clearly antedated the florid symptoms. Indeed we did not start serious research until a possible solution to this objection occurred to us. This struck us when considering the man who had stayed at home to await an operation. He had apparently done so for reasons clearly independent of the schizophrenic illness: it was his doctor who had insisted that he remain at home to rest. If we were to look only at events that could be argued on logical grounds very likely to be independent of any insidious onset of the disorder, there was hope of a solution. We therefore classified events as *independent* which were apparently imposed upon the subject and which were for all

Table 1 *Percentage with at least one event in the four 3-week periods before onset (schizophrenic patients, n = 50) and interview general population, n = 325*

	3-week periods before onset/interview			
	(furthest) 4th[b] %	3rd[b] %	2nd[b] %	(nearest) 1st[a] %
	Independent events			
1. schizophrenic patients	14	8	14	46
general population	15	15	14	14
	Possibly independent events			
2. schizophrenic patients	16	10	6	22
general population	6	5	5	5
	All Events			
3. schizophrenic patients	30	18	20	60
General population	21	20	18	19

[a] p<.001 in all three groups
[b] no differences are significant

practical purposes outside his or her control: for example, learning of a father's serious illness, or discovering a burglary.[6]

The classification of 'independent' events excludes many possible precipitating events and therefore can only give a minimal estimate of the role of such factors. We therefore also classified as 'possibly independent' (of the disorder) similar events about which the same logical claims could not be made, but, again, about which there was no evidence to suggest they had been related to unusual behaviour of the subject. They mostly comprise the acquisition or loss of opposite-sex friends or changes in job (although loss of job would, under certain circumstances, be rated as 'independent', e.g. when a whole firm closed down).[7]

Since the association between events and onset of schizophrenia was equally strong for both 'independent' and 'possibly independent' events the possibility that our results had been influenced by the insidious onset of the illness could be discounted (*Table 1*).

Three sources of contamination

So far we have dealt with issues of methodology and life-event research in a somewhat haphazard fashion in terms of the development of our own thinking. It is time to discuss in a more systematic way the major methodological criticisms that can be levelled at such research. Some of the issues already discussed will be dealt with again but now within a more general framework.

One of the troubles of many definitions in social sciences and psychiatry is that they are circular and self-defeating for a causal enquiry. If we define 'endogenous' depression in terms of lack of precipitating events we are making assumptions that can make it extremely difficult to demonstrate that the effect does exist – that 'endogenous' depression is in fact linked to events. Similarly, if we decide to define crises in terms of untoward reactions there will by definition never be a crisis without such an outcome. How can we show this if we have already assumed it?

One way of avoiding the self-defeating nature of such definitions and the confusion of 'dependent' and 'independent' variables is to distinguish a *unit* of study from its *qualities* (Parsons, 1949: 27–41). While a unit can be thought of by itself (a family, a journey), it also has qualities that can only be conceived as existing as part of it (a happy or unhappy family, a tiring or relaxing journey). Circularity is avoided if we do not assume a one for one relationship between the two – that a life-event always involves changes in routine or always leads to tension. As a fuller example, let us assume that we wish to examine the link between change of job and onset of physical illness. 'Change of job' is the *unit* of analysis and we must keep from its definition anything that might follow from it (e.g. anxiety resulting from the change). We may already have an idea of what it is that is important for our problem – say anxiety arising from the change, the demand for new skills, and the like – but this must still be excluded. However, it is possible to take account of phenomena such as anxiety as possible *qualities* of the *unit* and their role as possible intervening variables can thus be examined.[8]

This approach means we can collect data systematically without committing ourselves to a final decision as to what constitutes 'stress'. It also, as will be seen, helps to solve a number of difficult methodological problems. It has, however, a significant corollary: it is essential that unit and quality are not only kept separate in the definition of a life-event but *at all stages of their measurement*. Although we may have defined life-events entirely without reference to the emotional upheaval that followed them, knowledge that incidents were followed by psychiatric disorder may be illegitimately allowed to influence what is counted as an event. There are many ways in which bias during measurement might occur.

We have already discussed one of the best large-scale, survey-type enquiries of mental disorder, done in Manhattan. Standard questions such as 'when you were a teenager did you have disagreements with your parents . . . often, occasionally, rarely, never?' were put to a random sample of people; and an overall score based on many such items concerned with past stress was found to be highly related to the presence of psychiatric disorder (Langner and Michael, 1963). The difficulty in accepting the association as causal is that it is possible, perhaps likely, that the meanings which the respondents attached to past events were influenced by their present psychiatric state; for example, the depressed may well see their pasts in a more unfortunate light, that is, they may reconstruct the past in the light of their present mood.

An example of particular relevance is provided by research published by Stott in 1958 showing that mothers of mongol children reported that they had had more shocks during pregnancy than had mothers with normal children. He concluded that socio-emotional factors were important in the aetiology of mongolism. However, work published soon afterwards indicated chromosomal abnormalities as the distinguishing feature of mongol children and this suggested that the interpretation was almost certainly wrong (Polani *et al.*, 1960). The obvious explanation for the association was that the mothers had been searching for reasons to explain their tragedy and because of this were likely to recall shocks or to define quite ordinary events as traumas where mothers of normal children would not. In other words, they assigned a meaning *after* the birth of their child to what happened during pregnancy which they would not necessarily have considered noteworthy *prior* to the birth.

Such reworking of the past can obviously play havoc with aetiological studies. In terms of our discussion, *defining* a life-event separately from possible consequences is not enough if they are allowed to influence each other in the process of *measurement*. The unit (shock) and its possible consequences (mongolism) appear to be causally related probably because they have been confounded during measurement.

The importance of this issue can be illustrated by considering the Holmes-Rahe measure of life-events which has dominated research in the field in recent years (1967). The instrument – the Schedule of Recent Experience (SRE) – has significant accomplishments. Perhaps most impressive has been its use to predict rates of illness in longitudinal studies (Rahe, 1969). The trouble comes in interpreting whether events have played any kind of causal role.

Measurement of life-events by the SRE schedule has two stages:

Stage 1: the development of weights

The investigators first carried out a calibration study. Subjects completed a questionnaire in which they were asked to allocate a score to forty-four brief descriptions of events in terms of the amount of social readjustment required. They were told that adjustment should be seen as the degree of rearrangement involved and length of time necessary to accommodate to the event, regardless of its desirability. The first event, marriage, was given a value of 50 – bearing this in mind, the subjects went on to give values to events such as 'troubles with the boss', 'death of spouse', 'major change in the health or behaviour of a family member', and 'major change in the number of arguments with spouse'. In this way life-change unit scores were calculated for forty-two life-events. Each of these sets of scores were then averaged and a new score allocated, ranging from 100 (death of spouse), 50 (marriage), to 11 (minor violations of the law).

The descriptions used to rate degree of readjustment were exceedingly brief. A person simply 'begins or stops work'; we do not know whether the change is forced or voluntary, whether due to the birth of a baby, a husband's antagonism, or winning money in a lottery. Does it mean losing important ties or the need to make new ones? Is the change the first or has it occurred many times before? Because of the briefness of the descriptions raters are bound to have to call upon their own experience. The avowed purpose of the approach to avoid issues of 'psychological meaning, emotion and social desirability' is thus not met; moreover, because the descriptions are so brief there is little control over the way such experience is drawn upon.[9]

Stage 2: use of the schedules

When used for research purposes the SRE questionnaires are filled out and the *averaged* weights from the calibration study used to score events. A total life-change score is obtained for each respondent based on his or her answers as to whether the events have occured (most usually in a six-month period). The item 'changes in health in a family member' is, for instance, given a score of 44 – this is a relatively high score, marital separation has a score of 65. But although the score for each event never changes, it is left quite open to the respondent to interpret what is meant by such questions. Just *what* is a change of health and just *who* is a family member? There is bound to be a variety of interpretations but the same life-event score of 44 is given to anyone checking the item. Instead of avoiding the issue of meaning, the investigators have come full circle and have no control over the way personal meaning influences their scores.

We are not in principle against trying to obtain average scores. *Our criticism of the SRE schedule is that it is far too vague in specifying the situations. The way in which each subject understands the brief account of each life-event must vary; and there can be little idea how to interpret results that show associations between life-event scores and illness.* In spite of appearances the research has not provided a convincing case for a causal link between life-events and illness.[10]

Such an approach cannot rule out the presence of two kinds of error. The first is essentially random; since the investigator in his measurement procedure is not placing like with like, the whole quality of research will suffer. This is a matter of sound data collection which we have already discussed. It is the second, the systematic biases that might well stem from the kind of procedures employed in the SRE, which are crucial for the present discussion; because of the open-endedness of the questions there is a considerable risk that the illness, or factors involved in bringing it about, will influence answers to the questionnaire. Cause and consequence may be related to the unit not because of shortcomings of definitions but because of possible bias in the measurement procedure itself.[11] In the SRE a correlation between events and illness may be produced by a confounding factor raising or lowering the threshold of either (i) what is considered worthwhile to report, or (ii) the range of persons borne in mind when reporting a particular event. For instance, under certain circumstances a person may be more likely to report a quite trivial illness; or, leaving aside severity, be more likely to report illness occurring to a wider range of kin than he would usually consider in answering such a question. We have already, in the example of mongolism discussed the way contamination can occur because of the *emergence* of meaning. The past, present, and future are not distinct in their influence on behaviour. Past experience can influence the definition of the present; but inferences about the future can also influence an understanding of past events – new meanings may emerge (McHugh 1968). Bartlett (1932) many years ago coined the phrase 'effort after meaning' when studying such behaviour. Such processes can also influence the reporting of central life experiences and this is a particular danger in studying depression, since grief is especially likely to involve 'reworking' the past.

Much of the research with the SRE schedule is retrospective and because of the very general nature of its questions about events is particularly open to such *direct contamination* through, for example, 'effort after meaning' on the part of the respondents. This is illustrated in *Figure 1*. The effect can occur as a result of either differential reporting by the subject or of differential rating by the investigator – referred to as R in the figure, standing for a rating /reporting effect. Since X (say the event) occures at time 1 but is not measured until later, time 2, its measurement can be affected by R's knowledge of the illness Y. Time of occurrence (top line) is shown separately from time of measurement (bottom line). Such contamination means that an investigator cannot claim that a correlation between X and Y represents a causal link – in this instance that life-events bring about illness.[12]

However, there have been a number of prospective studies; although direct contamination in these is no longer possible because of the nature of the questions, *indirect contamination* is unfortunately still

Figure 1   Direct contamination

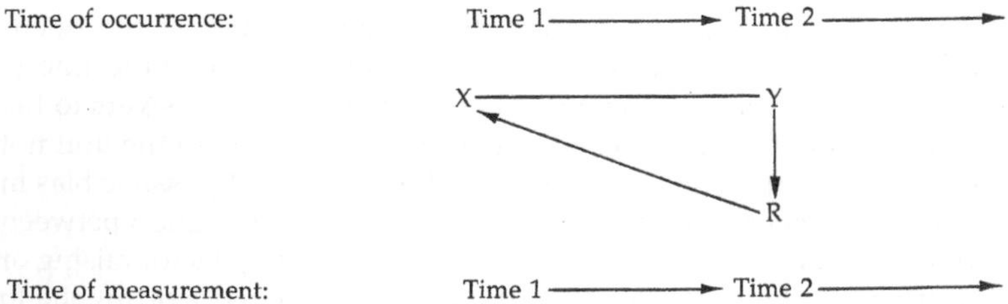

Time of occurrence: Time 1 ⟶ Time 2 ⟶

Time of measurement: Time 1 ⟶ Time 2 ⟶

likely. Such an effect is illustrated in *Figure 2*. Assume, as an example, X (event) is measured by investigator R before Y (illness) has occurred. Direct contamination must be ruled out as R does not know of Y when X is measured. But the measurement of X in the figure is influenced by, say, whether or not the subject is anxious, A, and it is in fact A and not X that is causally linked with Y. It follows that without A the correlation between X and Y would disappear. Contamination therefore is still present in spite of the prospective design. There are other ways this could come about. It is possible that a general high level of anxiety leads to *both* illness and a greater tendency to report life-events. It is well established that generally worded questionnaire items are particularly subject to response-sets (e.g. Berg, 1967). This means that the questionnaire items systematically pick up a characteristic of the respondent other than that which it is hoped to study. It is not at all far-fetched to suggest that in the use of the SRE schedule factors, such as anxiety level, influence reporting of events and experience of the physical illness studied. Indeed the items of the SRE schedule are so general that it may well function as a measure of 'mood' or 'personality'. The important point is that X and Y appear to be causally linked only because A is causing both of them.

Figure 2 Indirect contamination

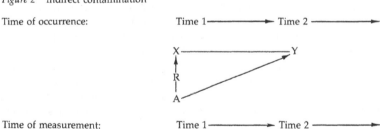

Time of occurrence: Time 1 ————————→ Time 2 ——————————→

Time of measurement: Time 1 ————————→ Time 2 ——————————→

There is a final source of contamination, which is particularly relevant to research, which specifies 'stressfulness' in its questioning about events and thereby makes it part of the unit of measurement rather than just one of the qualities an event may have. Even if life-event *scores* are not subject to either type of contamination, conclusions may still be invalid because the *experience* of life-events as stressful is influenced by a third factor that also influences the rate of illness. The two forms of invalidity discussed so far concern measurement, but the question here is whether the correlation between X and Y does not represent a causal link because a third variable, A, influences both and produces a *spurious* link as shown in *Figure 3*:

Figure 3   Spuriousness

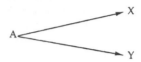

This kind of invalidity may occur even if *the measures are completely accurate*. Erroneous conclusions, for instance, may be made even if life-events were experienced as 'upsetting' in the way described by the respondent. Accurate description of the stressfulness of a life-event would not avoid false conclusions if a third and prior factor influenced the subject's *experience* of stressfulness of the event and the illness itself. For example, a person's high general anxiety level may lead to both a greater chance of illness and a greater tendency to experience life-events as markedly stressful. In such a case a conclusion about the existence of a causal link between markedly stressful events and illness would be misleading. The correlation between X and Y is not causal since it has been produced by the prior factor A; and the only way to sort this out would be to control for the component of the measure of life-events that was due to the personality trait. Again the SRE schedule is open to this possibility. A recent account of its use in a prospective study of 4,463 naval personnel does nothing to allay suspicion about the presence of either indirect contamination or spuriousness (Rahe, Gunderson and Pugh, 1972). Life-changes and anxiety both have small associations with subsequent illness (.07 and .15 respectively); but the correlation between anxiety and life-events themselves is a good deal greater (.32). There are several possible interpretations. It is possible that life-events are of causal significance and anxiety merely an intervening variable linking life-event to illness. But equally life-events may be irrelevant. A high life-change score may simply be the result of anxiety. While it is not worth speculating on such possibilities without additional data, the results do underline the argument that the SRE schedule has such serious flaws that its conclusions could justifiably be discounted by any critics.

This discussion should have made clear the full significance of the separation of unit and quality both in definition of life-events (what the investigator intends to measure) and in measurement (what he actually ends up rating); the procedures described in the London measure deal with all three sources of validity. Life-events are measured without relying on what the respondent said about his or her reaction to the event. In *measurement* as well as in the *definition* we exclude consideration of the reactions to the event. Further, by the detailed definitions of the thirty-eight life-events and the persons who are covered, there is strict control of what the investigator is able to include. By the use of standard questions (and suitable probes) about the occurrence of particular life-events and the avoidance of questions about reactions to events, it can be established whether certain events occur irrespective of how a person felt about them or of the inter- viewer's judgment of what part they may have played in the onset of the psychiatric disorder. The approach therefore controls possible contamination stemming from both respondent *and* interviewer.

The approach for all its strengths, however, has a devastating dis- advantage: it treats essentially all similar types of 'event' such as births as alike. It is strong methodologically but weak theoretically. It allows us to be reasonably confident about the presence of a causal link but at the expense of treating a wide range of events as alike that are not alike. The birth of a child does not mean the same thing for all women.

5 Meaning

This is the last of our preparatory chapters. The research with schizo-phrenia took little account of the nature of life-events – merely that they usually disrupted ongoing activity and led to a variety of emotions.

For schizophrenia it had made some sense to treat events as alike, but this was surely unlikely to pay off with depression. We had no alternative than to make an attempt to take account of the full variety of events, although doing our best to retain the methodological gains outlined in the last chapter. But before we outline what we did, why should we think of depression in this way?

First, it seemed absurd to separate its aetiology entirely from the kind of experiences capable of provoking ordinary experiences of depression. Since we began our work Aaron Beck has emphasized the parallel between the way in which emotions follow cognitions in ordinary life and in psychopathological states, and the importance of cognition – the way we look at the world – for the understanding of clinical depression. He has formulated his view in terms of a cognitive triad: a negative conception of self, a negative interpretation of life's experiences, and a nihilistic view of the future, and argues that the typical bodily and emotional symptoms of clinical depression arise from such an appraisal – from this cognitive triad (Beck 1971). We agree and in later chapters argue that feelings of hopelessness are the core of clinical depression. These feelings usually occur in response to some external change, although the possibility that such feelings of hope-lessness occasionally occur without an obvious external stimulus should not be ruled out. A somewhat similar theme treating depres-sion as an expression of a state of hopelessness, helplessness, and powerlessness, can be found in a number of writers, although it is not always entirely clear how far proponents of such a view of depression distinguish cognitions developing after onset of depression from those before (Bibring, 1953; Lichtenberg, 1957; and Melges and Bowlby, 1969).

Aaron Beck goes further and suggests that the difference between normal and abnormal reactions to the environment lies in the degree of correspondence between the conceptualization and the stimulus. 'In psychopathological states perseverative faulty conceptualisation leads to excessive or inappropriate affective disturbance' (Beck 1971: 495). There is, in other words, something wrong with the person in the first place. We believe that this is an unnecessary stipulation. Depression may also come from entirely accurate conceptualization, the 'fault' lying in the environment rather than in the person. We can envisage a society where the quality of life is such that a majority experience clinical depression at some time in their lives and another society that is so 'protected' that relatively few do so. It is clear that the ratio of faulty to unfaulty conceptualizations preceding these depressions is likely to be different in the two populations. Those developing depression in the less 'protected' environment are more likely to do so without obviously unusual conceptualizations. This view suggests that responses to the environment need to be studied as part of a broad investigation of clinical depression in a total population; it calls for research in which the guiding principle is first to explain as much as possible in terms of everyday experience in that community.

What then is the disruption that everyone agrees life-events can bring and whose meaning we must capture in our measures?

The disruptiveness of life-events

Life-events usually entail change and this they do to lives built about routine. Even at Auschwitz things that happen occurred against a background of routine, which broke the prisoners' day into just manageable bits:

> 'A day begins like every other day, so long as not to allow us reasonably to conceive its end, so much cold, so much hunger, so much exhaustion separate us from it: so that it is better to concentrate one's attention and desires on the block of grey bread, which is small but which will certainly be ours in an hour, and which for five minutes, until we have devoured it, will form everything that the law of the place allows us to possess.'
>
> (Levi, 1959: 49)

The significance of life-events must be sought, we believe, in this interplay of the exceptional and the usual. Razumov in Conrad's

Western Approaches, after a day of shattering experiences in which he betrays a man who came to him for help, arrives home pondering how his gateway has stayed the same:

> 'The sense of life's continuity depended on trifling bodily impressions. The trivialities of daily existence were an armour for the soul. And this thought reinforced the inward quietness of Razumov as he began to climb the stairs familiar to his feet in the dark, with his hand on the familiar clammy banister. The exceptional could not prevail against the material contacts which make one day resemble another. Tomorrow would be like yesterday. It was only on the stage that the unusual was outwardly acknowledged.'   (1963: 44)

But the exceptional may also deny to us this sense of reality and security. Tolstoy, in his short story, 'The Death of Ivan Ilyitch', describes how the daughter of the dying Ivan Ilyitch comes to his room dressed for a party 'with her exuberant bosom swelling in her stays and with traces of powder on her face'. The family gather about him and daughter and mother have a quarrel about who has mislaid the opera glasses. Tolstoy describes in harrowing detail Ivan Ilyitch's struggle to relate his pain and possible coming death to this everyday world – a world that no longer brings him comfort. The more his thoughts touch on his life the more dubious seem its pleasures: 'My marriage – so unexpected, and disillusionment and my wife's breath, and her sensuality and hypocrisy! And this dead service, and these labours for money; and this one year, and two and ten and twenty, and always the same thing.'

With change we risk, at least temporarily, losing the sense of life's reality. Tolstoy's story illustrates something else: crises may raise fundamental questions about our lives. They focus our attention on the present and since this is the visible outcome of our past – our choices, commitments, and mistakes – we may come to question what our life might have been, what it is about, and what it will become. A son leaving home may produce for his mother alarming thoughts about the hollowness of her marriage and how she is to cope with it without him. Indeed, anticipation of change may be enough – simply news that her son is proposing to emigrate. The turmoil produced by a life-event can therefore be as much about the routines of life as about the crisis itself – as much about her marriage as her son. An apparently innocuous event may at time be enough to do this. One woman in Camberwell who had been divorced eight years was quite certain that she began to worry endlessly about the loneliness and pointlessness of her life when her sixteen-year-old daughter returned from a summer holiday. 'I missed her. When she came back she was much more grown up and I felt I had lost her and I could realize then for the first time that one of these days I would lose both of them. It made me realize just how lonely I was and how I depended on their ways.' This woman, Conrad's Razumov, and Tolstoy's Ivan Ilyitch all reacted differently to thoughts about their daily lives; for the woman it brought despair, for Razumov comfort, and for Ivan Ilyitch resentment and confusion.

Murray Parkes has provided important insights into the effect of events in terms of the impact on a person's 'assumptive world'. Changes are important in so far as they alter assumptions a person has made about the world: about personal material possessions, the familiar world of home and place of work, and the individual's body and mind in so far as he can view these as separate from himself (1971: 103). The importance of such a formulation (to which we have not done justice) is that it makes clear how we can lose what we have never had: ideas of what we might possess or might become – hope of promotion, a child, someone's love. Indeed a crisis or change is probably only ever significant if it leads to a change in thought about the world. Nor is it just a matter of changes in thought about the external world; man has a *self* to which he reacts and on which he reflects. Change can occur in self-conception in response to some external stimulus with no alteration in outward behaviour. A husband's discovery, unknown to his wife, that she once had an affair may radically change the ideas he had held of his marriage and of himself, although nothing changes otherwise in his relationship with his wife.

Life-events and depression

It was with this formidable complexity in mind that we set about developing our basic measure of events. In the earlier study only scanty information was collected about each event and, as was made clear in the last chapter, this was ignored when we came to our analysis. Incidents once classified as 'events' were treated as equivalent as far as severity of threat, disruption, and the like were concerned. We now needed in some way to bring meaning back without the risk of circularity that comes when events are classified according to accounts of personal reactions to them.

In terms of collecting material, we first recorded events in exactly the same way as in the schizophrenic study. It was then that we made changes. The interviewer went on to cover, in as informal a way as possible, a lengthy list of questions about what led up to and what followed each event, and the feeling and attitudes surrounding it. We were interested not only in what happened but in what it *meant* for the woman – in the sense of the thoughts and feelings she had before, at the time, and after the event. The questioning was standardized only in the sense that there was a list of fairly detailed topics to be discussed. The ratings were still, however, highly standardized in order to be able to make comparisons between individuals. It was just this combination of flexible understanding of the individual and her milieu with systematic measurement that we hoped would close the gap between the clinical case history and the epidemiological approaches. For example, we questioned about worry before the event: 'After you *knew* it was going to happen, but before it actually happened, did you worry at all? What about? When did you start? How much did you worry? Did you talk it over with anyone? When? Did it affect your sleep? Anything else? For instance, were you restless; did you want to smoke a lot?' The interviewer encouraged the woman to talk at length and in the light of the picture that emerged questions could be omitted and others added as thought fit.

The interview was tape-recorded and the tapes were later used to complete twenty-eight rating scales covering each event. They dealt with (i) basic characteristics, (ii) prior experience and preparation, (iii) immediate reactions, and (iv) consequences and implications. The scales took two years to establish and several hundred depressed patients and close relatives were seen in the course of the developmental work. Most emphasis was placed on obtaining a full account of the situation at the time of the event. While the material was obtained from the subject, it must be emphasized that it was *the interviewer who carried out the job of measurement*. For example, there were two measures of the length of warning of the event. A 'specific warning' was defined by any cue that predicted its *definite* occurrence, regardless of whether this allowed its timing to be anticipated by the subject, and a 'general warning' by anything that gave the subject some idea that the event would occur, without necessarily definitely predicting its occurrence. In addition to such definitions there was a commentary and examples to act as a guide.

In the interviews vague statements were not enough; the interviewer had to do her best to obtain clear evidence – not that a woman had 'known for some time' but that her son had *said* the day after Christmas he was thinking of emigrating. Close attention had to be paid to the notes developed for each scale. The interviewer knew, for instance, that a 'specific warning' involved the person being made aware that the event would occur at some time; the timing of its occurrence did not have to be known. Where the reverse occurred (for example, for someone waiting to hear an examination result) a 'general' and not a 'specific warning' was rated. Such points had to be borne in mind both during the interview itself and while listening to the tape recordings. Inconsistent accounts of what had occurred were sometimes given by the same person. One woman, for instance, said in response to a direct question that her father's death had been completely unexpected and yet, earlier in the interview, had talked about the warning the doctor had given her that he might die. In such instances the interviewer took account of what the woman *probably* experienced in the light of all that she had been told. The woman just mentioned was rated as having had a 'general warning' of her father's death. Of course, such interpretations of what-any-similar-woman-probably-would-think-in-the-circumstances would at times be wrong about a particular woman; but once this is accepted advantages are considerable. We could avoid, for example, becoming involved in the investigation of 'denial'. We assume that, if a woman was able to tell us certain things about what had occurred (e.g. that the doctor had discussed her father's likely death), that in some way she would have had to deal with the 'fact' and this should be reflected in our measures. In the early stages of our work we did develop more complex ratings to deal with this issue but, as our work progressed, we dropped them as we rarely came across the kind of blatant discrepancy we have just described.

Ratings were therefore always based on what we were told but occasionally we went *beyond* this to rate what most women would probably have experienced in similar encounters. A woman who told us that she had noticed several things about her husband's health before his serious illness (e.g. lack of energy and difficulty in swallowing) would be considered to have had a 'general warning' of the illness irrespective of what she had told us about how she had interpreted the signs. But these were relatively minor issues; we still faced major problems surrounding the issue of meaning. As was made clear in the last chapter, measures based on what people say events actually meant for them inevitably create serious difficulties in a causal enquiry. It is difficult to rule out the possibility that the association between event and onset is the result of some measurement artefact. We also outlined a radical solution – to record events irrespective of how people said that they felt about them. But how were we to deal with these problems now that so much more about each woman was known?

The meaning of life-events

Henry VIII's fifth wife committed adultery (or at least was sufficiently indiscreet to make it appear that she had). The King, from contemporary accounts at the disclosure of Katheryn's blemish, was 'pierced with pensiveness' and moved to tears before the assembled Council. The French Ambassador wrote in a letter to his own court:

> 'The King has wonderfully felt the case of the Queen his wife and has certainly shown greater sorrows at her loss, than at the faults, loss or divorce of his preceding wives. It is like the case of the woman who cried more bitterly at the loss of her tenth husband than at the deaths of all the others together, though they had all been good men, but it was because she had never buried one of them before without being sure of the next: and as yet this King has formed neither plan nor a preference.'

At this distance the interpretation rings true – and touches poignantly on the meaning of the news for the King. Perhaps for the first time one of his wives *had* been unfaithful and had caught him unprepared. The Ambassador relates the events to the King's plans and preferences (or rather his lack of them). McCall and Simmons (1966) remind us that until we have made out the meaning of a thing *vis-à-vis* our plans, we have no bearings; we cannot proceed. An essential element of meaning therefore concerns a person's plans of action.

The ambassador's report rings true because he relates the incident to what he knew of the present and the past *behaviour* of the King, the way of life at the court, and thus to the King's presumable plans. It is therefore unnecessary to see the measurement of meaning as inevitably dependent on a person's own account of his feelings and actions. Clearly, this is desirable – but if, as in our present case, it is suspect for methodological reasons, a full account of past behaviour and circumstances surrounding an event will enable us to make, in the majority of instances, a reasonable estimate of the meaning of an event. We use the term reasonable as sociologists, in the sense that the aggregate results for a number of individuals will approximate to the truth and, most important, be free of the kind of systematic bias that vitiates hope of explanatory enquiry; we are not competing here with the poet, biographer, or novelist. Alfred Schutz takes a similar position when he writes of the use of commonsense experience of the world:

> 'But the world of everyday life is from the onset a social cultural world in which I am interrelated in manifold ways with fellowmen known to me in varying degrees of intimacy and anonymity. To a certain extent, sufficient for any practical purposes, I understand their behaviour if I understand their motives, goals, choices and plans originating in *their* biographically determined circumstances. Yet only in particular situations, and then only fragmentarily, can I experience the other's motives, goals etc. – briefly, the subjective

meaning they bestow on their actions, in their uniqueness. I can, however, experience them in their typicality. In order to do so I construct typical patterns of actors' motives and ends, even of their attitudes and personalities, of which their actual conduct is just an instance or example.'   (Schutz, 1971: 496)

Schutz' work has influenced recent schools of phenomenological sociology whose position might be construed to be inimical to the approach we will outline. In contrast to Schutz many sociologists have been castigated for their uncritical use of commonsense meanings in order to categorize social phenomena. (It will be remembered that in the first chapter we asserted that measurement was by far the weakest component of the survey approach to aetiology.) Durkheim is among the prominent sociologists who have been found wanting. He has been particularly influential because he did not simply relate rates of suicide to factors such as sex, marital status, and religious affiliation, but used such evidence to develop theoretical ideas about the effects of various kinds of social bond on the individual. For Durkheim, men and women responded differently to experiences such as marriage, widowhood, divorce, and childlessness because, according to his commonsense judgment, they *meant* different things to the two sexes; but he never established this by interviewing individual men and women. The dispute therefore between 'phenomenologists' and 'positivists' is not about the use of commonsense observer judgments – everyone makes these – but how much information is required about the individual in order to make them. To take another example, Durkheim saw the higher rate of suicide among the more educated in nineteenth-century Europe as due to the lessening importance of traditional values with increasing industrialization. But he recognized that there were exceptions. For instance, Jews as a group had a low rate of suicide in spite of being well educated and more involved in industrialization than some other groups. He reconciled these anomalies by special arguments – in this case by asserting that education was, for the West European Jew, a way of identifying with traditional values. In other words, education had different meanings for a member of a minority group and for a member of a majority group.

Jack Douglas in *The Social Meaning of Suicide* makes a simple yet devastating criticism: that Durkheim supplied such interpretations, imposed such meanings on others, from his own experience, and made no serious effort to document them by independent enquiry. He never established whether education had a different meaning for minority groups. We used the word 'devastating' not because of the impact on Durkheim's reputation, which is impregnable for many reasons, but because such speculation about the meaning of experience to others is essentially what has been done in the hundreds of studies of all kinds of conditions that have followed Durkheim's.

If the possibility of this kind of bias is accepted (and it is only one of a number of possible biases) very little large-scale sociological work is left unscathed; for most of it, if not based on the investigator's own judgment about meaning, has used relatively superficial questioning of respondents and has not dealt at all seriously with the possibility of bias. In the general enthusiasm to put the sociological house in order there has even been suggestion that the job of measurement is hopeless – since meanings are never directly given by situations, general statements cannot be made about them. We see the matter as a good deal less fundamental although we do not deny the cogency of the criticism. The matter hinges on the point at which we are willing *as investigators* to begin constructing Schutz's 'typical patterns of motives and ends'. Schutz leaves no doubt that we as investigators must build on knowledge of typical patterns established in our daily lives. An investigator cannot be in the subject's position in the same practical sense but, like the ambassador, we must understand events by taking account of as much of the surrounding 'biographically determined circumstances' as possible.

Our solution to the problem of meaning follows the spirit of Schutz's argument and has two main components. The first we have already outlined: we excluded any consideration of what a woman said she felt. However, in order to meet the objections concerning arbitrariness and superficiality, we collected background biographical material about each event in considerable detail; and developed twenty-eight scales to deal with aspects of each event (e.g. its expectedness, amount of prior experience, amount of support available to the subject). We used some of these to make a judgment about the likely meaning of the event for the average person in such circumstances without considering her personal reaction to the event and, in this way, eliminated the sources of possible contamination discussed in the last chapter. We did this by developing what we called contextual scales in contrast to scales of self-report. The most important concerned threat.

Contextual measures of threat

The threat scales measured the degree of threat or unpleasantness of each event at two points in time. The consequences of an event, such as unexpectedly having to deliver a neighbour's baby in the middle of the night, are usually resolved within a day or so. Others, such as the discovery of a daughter's repeated thefts at school, have much further implications. *Short-term* threat is that implied on the day it occurred or soon after, and *long-term* threat is that implied by the event about one week or more after its occurrence. Therefore the woman delivering her neighbour's baby would experience only short-term threat but the woman learning of her daughter's thefts would be likely to experience both short and long-term threat. By the end of the week she would still have to live with the implications of what she had learned about her daughter.

We have already discussed the problem we faced in developing such scales: since in the course of discussing each event we inevitably learnt a great deal about how each woman felt and reacted we risked introducing possible bias in our ratings. To deal with this we developed *contextual measures of threat* which deliberately excluded any consideration of what a woman told us about the way she had personally reacted to the event. We wished these contextual measures to retain an important, perhaps crucial, element of meaning while ignoring what we had obtained by way of self-reports of threat and unpleasantness.

In addition to the two contextual scales we also made parallel ratings based on what the woman told us she had felt. There were therefore four scales, each rated on a four-point scale of severity of threat – 'marked', 'moderate', 'some', or 'little or none':

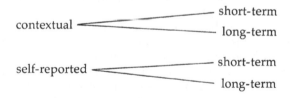

The contextual and self-reported scales were kept apart by the interviewer whilst reading to other members of the research team an account of the event and its surrounding circumstances. This account left out any mention of the woman's reactions to the event including whether or not she was psychiatrically disturbed. The rating was then made by the rest of the team, independently and without discussion, using their judgment of how much threat such an event would involve for most people in biographical circumstances like those of the respondent.

The raters were helped in three ways. First, there were a series of anchoring examples to illustrate the four points on each scale. Second, a rating was followed by a discussion about any discrepancy, and a final rating agreed. Inter-rater agreement was high, and these discussions undoubtedly helped to establish and maintain this. Third, fairly 'standard' ratings were applied to events such as death and childbirth. These were not subtle and on the whole we kept strictly to them. All deaths of close relatives were rated on the highest scale point of threat (except in rare instances – for example, the death of a mother who was eighty, who lived in South America, and who had not been seen for twenty years was rated lower). We had a convention also that childbirth was only rated high on long-term contextual threat when it occurred in obviously difficult circumstances such as poor housing, acute financial shortage, or very poor health of the mother. These we considered to be integrally part of the context of the birth and therefore relevant to its degree of threat. The death of a parent antedating the birth would not be relevant to the context; for even though the new mother might herself repeatedly refer to the close juxtaposition of the death and the birth as having caused even more upset than she thought she would have felt with either singly, according to our rating the earlier event would not be part of the context of the second one. The rating was based on our view about women's usual plans and expectations at the time of birth; in our geographically mobile society the presence and support of a husband at the time of a birth is expected in a way in which that of a parent usually is not. We might, however, have made exceptions: a woman whose husband, although in no way estranged, was often away for weeks at a time on his job might plan, in the absence of a substantial income, to continue her job soon after the birth, leaving the new baby with her mother-in-law who would receive no payment for this. The mother-in-law's unexpected death six weeks before the birth now becomes part of the context of the birth in the sense that it crucially affects the young woman's plans and life-style; she may not be able to afford an au-pair or find a suitable baby-minder, and so now she may be unable to continue working, with all the attendant financial problems. If these were serious enough, the birth might now be rated threatening, whereas it would not have been so without the death. The converse, however, did not apply; a separated woman, however rich, with the house in her sole name and an income from the Stock Market, with an au-pair and a doting grandmother, would still have been given a rating of moderate threat for her childbirth just because she was separated, and because there is still some conventional expectation that a birth should occur in a two-parent context. There was thus a slight imbalance in our estimates of threatfulness; for while we might raise the rating of threat above the standard rating for that particular type of event in the light of other circumstances, we would not lower it beneath the standard rating, despite other circumstances which might seem to mitigate its impact. In this particular example the threatfulness of a birth in a single-parent family could not be mitigated by the financial and social support, even though the threatfulness of a birth in a two-parent family could be increased by the removal of financial or social support. If this imbalance introduced bias, it was a bias in the direction of an *underestimate* of the causal link between threatfulness and onset of disorder; for it would be among women whose plans were less threatened than average for whom we were not lowering the threat rating, and, if there was a causal link between threat and depression, they would be expected to be, if anything, less depressed just because their plans were less threatened. They would thus be expected to be in the comparison rather than the depressed group. Not lowering their threat ratings might be expected to have, if anything, raised the rate of threatful events in the comparison group and thus reduced the size of the association between threat and depression.

To summarize: the contextual measures of threat were made in three stages. First, the event was obtained by a method that ignored the respondent's judgment of its impact on her (as in the schizophrenic study). Second, the interviewer collected extensive background material about the event. Third, the rating was made by people not involved in the interview, taking into account only biographically relevant circumstances surrounding the event and how they thought most people would react given this configuration of factors. Since self-reports of threat were controlled both at the stage of enquiry about the event itself and also at the later stage of rating threat, we believe we much reduced the risk of all three kinds of invalidity outlined in the last chapter and yet managed to take account of the meaningfulness of events – in the sense of their relevance for goals and plans.

The long-term contextual threat scale has proved to be the measure of crucial importance for understanding the aetiology of depression and we will therefore spend less time in describing the remaining measures. Rather than describing in detail each of the additional scales we outline two events that happened to one of the women living in Camberwell, giving in footnotes the full scales and the ratings made.

Two events

Mrs Smith was fifty-four, had been widowed for ten years and when seen had no psychiatric symptoms. On the death of her husband she had moved from Wales to London and had worked for some time as a supervisor in a local factory. Her daughter who had lived in London at the time now lived some fifteen miles to the north. Two incidents that happened to Mrs Smith in the twelve months before interview were judged to be events in our terms. The first was a move from a furnished to an unfurnished flat. The furnished flat had had many shortcomings, but she had been living in it since she moved to London. It shook at night from the railway behind, and sharing a bathroom had many inconveniences. She happened to hear from a friend that they had an empty unfurnished flat in their house. They did not want much by way of rent.

'I wondered what to do. I didn't really have enough money to furnish it. I thought I would be more or less obliged to them ... but there was the garden ... it was quite a worrying time wondering what to do for the best. If I had stayed where I was I might in time have got a council flat; it was due for redevelopment. But they had put the rent up and many things were wrong ... It is different now sharing a bathroom with friends. I had to think a bit about it. It did worry me at the time what was the best thing to do. I came to look at this place ... ooh the damp ... really it was a state ... should I take it or not. My friend had just mentioned it – I had not entertained it ... When I had decided to take it, I thought, had I done right, had I done wrong; it was so handy for the shops in the old place. I've got quite a trail now. I didn't like where I was but I had just done it up.'

The focus of this event was Mrs Smith herself (A). She had clearly worried a good deal about the move (B). There had been a great deal of cleaning and decorating to do, but she conveyed that overall she had been pleased once she moved, especially by the greater privacy that she had. She said that before the move she had worried that she would not be able to have her father who still lived in Wales to stay. 'There are too many stairs and nothing for him to watch out of the window' (C,D,E,F,G).

She said she thought about it for two weeks and then decided to take the flat and had moved out two weeks later (H,I). By the end of the week she conveyed that she still had somewhat mixed feelings about the move – in particular, although it was only ten minutes' walk from her old place, she saw less of her neighbours and friends. She said she had missed one neighbour who was a friend but she had 'had a busy year' (she had made new friends) (J,K,L,M,N,O). During the move she saw friends and she got on very well with her friends downstairs: but although they were some help she did most of the cleaning and decorating herself (P).

The second event occurred almost six months later and was an altogether more disturbing affair. Mrs Smith mentioned it only in response to a final question we put to her about possible events: *'Whether anything disappointing had happened in the last 12 months?'* After

A *Focus of event*
① Subject
2 Other person
3 Subject *and* other jointly involved
4 Material object including pets

B *Emotional preparation for the event*
1 Marked worry/anxiety
② Moderate
3 Some
4 Little or none
5 No opportunity

C *Immediate positive feeling*
1 Welcoming – major emotional
   investment
2 Welcoming
③ Some positive feeling
4 Nil or very little

D *Immediate negative feeling*
1 Marked – major emotional investment
2 Marked
③ Some negative feeling
4 Nil or very little

E *Immediate feelings of anxiety*
1 Marked
2 Moderate
③ Some
4 Nil or little

F *Short term threat or unpleasantness:*
   self-report
1 Marked
2 Moderate
③ Some
4 Little or none

G *Short-term threat or unpleasantness:*
   contextual
1 Marked
2 Moderate
③ Some
4 Little or none

H *General warning*
4 weeks

I *Specific warning*
2 weeks

J *Long-term threat/unpleasantness:*
   self-report
1 Marked
2 Moderate
③ Some
4 Little or none

K *Long-term threat/unpleasantness:*
   contextual
1 Marked
2 Moderate
③ Some
4 Little or none

L *Interaction change in any close tie: increase*
1 None/little
2 $< \frac{1}{2}$ previous
③ $> \frac{1}{2}$ previous
4 New contact

M *Interaction change in any close tie: decrease*
1 None/little
2 $< \frac{1}{2}$ previous
③ $> \frac{1}{2}$ previous
4 Total loss contact

N *Change in routine*
1 Major
2 Moderate
③ Some
4 None/minimal

O *Expected time duration of N*
0 Little or$< 1/52$
1 Probably 1/52 – 2 months
2 Probably 2–4 months
3 Probably 4–6 months
4 Probably < 1 year
⑤ Probably 1 year +

P *Reported positive support*
1 Marked
② Some
3 Nil

a second or so delay, she said, 'I was not told about my daughter's wedding' and then spoke for a considerable time with little or no prompting. By the time she stopped, the interviewer found she had almost all the material she required to make the twenty-eight ratings and only needed to ask a relatively small number of additional questions – this is a common experiences in the interviews particularly about important events.

The daughter had confided in a friend of her mother's about her decision to bring the date of the wedding forward. Mrs Smith knew of her daughter's intention to get married that summer and had telephoned her daughter the week before she went on holiday to discuss the plans for the wedding. She asked her daughter to telephone her the day she expected to return to let her know how things were going. Her daughter did not phone, however, and Mrs Smith assumed all was well and that her daughter intended to stick to her original arrangements for the wedding. Then, a couple of days later her father in Wales telephoned and told her that her daughter had changed the arrangements and had married the day before. Her initial reaction was mainly disappointment but, as she considered the fact that no-one had bothered to inform her, especially her friend to whom she had been so close, she began to get annoyed.

> 'I think I'll 'phone up to see what's going on, I said to myself. My friend answered. She was not herself – her tone! She spoke like a stranger! I started to get a bit annoyed and said to her I thought you were my friend and you didn't tell me? She said she didn't want to interfere – I said what do you mean by interfere . . . I said I feel so upset about this that I think I had better put the 'phone down before I say anything I'll regret . . . and it's been like that ever since.'

(This had been three months before interview.) A few days later she telephoned again and her new son-in-law answered. He said, 'Everybody was there that mattered' and 'it came out that there was a lot of bad feeling 'cause they thought she hadn't been concerned enough about the wedding and had gone off on holiday'. She also spoke to her daughter who made it clear that she felt her mother had not been taking enough notice of her.

> 'But I didn't like to be one of those mothers always on the doorstep . . . she had her own definite plans about the wedding being quiet with just a few friends. I just didn't think she'd want her mother fussing around her. She's not that type. It came out that I was always out enjoying myself and that this was what it was all about . . . I was upset but it was over quickly. I can't understand it.'

Did it come as a shock to you? 'It did, it did. I was rather taken back by it all.' *Do you think it will get better?*

> 'I think it will. I think once my friend sees less of her . . . It did hurt a little bit, but let's say when you've had bad bumps like this before you can cope with it . . . at the time it did hurt. But I've got over it and it's not as though I'm out of touch – my father tells me how things are. I hope she'll [i.e. her daughter] 'phone soon and then it will be over . . . I don't think I've done any wrong . . . with your daughter you can forgive but with someone else you don't have to – I just think it was a mean thing to do. I'm not bitter: I was surprised and hurt. I'm sure I'll make it up.'

While we made no attempt to explore the underlying dynamics of the incident we did try to plot its obvious manifestations. The main incident was not being told of the wedding and this had within a day or so led to a break with both her friend and her daughter.

The focus of the event was again Mrs Smith because only she was involved in hearing the news. The fact that her daughter was involved in the main incident was irrelevant(A).

There was not a great deal of warning or preparation (G), but she said that her daughter had been slightly strange for two months and in retrospect at least she thinks that things had come on for about two months. Her daughter had not telephoned her as often (usually they telephoned each other at least every other day) (H). On the day the event occurred we did not think she had much preparation or anticipation (Q). She had no previous experience of such a crisis but she and her daughter had had several times of not speaking to each other before. The last time had been about two years earlier: this in the end had cleared up and they had then got on well together (R). She had

A *Focus*
① Subject (see earlier footnotes when full scale not given)

I *Specific warning*
Nil

G *Short-term threat/unpleasantness: contextual*
② Moderate

H *General warning*
2 months

Q *Expectedness of event on day of occurrence*
1 Totally unexpected
② Some anticipation – minimal cues
3 Some anticipation – definite cues
4 Expected

5 2 or 3 but important aspects expected
6 4 but important aspects expected

S *Immediate feeling of anger*
① Marked
2 Moderate
3 Some
4 Nil or little

R *Prior general experience or special knowledge*
1 Prior experience very similar event
2 Much experience similar events
③ Much experience of somewhat similar events
4 Some experience similar events
5 Some experience of somewhat similar event
6 Nil

B *Emotional preparation for event*
② Some worry

D *Immediate negative feeling*
② Marked

E *Immediate feelings of anxiety/upset*
① Marked

F *Short-term threat/unpleasantness: self-report*
② Moderate

J *Long-term threat or unpleasantness: self-report*
③ Some

K *Long-term threat or unpleasantness: contextual*
② Moderate

M *Interaction change*
④ Total loss

N *Change in routine*
④ None/minimal

O *Expected time duration of N*
⑧ Uncertain

T *Commitment to lost person*
1 Clearly higher than average
② Average
3 Clearly lower than average

U *Control of implications*
0 Quite unclear
1 Apparently no chance of control
2 Apparently little chance of control
③ Apparently some chance of control

4 Marked chance of modifying or avoiding consequences

V *Need to make important and specific decision as consequence*
1 Major importance
2 Moderate importance
3 Some importance
④ Nil of importance

W *Role changes*
1 Role change
2 Commitment to future role change
3 Both 1 and 2
4 Important change in self-image only
⑤ None

X *Fulfilment of major aspiration*
1 Aspiration made impossible or invalid
2 Major hindrance
3 Some hindrance
4 New important aspirations/
5 Major help
6 Some help
7 Significance unclear
8 Irrelevant
⑨ Confirms previous failure in important area of life

Y *Turning Point*
1 Major+
2 Major
3 Moderate
④ None

P *Reported positive support*
1 Marked
② Some
3 Nil

worried a little prior to the crisis as she thought her daughter had acted a little unusually and she had been a little concerned about this (B). But we established nothing by way of 'practical' coping in anticipation of the event or dealing with its antecedents. (She said she was not the sort of mother that would want to impose anything.) She felt angry at her friend and was generally upset (D,E,S). Both contextual and self-reported ratings of threat on the day of the crisis were rated quite high (F,G). The long-term threat ratings were, however, of more interest. By her own account she had not been greatly distressed once she had got over the immediate event. Although she might in retrospect have played down her feelings, her account was highly detailed and convincing and we had no hesitation in rating the *self-report* scale threat (J) lower than the *contextual* (K). In other words we had in effect judged that most women would have felt more threat than Mrs Smith reported she had felt. By the time of our interview she had not seen her daughter or friend for three months (M,N,O). The interviewer thought she was not in any way unusually involved or committed to the relationship with either her daughter or her friend (T); and considered she had some chance of controlling the consequences of the event (U). (There is also a self-report part to this scale concerning control and Mrs Smith considered she had 'no chance of controlling the circumstances' as far as her friend was concerned.) We did not think she had had any important decisions to make following the event (V) nor that it involved, in our terms, a change of role or important change in self-image (W). It might be expected that many women would have felt some sense of failure in their capacity as a mother – albeit with an adult daughter. It was a difficult rating to make and depended on more judgment than we liked. But Mrs Smith, as far as we could tell, did not see herself to blame in any way, and because of this we did not record any change in self-image. However, on another scale we did consider the event to reflect some kind of failure (X). It did not however qualify as a 'turning point' in her life. For this the event must necessitate not only a reassessment of future plans but general purpose in life. Expectations for the future are removed and made invalid (Y). Taking account of what had happened with her daughter in the past we did not think that this had occurred. Finally we considered that Mrs Smith had got a certain amount of support during the crisis. Her father had been helpful and had kept her in touch with what had been happening to her daughter and son-in-law and she had many friends to talk things over with (P).

The estimates of reliability and validity described in the last chapter were equally encouraging for these scales. There was, for example, 92 per cent agreement about the occurrence of long-term markedly and moderately threatening events which form about half of the events in the patient series and a quarter in the community sample. (In the next chapter we see that these categories contain all the events important in provoking onset of depression.)[1]

In this chapter we have described the way in which we tried to rescue meaning from the oversterilized instrument developed for the schizophrenic study. Rather than rejecting our first solution we extended it by developing ratings of various 'qualities' of the events as originally defined, but in the contextual scales still excluding consideration of emotional reactions of the respondent to the event and its consequences. First we took meaning out of our measure to avoid contamination and then in order to avoid being arbitrary and facile brought it back in the various descriptive scales.

6 Life-events and depression

We can at last turn to life-events and the aetiology of depression. We will first present some basic results.

Basic results

If a particular class of event plays a causal role it will be significantly more common among the depressed patients than non-depressed women living in Camberwell.[1] As it turned out it is only events with marked long-term threat, or moderate long-term threat, focussed on the woman herself or jointly with someone else, that have a higher rate and therefore appear capable of playing a causal role. We call these events *severe*.[2] (We assume that possible sources of invalidity have been ruled out.) The distinction between long- and short-term threat is central – it will be recalled that the threat of the latter sort has largely cleared up within a week of occurrence. Events threatening only in the short-term, however painful or outrageous, do not seem to bring about depression. This basic result occurred among all groups of depressed women.

Findings are summarized in *Table 1* and examples of severe and non-severe events given in Appendix 3. Severe events are relatively rare, forming only 16 per cent of the events occurring to normal women, but they are almost four times more common among patients. There is no other difference: if anything, normal women have a slightly higher rate of non-severe events. Results for onset cases are close to those for the patients.[3]

So far we have ignored the fact that we asked about events for as long as a year before interview. It raises the question whether recall of events over such a period has in any way influenced results? Quite important events can soon be forgotten. Cannell and his colleagues (1961) using an interview with standard questions have shown fairly marked under-reporting of episodes of hospital care when they interviewed patients one week to one year after their discharge. In *Figure 1* we have therefore plotted the frequency of life-events for patients and normal women in the sixteen three-week periods before onset or interview – forty-eight weeks in all.[4]

Table 1   *Rate of events per 100 women before onset for patients and interview for normal women by long-term contextual threat and focus*

	patients	normal women	ratio patient/ normal women
	(n=114)	(n=382)	
marked long-term threat: any focus	72	15	4.83
severe event	115	27	4.27
moderate long-term threat: subject/joint focus	43	12	3.50
non-severe event	175	191	0.92

Note: The average length of time before onset for patients was 38 weeks and the rate for normal women is therefore based on a 38-week period.

The first thing to note is that there is *no* fall-off at all in the reporting by women in Camberwell of severe events with the length of recall (*Figure 1B*). This is quite contrary to a finding by Cannell and his colleagues that admissions involving more threatening diseases and treatments tended to be under-reported as distance from interview increased. However, on another point, our results do agree with Cannell's: he reports that a stay in hospital of more than four days was more likely to be mentioned when degree of threat is controlled, presumably because such episodes involved greater disruption and were therefore easier to recall. Similarly we found that less threatening events (and presumably therefore events of lower salience) were less often reported further away in time. However, even here the women show no fall-off in the reporting of events occurring within the first thirty-three weeks before interview (*Figure 1C*).

After the thirty-third week the rate of non-severe events is reduced by about one third. Incidentally this amount of fall-off is enough to explain the slight excess of non-severe events occurring to normal women. For patients we have been dealing with an average period of thirty-eight weeks before *onset*, with interview a few weeks later, making the length of recall seventeen weeks longer than for normal women. If allowance is made for this the corrected rate of non-severe events for patients is 194 per 100 which is almost the same as the rate for normal women.[5]

Our conclusions are therefore unlikely to have been influenced by problems of recall. There is no tendency for severe events to be less

Figure 1   Rate of events in 16 three-week periods before onset (patients) or interview (normal women) by severity of threat

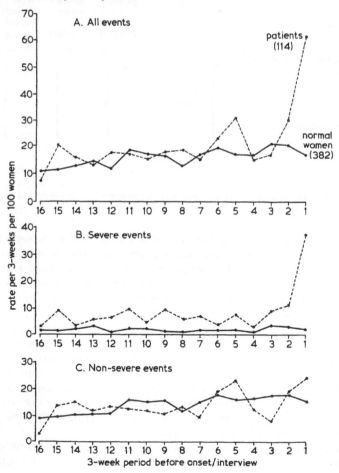

frequently reported and the under-reporting of non-severe events is of no significance, since fall-off is identical for patients and normal women. In any case the latter involve no aetiological effect. The validity of the life-event instrument is therefore confirmed – not only is there a high level of agreement between different respondents about the occurrence of particular events, there is surprisingly little fall-off in the reporting of events over a year.

The overall frequencies we have used so far tell us there is a causal effect but nothing about *how many* persons are involved. For this we must consider *proportions of women experiencing at least one severe event*. Sixty-one per cent of the patients had a severe event compared with 20 per cent of normal women (p<.001). The onset cases among the 458 women in Camberwell supplied a valuable independent check: 68 per cent had a severe event before onset (p<.001).

Three quarters of the severe events occurring to patients and women in Camberwell were rated as 'independent' and the rest 'possibly independent'. When considered separately, both types of event showed the same order of association with onset of depression, suggesting, as in the schizophrenia study, that the 'bringing on' of events due to woman's incipient disorder had not been a significant source of bias.[6]

Severe events and loss

Given that it is severe events that bring about depression, what is involved? Do the events have anything in common. The notion of long-term threat is rather abstract. Can any more be said?

Reading through the descriptions of events leaves us in no doubt that loss and disappointment are the central features of most events bringing about clinical depression and these are, of course, just the kind of events that would be expected to produce feelings of depression. Long-term and not short-term threat is important because it correlates closely with the experience of loss if this is seen to include: (i) separation or threat of it, such as death of parent, or a husband saying he is going to leave home; (ii) an unpleasant revelation about someone close that forces a major reassessment of the person and the relationship, such as the loss of one's conception of a relationship after finding out about a husband's unfaithfulness; (iii) a life-threatening illness to someone close; (iv) a major material loss or disappointment or threat of this, such as a couple living in bad housing learning that their chances of being rehoused were minimal; (v) an enforced change of residence, or the threat of it; and finally (vi) a miscellaneous group of crises involving some element of loss, such as being made redundant in a job held for some time, or obtaining a legal separation. *Table 2A* shows this in numerical terms: about threequarters of severe events occurring to patients and onset cases involved such a loss. Essentially the same holds when the proportion of *persons* with at least one severe event is considered – 79 per cent of patients and 88 per cent of onset cases who had a severe event had at least one involving loss. These figures would be even higher if we had included events such as a hysterectomy, which might be argued contain some elements of loss.

Table 2   *Types of loss or disappointment involved in the severe events among patients, onset cases, and normal women — period before onset of depression taken*

	patients (n=114, 38 weeks)	onset cases (n=37, 38 weeks)	normals (n=382, 1 year)
A *overall occurrence of loss*			
total severe events	130	37	141
total persons having a severe event	70	25	96
percent of severe events which involve 'loss'	72%	78%	70%
percent of persons with a 'loss' among those with a severe event	79%	88%	72%
B *types of loss* loss: separation or threat including deaths	37	14	47
loss: major negative revelation about someone close	9	3	1
loss: life-threatening illness to someone close	16	1	23
loss: material loss or disappointment or threat	11	5	9
loss: enforced change of residence or threat	5	6	4
loss: miscellaneous crises	15	2	15
non-loss: miscellaneous crises	27	5	20
non-loss: illness to subject	10	1	22

By comparison events high on short-term but not on long-term threat very rarely involve loss. Half of those occurring to patients involved illnesses or accidents whose threatening implications had largely cleared within the week; five of the remaining twenty-four involved contact with police or the courts, five births with some kind of physical complication, three witnessing serious accidents, three direct involvement in the death of someone who was not a close relative or confidant, and the remainder were a small number of crises such as witnessing a fight in a pub in which an acquaintance got hurt with a broken glass.

Table 2B lists severe events by six different types of loss. 'Separations' made up about a quarter of the total occurring to patients. (A third were deaths and the rest separation from either a husband, boyfriend, confidant, or child.) Those occurring to onset cases were similar: in most instances there was complete loss of contact although in a few it was not totally lost – a son, for example, going to live in Scotland, leaving his widowed mother without nearby relatives or friends. 'Separations' occurring to normal women were not on the whole as dramatic. Most involved moves of confidants; only a quarter involved loss of a boyfriend or of someone living at home compared with three times this for the depressed group – p<.01.

While 'separations' were on the whole more unpleasant for depressed women, other types of severe event did not appear to be so. To complete the list: the ninety severe loss events occurring to patients included nine 'unpleasant revelations' about someone close. All involved a major reassessment of another person such as learning that a child had been recommended to attend a special school because of his backwardness. Most came as a surprise – five women found out about their husband's infidelity and one that her daughter had been stealing from home for some time. A further fourteen of the ninety involved 'life-threatening illnesses' to someone close, eleven threat of or actual loss of a job, hope of a house or an important possession, five enforced rehousing or threat of it, and fourteen miscellaneous crises involving an element of loss or disappointment.

Given that severe events mainly involved loss and disappointment, their relationships with the various descriptive scales are much what would be expected. Anxiety and depression were common as immediate responses; there was usually little chance of controlling the consequences of the event and so on. More interesting are the descriptive scales that failed to show any association. Among patients and onset cases the severe events, when compared with *other* events, did not involve a significantly greater amount of change in day-to-day routine, amount seen of a person, length of warning, amount of increased contact with others, or amount of time that changes in interaction or day-to-day routine might be expected to last. The message is again that it is loss and disappointment rather than change as such that is important.

An element of disappointment was probably present in all severe events and for some it was clearly the dominant feature – a woman, for instance, who was told that her son's dislocated hip 'had gone again' after she had been allowed to believe that the third operation was going to be the final one. Most severe events concerned an actual loss, or disappointment – events involving intimation of some future incident were much less common. If we exclude from consideration the fourteen events involving life-threatening illnesses to someone close, only eighteen of the remaining 114 severe events occurring to patients involved *threat of loss* and this is only increased to a quarter of the total twenty-eight if physical illnesses occurring to the patient herself, such as being told she needed a serious heart operation, are included as threats of loss.

We will discuss more fully the fifteen patients with a non-loss severe event when we deal with long-term difficulties in a later chapter; but it is perhaps worth noting here that at least two of the fifteen probably did experience these events as a loss or disappointment, although our rules did not allow us to rate them as 'loss'.

One woman became pregnant, completely unexpectedly, after a childless marriage of eleven years. She had arranged her life on the assumption she would not have children – particularly her job (to which she wanted to return immediately after the birth) and her home in a small flat. The change probably represented a major threat to an entrenched and rewarding way of life, although she did not hint at this. The other woman with a severe non-loss event in fact developed depression after another incident not even included as an event: her handicapped son losing his third job in the year. Our 'rules' prevented us from including this event although it was clearly of major significance to her. (We include as 'events' only loss of a job to the subject herself or the 'chief breadwinner'.)

Although it raises an issue that deserves a more detailed exposition than we can give without losing the thread of the analysis, it is interesting that these non-loss severe events seemed to have occurred relatively more often to patients whose symptoms included a marked anxiety component. We return to this when we deal with the topic of symptom formation in chapter 14.

Additivity of events

So far we have discussed single events and the way they may relate to a person's assumptive world. But events by no means always come alone, and it is commonly assumed that the chance of illness is increased by the occurrence of more than one event. The Holmes-Rahe instrument assumes that in some way the effects of life events are additive and builds this notion into its measurement by allotting each respondent a total stress score which is the sum of the weighted scores for each of his life-events. Total stress scores are then related to illness. This can lead to the comparison of individuals in ways that strain credulity. For example, a young man who has recently been awarded a scholarship at Oxford could gain a total score of 79 (end of formal schooling = 26, plus outstanding personal achievement = 28, plus a vacation = 13, plus Christmas = 12) whereas a man whose wife has left him would have a score of 65.

The Holmes-Rahe approach assumes, as already discussed, that everyday life is itself stressfull. Even if this is ignored and only clearly 'upsetting' events considered, it is important to demonstrate and not simply assume the presence of additivity. This to our knowledge has not been done.

The most straightforward way to consider this question with our own material is to compare severe events occurring to depressed and normal women among those *with at least one severe event*; the question can then be put in terms of whether risk of depression is greater following more than one severe event. If, when those with a severe event are considered, depressed women have a greater proportion with two or more severe events, there is evidence that multiple events do increase risk of breakdown. *Table 3A* suggests that there is some increase in risk, but only for those with three or more severe events: of those who had had a severe event, 21 per cent of depressed women had three or more severe events compared with 8 per cent of normal women. The proportion having two or more are almost identical. The effect is therefore a modest one: at most only one in eight of the depressed patients and onset cases are involved in such an effect.

There is however, another way of looking at the question. Some events can be experienced as forming part of a single calamity and if we are interested in 'additivity' there are two reasons for treating such events as 'one'. First, there must be some uncertainty about how many 'events' are best seen as involved. Consider learning a husband has cancer, his entering hospital, and his death soon after. Is it perhaps somewhat artificial to include them as separate events? There is certainly not the same ambiguity about number of 'events' in the case of a woman learning that her brother has died and soon after that her son is going to emigrate. Second, and more important, are considerations arising from the way we have measured contextual threat. If a woman had separated from her husband, a birth some months later would be rated as severely threatening just because her husband had left. We have therefore often taken account of the influence of certain severe events on each other *at the stage of measurement*. The birth was only rated severe because of the separation; and to the degree we have been successful in taking account of the implications of such 'related' events for each other, it may well prove superfluous then to 'add' them when we come to our analysis. The job of 'adding' has already been done. It therefore seems more sensible to count such 'related' events as 'one' and then see what evidence there is for additivity.

Table 3 *Number of severe events before onset for those patients and onset cases with at least one severe event and in the 38 weeks before interview for normal women – A. counting all events, and B. counting only 'unrelated' events*

	Number of events					
	1		2		3	
	%		%		%	
A *All severe events*						
patients (70)	60	(42)	17	(11)	23	(17)
onset cases (25)	60	(15)	28	(7)	12	(3)
patients and cases (95)	60	(57)	19	(18)	21	(20)
normal women (75)	75	(56)	17	(13)	8	(6)
			For 3+ events, $p < .05$			
B *'unrelated' events*						
patients (70)	73	(51)	20	(14)	7	(5)
onset cases (25)	64	(16)	28	(7)	8	(2)
patients and cases (95)	71	(67)	22	(21)	7	(7)
normal women (75)	90	(68)	9	(7)	0	(0)
			For 3+ events, $p < .01$			

When severe events were considered in this way the association is, if anything, somewhat greater, suggesting that it is only 'unrelated' events that have an additive effect. Depressed women had more often experienced *two or more 'unrelated' severe events* before onset – of those with a severe event 29 per cent of patients and 9 per cent of normal women had two or more – *Table 3B*.[7] An analysis taking account of all types of severe event indicates that it is only multiple 'unrelated' severe events that increase risk of depression. We must add, however, that when seen in the light of results for events as a whole the effect is again modest. Only about one in five of the depressed women have two or more such 'unrelated' severe events.

We went on to examine the possibility that multiple *minor* events might contribute in some way to onset, either on their own or in conjunction with severe events, to increase risk of depression, but there was no hint that minor events played any role either on their own or combined with severe events.[8]

We draw two conclusions. That 'related' events do not 'add' is not surprising. As we have pointed out, the contextual threat rating takes into account biographical circumstances surrounding each event: the birth was rated severe because the woman's husband had already left her. If we have taken into account at the stage of measurement the way 'related' events influence each other, it is understandable that when we 'add' such events in the analysis we find no additional effect. All that is surprising is the apparent degree of success of our measurement of contextual threat in taking account of the meaningfulness of such events for each other. It seems probable that for 'related' events, only one (say the final death) is important in producing depression; but while this seems likely, it must be remembered that our method of measuring threat probably rules out finding an 'additive' effect should one exist.

This conclusion raises the further question of just where the 'context' of events begins and ends. The answer is perhaps rather lame: in the contextual ratings we take account of only *obviously* related factors. Bad news about housing is obviously relevant in rating the threatfulness of a pregnancy. Equally the death of a father will not be part of the context of hearing that one's son has been arrested; nor would we increase our rating of the threat of a birth because a woman had recently lost a friend. It follows that we must show great care in drawing conclusions about 'additivity'. We are unrepentant about this. It is difficult to think of an alternative and the approach does enable us to concentrate on the notion of additivity where it is theoretically most relevant – between 'unrelated' events.

The final question is, therefore, how to interpret the evidence that more than one 'unrelated' severe event increases risk of depression – albeit not by a substantial amount. There are four possible ways in which such events might 'add' to produce depression. The first by-passes the notion of consciousness. Regardless of the woman's aware-ness of the meaning of her experiences, the addition of another item of stress might prove the straw that breaks her resistance. The research with schizophrenia provides an analogy: a disturbing event probably has a greater chance of provoking onset in a home with high tension, the two factors being 'mechanically' added (Brown and Birley, 1968: 210). We think such *mechanical* additivity unlikely to have much rele-vance in the aetiology of depression. The other three ways in which events may 'add' all take account of the meaning of events; and do so with increasing degrees of complexity. The second involves a simple addition of distress by means of a *general appraisal*. It is as if the thought

'Oh God, yet another thing' is the final cause of the breakdown. Here we have in mind a series of quite distinct events – learning a son has been diagnosed dyslexic, a friend moving away, and a husband losing his job – although such a response might also occur in response to events forming part of a series – a husband's second heart attack. It is as though the proverbial camel's back would not break unless he realized that the load was too heavy. A third form of additivity rests on the particular implications of a first event for a second. (The argument is equally applicable to three or more events or to the relationship of an event with ongoing difficulties.) We have already suggested in discussing the contextual ratings that births occurring to women in a one-parent family are likely to be severe because of the social *context* of the women. Thus a husband's desertion would ensure that a subsequent birth later in the year would be rated as severe. The birth would be severe because of its implications for a woman living alone. Thus in the contextual threat ratings we assume a *specific appraisal* on the woman's part, which in this example is centred on the implications of the birth. (Of course, both general and specific appraisal might be at work in a particular situation.)

The fourth possibility is similar but the link between events is no longer contextual – in the sense that one event is directly and obviously involved in the roles and plans imposed by another event, as the husband's desertion imposed meaning on the later birth. In this fourth type of additivity the first event influences the second through its more individual personal significance. One of the patients developed a severe depression a few weeks after the birth of her first child. Several weeks earlier her father had died. His death was in no way part of the context of the birth in the sense we have used this concept – he, for instance, was not supporting her financially. But, for the woman, his death appeared to have been an ever-present part of the significance of having her first child; she could not stop thinking of how she had looked forward to him seeing his first grandchild and now he could not see it. It is possible that without the birth she might have weathered the death without a breakdown and that the poignancy of the combination of the two was crucial. However we did not attempt to take account of such *symbolic appraisal*. Although it would not have been impossible, we were not ready to face the formidable problems of interpretation involved.[9]

While the results we have so far presented come down clearly in favour of our emphasis on the meaningfulness of life-events, the finding that multiple 'unrelated' events appear to play *some* role in increasing risk of depression might be interpreted in terms of some *mechanical* reaction. While we will argue later that the impact of the social environment on depression is probably entirely the result of *general* or *specific* appraisal, we are clearly not in a position to assert that a mechanical process is *never* at work.

Short- or long-term effect

We have established that severe events can lead to depression and that under certain circumstances two or more severe events can increase risk of depression. We have so far left undiscussed the length of time over which the events can have effect. For example, Mrs Ferguson, a married woman of fifty-one with two adult children living at home, was one of the seventy-three women admitted as an in-patient. Her husband told her one day 'out of the blue' that he was having an affair. Before this she said she had no reason to think her marriage was not 'fine'. She said she had suspected nothing. Almost at once she said she felt depressed. She began to cry a great deal and did so every day. She felt life was not worth living and she thought carefully about various methods of committing suicide. She also began to feel guilty and in some way responsible for the failure of her marriage. She sweated a good deal and generally felt tense. These symptoms came on within a week or so of the event and for the next five to six months she gradually got worse. She had 'much less energy', her movements 'slowed up', and she lost interest in everything. She stopped going to evening classes the week after she learnt of her husband's affair and just sat and watched television although she was not really interested. She could not read and dreaded shopping as she 'knew she looked awful' and feared she would burst into tears if people asked her how she was. She ate much less; and in all she lost at least three hours sleep every night and felt at her worst in the morning.

Mrs Ferguson's depression came on quickly in response to an obvious crisis in her life. But matters were by no means always as clear as this – often women did not become *clinically* depressed for several months. Another of the seventy-three women admitted to hospital for depression developed her first clear psychiatric symptom thirty-one weeks after her husband had died of cancer and another developed her symptoms thirty-nine weeks after her son had been admitted to mental hospital after a drinking bout and having been largely unemployed for a year.

In terms of the overall frequency of severe events we have seen that patients have a greater number throughout the whole of the year before onset *(Figure 1B)*. While, as in the case of Mrs Ferguson, severe events are particularly common in the few weeks immediately before onset, they are three times more common even during the rest of the study period for patients than for normal women. Indeed we concluded in an earlier report that there is a possibility that a severe event can bring about depression as much as a year later (or perhaps longer) – see Brown *et al.*, 1973a. But in concluding this we ignored the fact that nearly half the patients with a severe event had more than one. This means that some of the patients with an event some way from onset will also have had one nearer onset. What is the implication of this for our evidence for the existence of a long-term effect?

Before we can answer this we must face the fact that where a patient has had more than one severe event there is no way of deciding whether depression was brought about by just one of them – and still less which one. (Although, as we have seen, we can tackle the question whether two or more severe events increase overall risk of depression when compared with that for one event alone.) How then can we conclude anything about the existence of a long-term effect if we have no way of deciding which events are involved? One way out of the impasse is to start by excluding the twenty-eight patients with more than one severe event. The issue surrounding multiple events no longer arises and there is no reason to believe that a long-term effect, if it exists, would not be equally present for patients with only one event. Using five nine-week periods before onset, a long-term effect for severe events is still present, but there is some hint that it may be restricted to the nine months before onset:

Table 4   *Nine-weekly periods before onset by proportion of patients with a severe event: patients with two or more severe events excluded*

37–45	28–36	19–27	10–18	1–9	(n = 86)
4.6%	6.4%	6.9%	6.2%	30.0%	

Equally significant is the predominant importance of the nine weeks before onset – over half the patients with one severe event had it within this short period.

One way to include the twenty-eight patients we have just excluded because they have more than one severe event is to deal with only the severe event nearest to onset, assuming for the present it was this one that brought about onset. Much the same result is obtained. The nine weeks before onset is again much the most important, almost two-thirds of the seventy patients with a severe event having one in this time (see *Table 5*).

Even if the single event furthest from onset is taken for these twenty-eight women, 44 per cent of the total seventy patients with a severe event had one in the nine weeks before onset. In the next chapter we will describe an index that allows us to quantify more precisely these results: but the overall implication is quite clear. Severe events usually lead fairly quickly to depression – most often within nine weeks and in the great majority of instances within six months. The existence of an additive effect does however suggest that we cannot entirely rule out the even longer term effects, though their overall importance cannot be great.

Table 5   *Nine-weekly periods before onset by proportion of patients with a severe event taking the severe event nearest onset for patients with more than one*

37–45	28–36	19–27	10–18	1–9	(n = 114)
5.0%	4.7%	7.1%	7.4%	42.0%	

Comparison of contextual and self-report scales

One of the major innovations of the depression study is the use of the contextual scales of threat, ignoring what women said they felt about events. This was done for the methodological reasons we have already given – we had no doubt that her reaction to the event, its meaning for her, was all important in producing depression. Since we also took account of any information we collected about how a woman said she felt about each event on the self-report threat scales, it is clearly of interest to examine the relationship of this scale to our other material. There was in fact a good deal of agreement between the self-report and contextual measures of threat for both patients and the general population. Results for the rating of events for long-term threat were:

Table 6   *Comparison of long-term contextual and self-report scales*

	patients before onset		total general population	
	%		%	
severe on both scales	32	(82)	14	(199)
severe self-report only	10	(22)	2	(33)
severe contextual only	5	(12)	2	(26)
non-severe on both scales	53	(116)	82	(1142)
	100	(232)	100	(1400)

The agreement between the two scales was somewhat lower for the patients than for the general population – agreement coefficients, taking account of association due to chance, are 84 per cent and 95 per cent respectively.

Although agreement between the contextual and self-report scales is high, there is *some* disagreement. It is noticeable that for the patients disagreement is almost twice as likely to be due to the report of threat being higher than the contextual rating. Do patients therefore tend to exaggerate the threatfulness of events? The only way we could examine this was to read through what we had collected and this gave a clear answer. There were twenty-two occasions when the patient's self-report gave the higher rating of threat. In thirteen there seemed to be no reason at all to doubt the patient's account of how she felt. There was simply a difference in the ratings.

In three further instances the contextual scale had clearly given too conservative an estimated threat, although the ratings had been correctly made by our standards. Our rules had not allowed us enough leeway in assessing the degree of emotional investment in a person or object who had been lost. For example in one instance the patient's brother's marriage had broken up. Both patient and husband gave the same account; she saw less of her brother and had been deeply upset. She had identified with her brother's plight, whom she thought had been badly treated by his wife. In another instance the patient's fourteen-year-old dog had died. She had been without doubt very involved. She 'missed him terribly' and 'really idolized the dog'. His photograph took pride of place on the mantelpiece in the living-room. But the 'rules' we had developed for contextual threat did not allow us to rate loss of a dog as 'severe'. In a further six of the twenty-two discrepancies, although there was no reason to doubt the patient's account of her feelings, the intensity of her response was probably due to the depression itself which followed within a day or so of the event, or to an 'over-reaction' because of a long-term neurotic personality. One woman, for instance, became disturbed very soon after the birth of her child; it was a girl and she had wanted a boy. She said that the baby reminded her of a child she had once fostered (and still missed).

The somewhat lower level of association of the patient scales could therefore be explained by a handful of instances where the patient's response, although accurately recorded, was due to the depressive disorder itself or some long-term 'neurotic' trait.[10]

These discrepancies can be viewed from a different perspective: can any of the events rated severe on self-report alone have provoked the patient's disorder? Taking a cautious view we felt that nine might well have brought about the depression; but, since in four instances the patient already had another severe event, our overall results are hardly changed. If the calculation is based on the self-report alone, the resulting differences between depressed and normal women are slightly less. Perhaps surprisingly, the softer measure does not change our conclusion.

These results, however, might raise a further question for some. Since the self-report ratings add so little to the contextual threat ratings, are not our criticisms of the SRE schedule of Holmes and Rahe misplaced? If our 'contextual' standards differ so little from peoples' self-reports of threat there is perhaps no need to worry that the answers given to the SRE may prove invalid in the way we discussed in the last chapter? In other words, should these results dispel our worries about the possible different thresholds people will have in answering whether they have or have not experienced 'legal trouble', a 'health difficulty', and so on during the year? We believe it would be quite false reassurance. Our criticism of the SRE is based on the procedure by which the data is collected and rated, and there is no reason to believe that in these respects our self-report measure is at all comparable to events obtained by the SRE. The fact that our contextual and self-report measures of threat were quite closely correlated is irrelevant given the differences between the two approaches to questioning and rating. The question in any case suggests a basic misunderstanding of methodological arguments. It is not that open-ended measures of life-events are necessarily invalid – simply that it is at present not permissible to rule out the possibility that they are.

Are other dimensions important?

Besides the two long-term threat scales there were a further twenty-six descriptive scales for each event. Did any of these relate to onset of depression, when long-term threat was taken into account? To check this we looked to see whether the severe events for depressed women differed from those four normal women on these other scales. We could in fact make fifty-two comparisons as both patients and onset cases could be compared with normal women. In only three of the comparisons were there statistically significant differences, all occurring between patients and normal women.

While the three differences are well within the limits of what would be expected by chance they are of some interest. Two concern the patients' emotional response. First, they somewhat more often reported marked negative emotion as an immediate response to the severe event than women in Camberwell (59 per cent and 41 per cent). Since they did not report more negative emotion to other events (9 per cent and 7 per cent), the difference is probably genuine. We also asked about three specific negative emotions – anger, anxiety, and depression – and it is only for the latter that patients differed. This is the second difference. Both differences are modest and hardly influence the overall conclusion that patients, onset cases, and normal women show a remarkably similar response to severe events.

The third difference concerned the length of general warning about an event. Patients were less likely to report a warning lasting for more than six months; and this held for severe and non-severe events. (For severe events 5 per cent of patients reported such a warning and 19 per cent of normal women; for non-severe events the proportions are 9 per cent and 19 per cent respectively). There are three interpretations: that patients underestimate the length of the warning that they had. Second, that a general warning is in some way protective; and third and most likely, patients tended to be more defensive and avoided recognizing signs of impending trouble for as long as they could. But once again the difference is a modest one. The upshot is that there is no evidence that any other than events severe on long-term threat are of aetiological importance.

The analysis also indicates that we were successful in applying identical standards when rating the threat of events occurring to patient and community groups. If rating had differed the severe events of depressed and normal women would have been expected to differ on more of the twenty-eight descriptive scales.

In this chapter we followed a general discussion of the nature of life-events with a detailed analysis of the events capable of provoking clinical depression. These usually involved a major loss or disappointment and we have argued that it is their effect on a woman's thoughts about her life that is critical. In a later chapter we suggest that it is the experience of hopelessness that brings about depression and in what follows we will explore some of the ways loss and disappointment can lead to such feelings. However before we do this we will discuss the nature of the link we have established. Just what kind of causal process is involved when a severe event is followed by depression?

7 The importance of events

The importance of the aetiological role of life-events can be judged in two ways: statistically and theoretically. The first asks how many depressed women have an event of causal importance; and the second the nature of the link? Do severe events, for instance, merely trigger a depressive disorder that was about to occur in any case? We will deal with each question in turn.

The size of the association

We have seen in the last chapter that 61 per cent of patients and 68 per cent of onset cases had at least one severe event before onset compared with 20 per cent of normal women in a comparable thirty-eight week period before interview. While the differences are substantial there is an ambiguity. Since severe events occurred quite commonly among women living in Camberwell some of the severe events occurring to depressed women must have been present before onset by chance. Subtracting the 20 per cent occurring to normal women from the proportions for depressed women will not correct for this as it ignores the fact that the probability of two independent incidents such as onset and event coming together by chance is the product of the probability of either of them occurring. This is the well-known multiplication law: if the chance of getting a 'six' when throwing dice is 1/6, the chance of getting two 'sixes' if two dice are thrown is 1/36 (i.e. 1/6 × 1/6). If event and onset are seen in this way a correction can be made for the chance juxtaposition of the two, and this will be smaller than the subtraction of the two proportions (e.g. 20 from 61 per cent). When this is done the proportion of patients with a severe event of *causal importance* is 49 per cent, indicating a substantial aetiological effect. (Throughout this book we will refer to this corrected proportion as 'x'.) Much the same results are obtained for the thirty-seven women in Camberwell who had an onset of caseness in the year: the proportion with a severe event of causal significance is 57 per cent.

In order to make this correction it is necessary to know the usual rate of severe events in the patient group: we cannot say how often a severe event is associated with onset by *chance* without knowing the usual rate of events. This clearly cannot be obtained by using the material for patients for the period before onset. Although the reason for this is intuitively obvious we will spell out the point with an example. Consider two ways of calculating the rate of *heavy drinking* among car drivers. One way would be to find out how long before a car accident a person had taken a large quantity of alcohol. Another would be to select the same people at some random point in their lives and find out when they last drank heavily. Two quite different rates would be obtained. Since it is known that drinking is related to car accidents, selecting individuals because of a car accident would mean that the time between heavy drinking and the point of interview would be on average much less than in the random time sampling. We would thus obtain more heavy drinkers using the first method. The distinction is so important that we label the two rates differently: (i) the measure obtained by random time sampling which, we believe, accurately reflects the rate of heavy drinking among drivers of cars we call the *true rate*, and (ii) that obtained by measuring backwards in time from a car accident we call the *conditional rate*. Because there is a causal link between heavy drinking and car accidents this conditional rate cannot, in any circumstances, be used as the true rate. The situation is exactly parallelled by life-events and depression. If there is a causal link, a selection of patients will in no sense provide an estimate of the *true rate* of severe events. It will be too high since the patients have been especially selected because they have just become disturbed.

We have already illustrated in the last chapter how a causal link between events and onset is inferred from the fact that the conditional event rate is elevated in some period prior to onset. We will refer to this as *the causal period*. If we go far enough back in time the *conditional rate* (i.e. the rate measured from the point of onset) should return to the *true rate* and it is in this way that we are able to identify the beginning of the causal period. For the schizophrenic patients this could easily be seen to be three weeks and the true rate calculated from the rate of events in the ten weeks before this. But for depressed patients it did not seem to have fallen to a lower level by the twelfth month and this raised the possibility that they had not returned to their true rate. We therefore have assumed that a completely random sample from a similar general population (matched for variables such as age, known to relate to the frequency of events) *experiences the same life-event rate as the patients* over their usual rather than their pre-disorder life span. We believe that this is the case for schizophrenic and depressive patients.[1] For schizophrenic patients there is direct evidence; for depressed patients the evidence is so far only indirect. We have already seen in the last chapter that non-severe events play no causal role in depression *(Table 1*, p. 101). If patients had a higher *true rate* of events, it would be reasonable to expect this to hold to some degree for all types of event and not just the small minority that are severely threatening from the long-term view. The fact that it is only severe events that differ suggests that the entire difference in rate of severe events is due to the causal role of these events and not to their higher rate in general among women who become depressed. That is, if we had gone back further in time their frequency would be the same as that of the community sample. (It will be remembered that in the last chapter there was some hint that by the thirty-seventh week before onset this had begun to happen.)

Nevertheless, it is possible that the patients as a group might have a somewhat raised rate of severe life-events over the whole of their lives. Some may cope less well than most – they might, for instance, more often have made obviously unsuitable marriages which led to a greater number of crises over the years. Such a process might produce a somewhat raised rate of life-events over a very extended period of time but would hardly produce such a sudden and large increase in the overall patient rate in the period preceding onset. A *slightly* higher true rate of severe events over the whole life span in the patient group would have no appreciable effect on the argument we develop and we are content to wait until the matter is settled by future research.

Meanwhile, since we have no data on events occurring to patients in the year prior to the year before onset, we cannot calculate directly a value for the true life-events rate for patients, and so we will use the data from the *total* Camberwell community sample. The logic of this comparison is that the true life-event rate for patients approximates the rate of the average woman of the same class and age in the community where they live. This means that for this estimate those who are psychiatrically disturbed in the general population are included, whether or not they have received medical attention. There is no reason to exclude them as their presence in the sample is not the result of selection of those with a recent onset. Indeed, it is essential to include them. Since life-events and onset of depression are causally linked (and most community 'cases' are depressed) they would, as a group, be expected to (and do in fact) have a greater proportion with life-events in the year prior to interview. Their exclusion would artificially lower our estimate of the true life-event rate of the average women in Camberwell.[2]

With an estimate of the true rate of events we are now in a position to estimate the proportion of onsets caused by events.[3] The proportion of patients with at least one event in the period, h, includes both the proportion of patients whose disorder was provoked by an event, x, and patients whose event and onset have been juxtaposed by chance. Therefore p, the proportion of the community sample having an event in a period of the same length as the causal period, gives the proportion of the patient group which would have had an event had the patients not been especially selected because of onset. Since $1 - x$ is the proportion of unprovoked onsets, $p(1 - x)$ is the proportion of patients with an event in the causal period which is *not* of causal significance. In other words $p(1 - x)$, using the multiplication principle for independent probabilities, is the proportion where onset and event are juxtaposed by chance. Therefore:

$$h = x + p(1-x)$$

Hence x, the proportion of patients whose onset was provoked by an event, is given by:

$$x = \frac{h - p}{1 - p}$$

For the present material on patients a thirty-eight-week period is taken for women in Camberwell because there was on average a thirty-eight-week period before onset for patients. The value of h is 0.614 and p is 0.249 and

$$x = \frac{0.614 - 0.249}{0.751} = 0.486$$

Therefore, as already stated, 49 per cent of patients had a severe event of causal importance. It is important to note again that this calculation requires the proportion with a severe event in the *total* community sample (i.e. including all those who are psychiatrically disturbed, taking in every instance the thirty-eight week period immediately before interview). It should be noted that in calculating the corrected proportion, x, for the *onset cases* in the general community, the *total* community is again used for p, and, as we have already seen, gives a figure of 57 per cent. The correction, of course, also allows comparisons to be made more easily. We have, for example, already referred in the last chapter to results for severe events based on the self report scale. For patients, 'x' for this scale is 47 per cent, compared with 49 per cent for severe events on the contextual scale and 54 per cent when events severe either on the contextual or self-report threat scales are taken. Comparable figures for onset cases are 53, 58, and 53 per cent respectively.

We will finally make a general point about the correction the significance of which will become clearer as we progress. The calculation of the corrected figure requires the proper identification of the causal period and its use to calculate the proportion of the disturbed group with an event in the same period, p. However, since the formula corrects for the chance juxtaposition of onset and events it can still be surprisingly accurate if a time longer than the causal period is taken – although a longer period will tend to reduce 'x'. For example, using the correct causal period of three weeks for the schizophrenic series gives an 'x' of 50 per cent, but if thirteen weeks is taken 'x' is still 45 per cent.

What kind of cause?

So far we have concluded that severe events, usually involving a major loss, bring about clinical depression both among patients and women in the general population. When the methodological procedures employed are borne in mind, the evidence for such a causal effect is good. But just what is meant by a causal effect? Most women who experience such events do not break down (only one in five of the women in Camberwell who experienced a severe event developed a definite depressive disorder). Since relatively few develop depression following a severe event, is it possible that such events merely aggravate a pre-existing tendency and that the women would have become depressed before long whatever had happened?

It can be said at once that the view is certainly at fault if it is not recognized that vulnerability to life-events may arise equally from the social environment. There is no justification at all for giving priority to hereditary or constitutional factors. The question ideally requires consideration of all bodily, psychological, and social factors possibly involved in leaving a woman vulnerable to life-events; something, of course, that is not possible – at least at present. Instead we have complemented a direct study of social factors predisposing women to depression (to be presented later) with an entirely different approach which, we believe, allows us to reach a conclusion about the nature of the causal role of life-events *by studying them alone*.

A triggering versus a formative effect

Two positions can be taken about the causal role of events: one emphasizes the importance of predispositional factors and plays down the influence of events. At most, events are seen as triggering something that would have occurred before long for other reasons. In terms of our discussion an event merely aggravates a strong pre-existing tendency. We refer to this as a *triggering effect*. An event for the most part simply brings onset forward by a short period of time and perhaps makes it more abrupt. The opposing position is that onset is either substantially advanced in time by the event or brought about by it altogether. The event is in other words of fundamental aetiological significance. We refer to this as a *formative effect*. Of course, triggering and formative effects are opposite ends of a continuum rather than entirely different processes.

A quite separate characteristic of the causal process is the time between an event and any onset it brings about. We have already discussed this in the last chapter and here again we shall, for convenience, simply divide what we see as a continuum, using *short-term* if onset always follows an event almost immediately and *long-term* if the causal period is long. The main purpose of referring to the distinction here is to make clear that it is quite separate from the difference between formative and triggering effects, which may be either short- or long-term. One cannot rule out a formative effect in a condition simply because the effect is entirely restricted to the three weeks before onset.

We have elsewhere discussed in detail an index developed to distinguish a triggering from a formative effect (Brown, Harris, and Peto, 1973b). The statistical argument can be found in Appendix 4. The index can be applied to any psychiatric or physical condition with a clear onset. Essentially it relates the proportion of those with the disorder with an event of causal importance (x) and the true rate of such events in a given period (r). It will be intuitively apparent that the higher the proportion of those with a disorder brought about by an event (x) and the lower the true rate of such events (r), the more important the events must have been in their causal role. The index itself translates this insight in terms of periods of time.

In order to develop the index it was necessary to assume that all the women who had the disorder and the event would have become disturbed in time *without* the event. The longer this hypothetical period the more important the causal effect – that is the more likely it was to be formative. The index is an estimate of the amount of time that would have elapsed before the postulated onset of the disorder if the event had *not* happened. This is why we call the index the brought

forward time (T_{BF}). The calculation is based on various assumptions –
for example, that all the women would have broken down without the
event – all of which have the effect of reducing the brought forward
time and thus underestimating the importance of life-events. If the
estimate of the brought forward time is large, we can conclude that the
effect is formative; if it is small, we can conclude that the effect may be
triggering.

The formula is:

$$T_{BF} = \frac{h - p}{r(1 - h)} \text{ . one time unit}$$

where r is the rate of events under consideration in the total community sample, h is the proportion of patients with at least one event
during the causal period and p is the proportion of the total community
who suffer at least one event during an equal period. The length of the
causal period is used as the unit of time.[4] Although a formative effect is
quite compatible with a short causal period when there are high values
of x and low values of r, it will be apparent that for given values of x and
r the longer the causal period, the more important the events will have
been in the aetiology of the disorder.

The value of T_{BF} allows us to choose between the two rival causal
hypotheses. If it is long, say twelve months, a triggering effect is
untenable. Since the assumptions underlying the model mean that the
index will be an underestimate, its magnitude is not intended to be
taken literally.

Thus, because the index underestimates, a T_{BF} of less than one year
may still be compatible with a formative effect, but one of more than a
year will always be a clear indication of a formative effect.

The usefulness of this formulation will now be illustrated for depression and for schizophrenia.

Depression and the brought forward time

In the previous chapter we showed that only severe events are capable
of provoking onset of clinical depression and it is these that must
therefore be used to calculate the brought forward time. The time is
1.95 years for the 114 depressed patients and a formative effect is
indicated.[5]

The brought forward time for the onset cases in the community can
be calculated in the same way (again using the *total* sample for the
thirty-eight weeks before interview, including all cases, to calculate
p and r). The brought forward time is 2.18 years, again indicating a
formative effect.

It is worth noting that an entirely different result is obtained if *all* events occurring before onset of depression are used. We saw in the last chapter that when only these are considered, the one clear-cut result is an increased rate of events in the three weeks before onset (see *Figure 1A*, p. 102). Fifty-one per cent of the patients had at least one event in this period and 20 per cent of the total community sample. The brought forward time based on these values is about ten weeks and a triggering effect therefore suggested. This underlines the over-riding importance of identifying the *type* of event that plays a causal role if the brought forward time is to be correctly estimated.

Schizophrenia and the brought forward time

We have already seen in chapter 4 that it is only events in the three-week period immediately before onset that appear capable of pro-voking a schizophrenic disorder. (Sixty per cent of patients had at least one event in this three weeks compared with an expected proportion of about 20 per cent.) The brought forward time of these events is ten weeks and a triggering effect is therefore indicated.

It is important to emphasize that this conclusion does not mean that the result is without practical or theoretical interest, or that other environmental factors do not play an important part in the onset of schizophrenia. In fact, the result is much what would be expected from current knowledge. There is evidence that schizophrenic patients living in 'difficult' or 'tense' homes are much more likely to relapse with florid symptoms and that the patient's ongoing level of arousal is likely to be a critical factor (Brown, 1959; Brown *et al.*, 1962; Brown, Birley, and Wing, 1972; Vaughn and Leff, 1976a and b). Life-events would be expected to act as triggers in a patient sufficiently aroused by the home situation to stand a high chance of relapse (Brown and Birley, 1968: 210).

Although we had not developed our ratings of threat at the time of the schizophrenic study, it seemed worthwhile to attempt to go back to our original data to rate what descriptive material we had about each event. We felt that we could make a reasonable estimate of contextual threat as long as we restricted ourselves to the long-term rating; but, since the information we used was much less detailed than in the depressive study, results cannot be any more than provisional.

Taking into account the degree of threat of events changes the original results surprisingly little. Differences were again largely restricted to the three weeks immediately before onset (*Table 1*). The most striking result is that events considered of 'little or no' long-term threat were often implicated in onset. This is just what would be expected if it is emotional arousal immediately following the event that is critical in schizophrenia and, of course, quite different from what happens with depression. A study by Jacobs, Prusoff and Paykel, (1974) has confirmed this distinction between the role of life-events in schizophrenia and depression; in a less well controlled study Beck and Worthen (1972) reached much the same conclusion.

Table 1 *Events in the 12 weeks before onset of schizophrenia by the severity of their threatening implications*

		percent with at least one event in the 3-week periods before onset (patients) and interview (normal women)				percent for the 12 weeks
		4	3	2	1	
1 All events	schizophrenia	30	18	20	60**	74**
	normal women[6]	19	23	24	25	49
2 Markedly long-term threatening events	schizophrenia	6	0	2	12**	16**
	normal women	0	2	1	1	3
3 Moderately long-term threatening events	schizophrenia	4	2	2	16**	20*
	normal women	2	4	3	2	11
4 Events of some or no threat (i.e. excluding 2 and 3)	schizophrenia	18	14	14	32**	54
	normal women	12	13	15	12	41

* p < .05
** p < .01

But the reanalysis did add something: there is some hint that if an event is severe enough it can influence onset of florid schizophrenic symptoms *outside* the three weeks. Sixteen per cent of the schizophrenic patients had a markedly threatening event in the twelve weeks before onset, which is three times the expected number. One patient, for instance, suddenly developed symptoms eleven weeks after her mother had committed suicide. Too much should not be made of this: numbers are small and the brought forward time is still only seven months, but it suggests a certain caution in accepting the role of events in schizophrenia as entirely 'triggering'.

Overall it seems most likely that the original conclusion is broadly correct – that events for the most part trigger florid schizophrenic symptoms in those already likely to break down for other reasons; and that such an effect is particularly likely when the patient is experiencing tense or difficult situations either at home or at work or in some key relationship. To this we must now add that events may at times have a formative effect. Some susceptible individuals might *never* have broken down with schizophrenia without the event in question. It is not difficult to imagine that some of the younger patients might always have remained somewhat shy and withdrawn but without ever experiencing a schizophrenic episode if it had not been for the particular event occurring at the time it did. The fact that half of all first admitted schizophrenic patients do not experience another episode for many years, if at all, is compatible with such an interpretation (Brown *et al.*, 1966).

Length of effect

In the last chapter we dealt with the length of time over which a severe event can have an effect in depression. Now we have introduced a method of calculating the proportion involved in a causal effect (x), it is possible to deal with the issue rather more neatly.

The importance of the nine weeks is confirmed if we calculate the proportion involved in a causal effect (x) just for this period. For patients it is 37 per cent, three-quarters of the original 49 per cent based on the thirty-eight weeks.[7] When six months is taken, almost the same proportion involved in a causal effect is obtained as for the study period as a whole (45 per cent versus 49 per cent). Results for onset cases in Camberwell are even more clear-cut: there is no indication that severe events outside the nine weeks before onset play any role in increasing risk of depression.[8] Given these results it might be asked why we have used the full thirty-eight weeks to calculate the T_{BF} for onset cases. We used it, instead of nine weeks, because of the patient results, but if the shorter period is used the result is the same – the T_{BF} for onset cases is, in fact, five weeks longer.[9] As already noted, using too long a causal period should not influence the T_{BF}.

A final point: we have so far discussed the causal period in terms of a raised conditional rate of events due to their role in onset. Our present discussion suggests that it may be useful to distinguish a *conditional period* over which the rate of events is raised in this way and an *effective causal period* in which most of the depressed women have had their provoking event. It is possible that some of the distant events play no direct causal role, although because multiple events can increase risk of depression this cannot be ruled out. However, an effective causal period is easily established by calculating 'x' corrections for periods of varying lengths before onset. On this basis we can conclude that severe events for the most part have their effect within six months of their occurrence.

Other research on life-events and depression

Many other published studies have looked at the role of life-events in depression but, as already noted, most have not met the minimal demands of an acceptable research design – a comparison group selected at random from the general population. The use of medical or psychiatric patients or relatives of the patients are inadequate. A study by Eugene Paykel and his colleagues at Yale University does contain an adequate comparison group and is in a number of ways comparable to the Camberwell survey. One hundred and eighty-five depressed psychiatric patients, about half of them out-patients, were studied. A comparison group was drawn from a sample of the same New Haven population.[10] The study met a number of the criteria we have discussed, particularly the use of a defined period before onset and an interview rather than a questionnaire. It can be considered in terms of the two criteria of the causal link which we have discussed – 'x' and T_{BF}. Like us, Paykel and his colleagues were concerned with the unpleasantness of events rather than the magnitude of social change involved in the event, but their classification of events as 'desirable' and 'undesirable' does not, as do our ratings of threat, take account of the particular circumstances of the individual. When correction is made for the chance juxtaposition of event and onset of depression (i.e. 'x') 33 per cent of the depressed population had an 'undesirable' event of causal significance, a result not greatly different from the 49 per cent obtained for the role of severe events in our patient series. It is also of interest that the 'undesirable' events frequently concerned 'exits' – death of a close family member, separation, divorce, family member leaves home, child's marriage, son drafted – a category reminiscent of our own 'loss' events. (For 'exit' events 'x' is 21 per cent.) The categorizations are probably a good deal less sensitive than those based on the Camberwell threat ratings. For instance, we would not include as a matter of course a child marrying and a son drafted as 'severe' events and Paykel apparently would not include as 'exit' events an incident such as finding out about husband's love affair. With this in mind the fact that the New Haven group obtained a figure that is two-thirds of that obtained in the Camberwell research suggests the robustness of the basic results.

It is also possible to calculate the T_{BF} index for the New Haven material. It is 2.7 years, for example, for the exit events. The index can be used in fact on any study giving 'events' for a patient and a suitable comparison group. A study by Parkes (1964) compared the proportion of psychiatric patients admitted to the Bethlem and Maudsley hospital during 1949–51 who had lost a parent, spouse, sibling, or child in the six months before the development of their illness, with an expected proportion based on the Registrar-General's mortality tables of 0.5 per cent. The T_{BF} is 2.5 years, again, like the New Haven study, indicating a formative effect. [11]

The picture that emerges from our data is that at least half depressive disorders are the result of the formative environmental effect of severe events – in some sense that onset either would not have occurred anywhere near the time that it did without the event or indeed might not have occurred at all. For schizophrenic patients life-events are as frequently implicated in onset but play a less central role – in the majority of cases they probably trigger an onset that might well have occurred soon in any case. [12]

Summary of argument

In the last two chapters we have outlined four steps which we have used to unravel the causal role of life-events. First, we have shown how time periods over which rates of events are elevated can be examined to establish a *causal period* in which events are capable of influencing onset. Second, and as an integral part of the first step, rates have to be examined for different *types* of event. We have found the degree of long-term threat to be crucial for depression but not necessarily for other psychiatric conditions.

For depression it is only events severe on long-term threat that are capable of provoking onset. They can act in this way for six months before onset – and perhaps occasionally for as long as one year. For schizophrenics a very much wider range of events is capable of bringing about an onset of florid symptoms but this is restricted to the three weeks before onset (although as we have seen marked events may possibly prove an exception to this). The third step takes account of the chance juxtaposition of events and onset in order to estimate the proportion of events involved in a causal effect – this was 50 per cent for schizophrenic patients, 49 per cent for depressed patients, and 57 per cent for women developing depression in the general community.

The outcome of these first three steps depends a great deal on the measures used and whether events and onset have been dated accurately.

The fourth and final step concerns the need to distinguish whether events play a triggering or formative role. We have based this distinction on the notion of how far the event has 'brought forward' the onset in time. The effect is triggering if patients are affected by events when they are likely to have an onset before long anyway and formative if they were affected by events when they would otherwise not have broken down for a long time, if ever, without that event.

It is possible to check for the presence of a formative effect by the use of the T_{BF} index. Because of various assumptions made in its calculation it provides a conservative estimate. For example, our calculations assume that all the severely threatening events we recorded inevitably lead to onset of depression. We therefore do not take the actual time of the T_{BF} index literally. A period of a year is quite enough to indicate a formative effect; and the T_{BF} of two years for the depressed women in Camberwell is enough to suggest that many of them might never have suffered onset at all if it had not been for the life-event.

The onset of schizophrenia seems in the majority of cases to have been triggered. Most of the patients would probably have broken down before too long for other reasons; but there was also some hint of the presence of a formative effect for a few of the patients. Because of the assumptions underlying the T_{BF} index, conclusions about a triggering effect must in any case be tentative; we can only be reasonably sure when we have found evidence for a formative effect.

8 Difficulties

Life-events occurring at a discrete point in time were by no means the only kind of adversity faced by the women in Camberwell. A woman living for three years in two small damp rooms with her husband and two children would not have been picked up by our measure of events unless her situation had led to some kind of crises in the year – say that plans to move to another flat had fallen through or she had become pregnant. There is clearly no theoretical justification for dealing with such situations only when they give rise to a crisis. To our knowledge one other research team had tackled the issue: Coates and his colleagues (1969) asked about relevant problems in a survey in Toronto, using a list developed by Elinson, Padilla, and Perkins (1967). However, other life-event studies usually include several items reflecting ongoing difficulties. The New Haven study for example, asked about 'major financial problems' and 'increase in arguments with spouse' and these accounted for as many as a quarter of the 'events' occurring to patients (Paykel, 1974: 139). But living in an overcrowded flat is not of the same order of experience as unexpectedly finding that your husband has not long to live; and it does not follow that a woman who has lived with distress and frustration for years will be at risk of depression in the same way as one who has just experienced major loss or disappointment. We therefore set out to develop a quite separate measure of ongoing difficulties and, as we will show, found certain types to be of aetiological significance.

Measurement of difficulties

We started by defining a difficulty as a problem that had gone on for at least four weeks. While those arising as a direct result of an event

occurring in the year had already been covered by the life-event measure, we had to start from scratch with those beginning in the year but
not resulting from an event (e.g. a husband who had increased his
drinking) and with those beginning outside the year irrespective of
whether they had begun with an event (e.g. a husband's poor health
that followed a serious car accident several years before). We started
with the idea of following the same method as with events. But we
were soon forced to accept that difficulties were too varied to be
covered comprehensively by a detailed list of specific questions. A
son's drug-taking, receiving unpleasant letters from a parent about
living with a man, a husband's impotence, a damp flat, and a daughter
withdrawn after a schizophrenic illness are just some examples of
problems occurring to women in Camberwell and their variety can be
multiplied a hundred-fold. A comprehensive list of questions to cover
them would be impossibly cumbersome. We therefore first asked a
series of general questions of the kind 'have-you-had-any-
problems-with?', deliberately couching them in terms of *what the
woman had been finding* unpleasant. They dealt with work, housing,
health, children, marriage, social obligations, friends, leisure, money,
neighbourhood, and general disappointments. In other words the
woman had to tell us what was troubling her. But, although the list of
questions was still quite a lengthy one, we added to each a number of
probes covering some of the more common difficulties we had met in
our exploratory work – about hours of work, difficulties with colleagues, travel, and so on. The specific questions also, of course,
conveyed the kind of things we wanted to hear about. The interviewer
always probed further if there was any hint that there was a difficulty,
although we found that the respondent usually made this clear from
the start.

Once a difficulty was established, the interviewer went on to collect
a good deal of 'hard' material about it – the state of repair of the house,
number of rooms, contact with social services, what the doctors had
said, degree of handicap, quarrels, and so on. She also established
when the problem had begun (often in doing so discussing events
outside the year). Finally, if it was not already clear from spontaneous
expressions of feelings, she explored what the woman felt. The interview schedule used for events and difficulties is reproduced in
Appendix 5.

While this approach ensures that accounts of difficulties were almost
always accompanied by expressions of worry or distress this was not
strictly necessary. A boy who had been caught several times stealing
from local shops would be rated as a difficulty for his mother even if
she did not admit to any worry. But too much should not be made of

this; in almost every instance a problem was also seen by the woman to exist. We would, in any case, probably take account of some of the reasons for such apparent lack of concern in rating severity. If the woman had come from a family who saw 'crime' as a way of life (there are some such families in Camberwell) we would judge her son's stealing in this light.

So far we have discussed the decision about the existence of a difficulty. As just indicated, we also took account of the broader social milieu in rating its *severity*. We followed here the same logic as with events, although *contextual severity* was now rated on a six and not a four-point scale. Ratings were made at the same weekly meetings of the research team, the interviewer withholding information from the rest of the team about the woman's subjective reactions and her psychiatric symptoms.[1] We found little trouble in deciding about 'objective' features to include in these descriptions. The bad state of repair of a house would clearly be 'objective' while unhappiness about living in Camberwell would not. One woman, who had not long before been forced to move from her house because she and her husband could not keep up with mortgage payments, expressed strong dislike about living in furnished rooms. Since this provided an unequivocal reason for her feelings we took account of it in defining the existence of a difficulty. And when it came to rating contextual *severity* we still excluded what she said she felt – merely reporting that one year before she had been forced to move to furnished rooms.

The distinction between 'objective' and 'subjective' is a device to deal with the possibility that women who are depressed will exaggerate the distress brought about by the trouble in their lives. As with the rating of events these procedures were grounded in methodological considerations, and again, once the contextual rating had been made from the 'objective' material, a second was made based on all that was known. However, this *general* rating was not, as with the self-report scale for events, a rating just of feelings. We repeated the contextual rating unless what a woman said she felt was clearly at variance with it.

To sum up. Worry about an engagement would not be counted unless there was something 'objective' involved – say vociferous family objections to it. In a similar spirit of caution complaints about the 'intangibles' of loneliness and past disappointments were omitted altogether – say the death of a woman's fiance twenty years before. If anything this led, of course, to an underestimate of the aetiological role of difficulties. But too much must not be claimed for the measure. Because we asked directly about the presence of difficulties it is impossible to rule out that respondent and interviewer were influenced by the fact of her depression, leading, if anything, to the *inclusion* of too many difficulties. Such initial bias would not be met by the subsequent care in making contextual ratings designed to safeguard the severity rating of difficulties once they had been established. But, as it turned out, we can be reasonably confident that there has not been significant bias. Bias, if present, should be equally apparent for *all* types of difficulty. But since women developing depression did not have more difficulties concerned with health than other women and had, in fact, only more of the relatively rare and serious difficulties, there was no suggestion of a generalized 'over-reporting'.

It is perhaps worth adding that we had the strong impression that depressed women were remarkably accurate in describing their lives *before they became depressed*. This is supported by the interviews with a close relative. For the first twenty patients a total of 130 difficulties were reported by *either* patient or relative, somewhat more than half being reported by both. (The detailed descriptions enabled us to match the same difficulties quite easily.) Most of the differences were due to the patient reporting a relatively minor difficulty not mentioned by her relative. Patient and relative agreed 86 per cent of the time about difficulties rated on the top three points of severity and, as will be seen, it was only difficulties of this severity that played an aetiological role.

Some descriptions

We made a number of other ratings about each difficulty and, as with events, developed detailed rules as a guide to interviewing and rating. Before going further we give brief descriptions of difficulties spanning the range of severity points covered by our measures. In the first six the contextual and general scales agree; in the last four they do not. (Further examples are given in Appendix 6.)

Point 1 (highest severity) on contextual and general scales

Mrs Ricks, her husband, their five children, and her mother live in a three-room flat. All the children sleep in one room and she and her husband in the living room. Her six-year-old daughter has a history of tuberculosis and Mrs Ricks worries about her sleeping in the same room with her brothers and sisters. (They are aged from one to ten.) They have to share a kitchen and bathroom with a family downstairs. Since they do not live on the ground floor, it is difficult to let the young ones go out to play. There has been a good deal of mix-up over rehousing and the local authority has told them that they will have to wait three years. All this worries her and it is on her 'mind most of the time'.

Point 2 on contextual and general scales

Miss Thomas is in her early twenties and still lives at home with her parents. Her father regularly gets drunk and gets on badly with everyone at home. He is generally unreasonable and not infrequently violent to her mother; the only time he talks to Miss Thomas is to 'shout when he is drunk'. She said she felt nervous of him all the time and generally upset about her life at home.

Point 3 on contextual and general scales

Mrs Smith is married with three children. She finds her eleven-year-old daughter difficult to manage: she 'lacks responsibility' and has been stealing from them for some time. It 'upsets her a lot' and she cannot tell whether it is 'a phase' or not.

Point 4 on contextual and general scales

Mrs Black says her neighbour downstairs is disturbed and caused them a good deal of trouble. He has, for example, put barbed wire round the front fence and pulled up the lino in the hall. He called the police when she and her husband last complained. They try to ignore him but she said she is 'fed up with it all'.

Point 5 on contextual and general scales

Mrs John's husband has some kind of liver complaint that caused recurrent jaundice. He has persistent mild symptoms but refuses to see a doctor about it. She worries 'quite a bit'.

Point 6 (lowest severity) on contextual and general scales

Mrs White in her early twenties suffers from headaches every few weeks, especially since she has been on the pill. They are often accompanied by a 'stabbing pain in the back'.

Point 3 contextual scale and point 2 on the general scale

Mrs Grey and her family were rehoused by the local authority after a wait of many years. Within a fortnight bad damp appeared and within nine months 'only the kitchen was free of it'. The local housing authority put off coming for six months. When they came they could do little and the family are now on the housing list again. The flat is not on the ground floor and there is nowhere for her two-year-old to play. The general rating was raised one point because of Mrs Grey's disappointment and distress, contrasting with her excitement and pleasure when she was originally rehoused.

Point 4 on contextual scale and point 2 on the general scale

Mrs Smith's marriage had been very poor all year. She is thinking of separation but is worried about the children. Her husband works long hours as a hospital doctor. She feels tired and lonely and tense, and has 'ceased trying' to sort out her marital problems. It was difficult in the interview to document just what were her 'concrete' problems despite the large number of standard probes (e.g. about quarrels, the sexual relationship, talking, leisure activity, financial independence); but she was very unhappy and dissatisfied.

Point 4 on contextual and point 2 on general scale

Mrs James' sister has very poor health. She used to visit her sister daily but has had a heart attack herself and cannot manage this now. Her sister has her own family for support but she worries very much about her and about her own inability to help.

Point 1 on contextual and point 4 on general scale

Mrs Barker has a long history of family problems. She was deserted by her husband, has four young children, and has manifestly failed to cope – has 'battered' two of the children who have been taken away from her and are at present in care. She reported these troubles in a very off-hand way and many aspects of the family's problems only emerged during the interview after much probing.

Difficulties and onset

Each woman in Camberwell had on average four 'difficulties': and about half had one of sufficient severity to cause, as far as we could judge, considerable and often unremitting distress.[2] But we will leave to one side for the present the distribution of suffering in Camberwell and deal with the role of difficulties in bringing about depression.

In order to assess the role of ongoing difficulties separately from that of life-events it is necessary to exclude just under 10 per cent of the difficulties beginning as a result of a severe life-event in the year. When *rates* are considered for the rest, the severity of the difficulty, its length, and whether it involved a health problem are related to risk of depression.

In the first Camberwell survey only difficulties (i) on the top three points of severity, and (ii) lasting at least two years, and (iii) *not* involving health problems were associated with an increased risk of depression. We called them *major* difficulties. The second Camberwell survey confirmed that these same difficulties were highly associated with depression. They form only 15 per cent of the difficulties occurring to the 458 women in Camberwell but are three times more common among depressed women than normal women, this holding for patients and for onset cases (*Table 1*). Since health difficulties are *not* related to depression we will henceforth distinguish *major difficulties* and *marked health difficulties* both rated on the top three scale points and lasting at least two years.

Table 1   *Rate of difficulties for patients, onset cases, and normal women*

	rates per 100			ratio of rates (1.0 = normal)		
	patients	onset cases	normal women	pt/ norm	case/ norm	pt + case/ norm
major difficulties	67.5	64.9	20.4	3.31*	3.18	3.28
marked health difficulties	21.1	13.5	17.8	1.19	.76	1.08
all other difficulties	287.7	300.0	253.4	1.14	1.18	1.15

* i.e. the patient rate is 3.31 times greater than that for normal women

These results point strongly to an aetiological effect. Differences are large and are similar for patients and onset cases – a welcome replication, particularly as neither show marked health difficulties to be important.

When we turn to the *proportion* of women involved, 47 per cent of patients, 49 per cent of onset cases, and 17 per cent of normal women had at least one major difficulty (p<.01). The proportions experiencing other types of difficulty do not differ. However, *Table 1* shows that other difficulties do have a slightly raised rate among patients and onset cases – although one that is only a fifteenth of that for major difficulties. Does this mean that they do after all also play an aetiological role? We will consider the question in two stages.

Eighty-five percent of these remaining difficulties were rated 4 to 6 on the 6-point contextual severity scale. We called them 'minor' although they could be upsetting enough. Over half of them concerned health but there is again no difference in the rate of health difficulties for patients or for onset cases compared with normal women. There is a somewhat raised rate when the remaining minor difficulties are considered. However, the difference is greatly reduced when women who already have a major difficulty are excluded.[3] (Women with a major difficulty often had one or two minor problems associated with it. A woman with an alcoholic husband might be rated not only as having a marital difficulty, but also a financial problem resulting from his drinking.) The difference seems therefore largely explained by the link of minor with more serious difficulties; there is certainly little or no convincing case to be made for their aetiological role in depression.

This leaves a small number of difficulties rated on the top three scale points of severity and lasting *less than two years*. When these are considered there is some hint that non-health difficulties among them play an aetiological role. However, since evidence is equivocal, we have continued to ignore them. This, if anything, slightly reduces the association between difficulties and depression.[4]

We have now shown that severe events and major difficulties can bring about depression and in the next chapter we consider how far they have aetiological effects that are independent of each other.

9 Events and difficulties

We now turn to consider the joint effect of the two provoking agents. Do they make independent contributions to the aetiology of depression? If so is a woman with both a severe event and a major difficulty more likely to become depressed than a woman with only one or the other?

Independent effects of severe events and major difficulties

As with events it is possible to correct for the chance juxtaposition of major difficulties with onset and this shows that 31 per cent of the patients and 35 per cent of onset cases had one of aetiological importance. The correction also shows that major difficulties do play an independent causal role. Sixty-one per cent of patients and 83 per cent of onset cases have an event *or* difficulty of causal importance compared with 49 per cent and 57 per cent when severe events alone are considered (*Table 1B*). *Table 1A* makes clear that the influence of events is about twice as great as that of difficulties and this is further corroborated by the thirty-four women attending general practitioners with a recent onset of a depressive disorder, 62 per cent having an event or difficulty of causal importance.[1] (Results for the small series of male patients were also similar.)

With this clear-cut result we can deal with the second question – the effect of having both provoking agents. Since event and difficulties both influence onset, what happens when they occur *together*? Does this raise the risk of depression among the women in Camberwell above that of an event occurring without a difficulty or a difficulty without an event?

Table 1A   *Proportion with at least one provoking agent in the period before onset for patients, onset cases, and general practitioner patients or interview for 'normal' and 'borderline' women*[2]

	psychiatric patients (n = 114)	onset cases (n = 37)	'normal' and 'borderline' women (n = 382)	general practice patients (n = 34)
	%	%	%	%
1 severe event alone	30 ⎫	41 ⎫	13 ⎫	26 ⎫
2 severe event *and* major difficulty	32 ⎬ 75	24 ⎬ 89	6 ⎬ 30	24 ⎬ 74
3 major difficulty alone	14 ⎭	24 ⎭	11 ⎭	24 ⎭
4 no severe event or major difficulty	25	11	70	26

Table 1B   *Corrected value (x) for the proportion involved in the causal effect*

	psychiatric patients	onset cases	general practice patients
	%	%	%
based on severe events	49	53	38
based on severe events and major difficulties	61	83	62

The additivity of events and difficulties

There is surprisingly little to suggest that having both provoking agents does much to increase risk of depression. Twenty-seven per cent of the women in Camberwell with both provoking agents developed depression in the year compared with 21 per cent who had one *or* the other but not both, a difference well below statistical significance. But this dealt with all severe events and major difficulties; there remained the possibility that those that are 'unrelated' might increase risk. To check this we extended the procedure used so far – inability to move from bad housing (difficulty) and the birth of a baby into that housing (event) being 'related' and counted only once; bad housing and loss of a friend being 'unrelated' and counted twice.[3] But even this did nothing to increase the size of the effect: 'unrelated' events and difficulties did not increase risk when they occurred together compared with events considered alone.[4]

Finally, there is the possibility that more than one difficulty can increase risk. This can be checked by considering only those with at least one major difficulty: patients in this group do have a slightly higher proportion with two or more 'unrelated' difficulties – 21 per cent and normal women 11 per cent – but the difference is not significant. Onset cases do not differ in any way from normal women and even for patients the effect disappears when those with multiple events are excluded.

It is therefore clear that there is unlikely to be more than a very small additive effect between major difficulties or between a severe event and major difficulty. But, as we argued when discussing events, since contextual ratings of threat take into account the meaning of provoking agents for each other, to a considerable degree their influence on each other is built into ratings of threat. If we take account of bad housing in considering the threat of a birth it is hardly surprising that the two do not show an increased association with risk of depression. The largely negative conclusion we have reached about the power of events and difficulties in combination to increase risk of depression only holds for those without any obvious meaning for each other – such as poor housing and death of a brother. (Although here, of course, we refer only to what is likely; for a particular woman they may have some symbolic significance.) When the approach is changed and the meaningfulness of provoking agents for each other is considered more directly they certainly do act together to increase risk. We give three illustrations. The first deals with pregnancy and birth and shows how they can bring about depression when an ongoing difficulty endows them with threat; in other words, how events and difficulties act together to increase risk of depression when they are meaningfully 'related'. This is followed by two, more complex, illustrations of the same point. In the first, although the phenomena may not be 'related' in any obvious sense, the event has its effect by highlighting the implications of a major difficulty. The final example concerns long-term marked health difficulties and shows how they increase risk of depression only when they give rise to a crisis.

Pregnancy or birth and onset of depression

Patients had a rate of pregnancy and birth events that was twice that of normal women. This association with depression has long been recognized and has been generally attributed by implication, if not by definite statement, to bodily changes associated with pregnancy (e.g. Kendell *et al.*, 1976). The fact that many reported feeling 'the blues' soon after giving birth has reinforced this kind of interpretation. An important physical component certainly appears likely in severe psychotic-like states arising within two weeks of birth (Paffenbarger, 1964). However, there is no reason why birth and pregnancy in general should be any exception to the principles we have been developing. Indeed, given the existence of *some* evidence for a physical component, it is a test case for the view that, by and large, clinical depression arises because of the meaningfulness of experience. As things turned out in our series there is *no* evidence that child birth and pregnancy *as such* are linked to depression. The high rate of depression associated with child birth and pregnancy was *entirely* due to those rated severe: only pregnancy and child birth associated with a severe ongoing problem played an aetiological role – *Table 2*. Among the seventeen patients with either a birth or a pregnancy in the year, five were living in grossly inadequate housing, five had very bad marriages where continued support for the new child was called into question, one was an unmarried girl who later had an abortion, and one involved a later miscarriage. While numbers are small, the result clearly suggests that it is the meaning of events that is usually crucial: pregnancy and birth, like other crises, can bring home to a woman the disappointment and hopelessness of her position – her aspirations are made more distant or she becomes even more dependent on an uncertain relationship.

Table 2 *Proportion of patients and normal women with (a) child birth and (b) an event associated with either pregnancy or birth in a 9 month period by whether a severe event was involved (period before onset for patients)*[5]

	patients (114)		normal women (382)		
(a) *threat associated with birth*					
severe	5.3	(6)	0.2	(1)	p < .01
non-severe	4.4	(5)	4.0	(21)	n.s.
(b) *threat associated with pregnancy or birth*					
severe	10.5	(12)	1.1	(6)	p < .01
non-severe	4.4	(5)	8.1	(31)	n.s.

Severe events without loss

While most severe events involve loss if this term is defined broadly, a fifth of the patients who had a severe event did not have one involving loss. It is clearly important to explore these apparent exceptions to the conclusion that loss is the central feature of events bringing about depression.

Eight of the fifteen were involved in a particularly threatening 'illness', some of which were pregnancies of the kind we have just discussed:

1 A serious asthma attack that led to a hospital stay of three weeks for a woman with an unsatisfactory marriage whose husband was often out of work and who gave her little or no financial support. (After onset of her depression and before her admission there had been a marked improvement lasting about a month while her husband was working away from London.)

2 An admission to hospital for high blood pressure five weeks before the birth of a child for a woman with an unsatisfactory marriage. She had some fear (not apparently unreasonable) that the child might belong to a man with whom she had had an affair.

3 A hysterectomy requiring a two-week hospital stay and three weeks in a convalescent home.

4 An admission to hospital for high blood pressure two weeks before the birth of a child. She said she was worried about her husband's ambivalence to the child and its effect on their marriage – the pregnancy had been totally unexpected after she had failed to conceive during eleven years of marriage.

5 An admission to hospital with high blood pressure two weeks before the birth of her child. She had been extremely worried about her bad housing and this had been accentuated by her pregnancy.

6 An admission following a major haemmorrhage due to a contraceptive coil. For many years she had had a great difficulty in finding suitable contraception – she had been told she could not take the pill. She stayed in hospital two days after a blood transfusion.

7 An admission to hospital for one week with pneumonia. While there, she was told that she needed a heart operation.

8 An admission to hospital for an appendectomy. Afterwards there were quite serious complications. She stayed in hospital about a week and was ill at home four weeks.

The remaining seven women were involved in a variety of events:

9 The birth of first baby for a thirty-four-year-old woman who had two adopted children. It was a painful and difficult birth. She had a very unsatisfactory marriage and the baby she said would require a great change in the routine of her marriage.

10 Being attacked in the street – by a man who tried to strangle her.
11 Joining the Salvation Army and moving to London, where she knew no one, from a small country town.
12 An unplanned pregnancy for a woman who lived in just one room with her husband and one child.
13 A son's first admission to mental hospital for alcoholism.
14 A son's discharge from mental hospital. (Onset, in fact, was one week after the son lost his third job which was a great disappointment: 'I had been trying for nine months to get him settled.' This was not included as an event since our rules specified that loss of job to others was only an event if the 'other' was the head of household.)
15 A sister leaving her husband and in great distress coming to stay with the subject. The patient had not grown up with her sister and there were difficulties in the relationship.

There are certain points of interest. Some of the events could be construed as involving loss. For instance, the woman who moved from a country town to join the Salvation Army and the woman who broke down a week after her handicapped son lost his third job. In all, nine of the fifteen (60 per cent) also had a major difficulty, a figure similar to that of the patient sample as a whole where 54 per cent of those with a severe event also had a major difficulty. But of the nine patients whose severe event led to a hospital admission, 78 per cent also had a major difficulty to which they returned on discharge. Four had highly unsatisfactory marriages and two had major housing problems. It seemed possible that when in hospital they saw their life at home in a clearer and more hopeless perspective. For five of the women onset occurred either while they were in hospital or on the day of discharge. The first woman we listed, for example, became clinically depressed while she was in hospital and then became steadily worse in the following nine months; and yet during this time she was almost well for the month in which her husband left home to work away from London. For some of these women a temporary period away from home may well have heightened their awareness of abiding disappointment in their lives. The theme of loss and disappointment could therefore have also been relevant for most of these fifteen women with a severe 'non-loss' event. Of particular interest is the possibility that the impact of an event, such as hospital admission, may not be through more obvious aspects of the crisis, serious though these are, but through setting a person's broader life situation in a new, or clearer, perspective.

Major health difficulties

This leads us to the third illustration. The failure of health difficulties, however unpleasant, to increase risk of depression has puzzled us, especially as severe *events* involving health crises were clearly capable of bringing about depression. One explanation is that chronic physical conditions such as cancer in a husband or a debilitating heart condition in the woman herself usually involve some kind of accommodation to the *threat* of loss of a close tie or the *threat* of loss of an active life for herself and that only a crisis, forcing a change in perspective, will bring about depression. This might be an actual loss (someone dying) or an increase in the threat of loss already implicit in the difficulty (her own second stroke). If this were true, certain deductions could be made: the marked health difficulties of patients, for instance, would be expected to have had an associated crisis in the year more often than the health difficulties of normal women. This proved to be so: 37 per cent of patients and 13 per cent of normal women who had a marked health difficulty, also had a severe event directly arising from the difficulty (p < .01). It also follows that, since major difficulties (by definition not involving health) are effective in producing depression in the *absence* of severe events, there should be no association between them among the patients. This is again confirmed – 10 per cent of patients having a major difficulty had an associated severe event compared with 15 per cent of normal women.

Yet a further deduction can be made. Since severe health crises can lead to depression, a raised rate of marked health difficulties would be expected among women with *chronic* depressive conditions. A health crisis is capable of provoking depression; if the depression should then persist, it would not be surprising to find that the health problem had also persisted – indeed, the difficulty might have played a role in *perpetuating* the woman's depression. The women in Camberwell with chronic psychiatric disorders did have a very high rate of health difficulties – marked difficulties concerning their own health were five times more common than among normal women and more minor ones nearly twice as common; marked health difficulties concerning others were three times as common and more minor ones nearly twice as common.[6]

Long-term health difficulties do not necessarily deprive a woman of hope. She, or the other person involved, is still alive and perhaps still active and receiving treatment. The very act of caring for someone may give a woman a sense of purpose – of doing something significant. A sudden crisis can change this – her own third heart attack or a return of her daughter's severe epileptic fits. Then the difficulty can turn into an experience of loss, disappointment, and hopelessness and it is profound hopelessness that, we believe, plays a vital role in bringing about depression. In this way, health crises can bring about depression by changing a subtle balance of hope and despair. As far as the excess among chronic psychiatric cases is concerned some of the difficulties concerning the woman may, of course, be the direct result of the psychiatric disorder. But a higher rate would in any case be expected just because health crises may have brought about the depression originally. To this it can be added that the ensuing feelings of despair arising from the illness may also help to perpetuate the depressive condition.

Reassessments

These illustrations also suggest an answer to another puzzle – why in the absence of a severe crisis a woman with a major difficulty that has already lasted for so long should become depressed at that particular time.

Earlier we discussed how the return of a divorced woman's sixteen-year-old daughter from holiday had an apparently devastating effect. It was on her daughter's return, the woman told us, that she 'could realize then for the first time that one of these days I would lose both of the children. It made me realize just how lonely I was and how I depended on their ways.' The assessment was not unrealistic. A major depressive disorder followed soon afterwards. The possibility is raised that when a woman has major difficulties, a quite trivial incident may at times lead to a fundamental reassessment of her life and in turn a depressive disorder. The lack of evidence for an *overall* excess of minor events among depressed women does not necessarily rule out this possibility. The kind of incident we have in mind is bound to be rare; and some, such as a daughter returning from holiday, may not have been recorded by us as 'events' at all. Rather than looking at the rate of all events, a more sensitive way of looking at the question is to consider whether minor events cluster in the few weeks just before onset – if minor events were to play such a role they would surely be expected to cluster here. There is indeed a tendency for depressed women (both patients and onset cases) with a major difficulty (and *no* severe event) to have a minor event just before onset. Twenty-seven per cent (6/22) had one in the first five week period before onset compared with 14 per cent (2/22) in the five week period before this. (The figure for 'normal' women is 15 per cent.)

Since numbers are small we looked at the further possibility that such events might at times 'bring home' to a woman the implications of a severe event that had occurred earlier in the year and that perhaps she had done her best to deny. There was again an association; the twenty-one patients with a severe event more than ten weeks from onset (and no major difficulty) more often had a minor event just before onset. Combining the two results, 35 per cent of the forty-three patients had a minor event in the five-week period nearest onset compared with 12 per cent in the previous five weeks (p < .05). Our descriptive material also suggests the presence of such an effect. One of the women, for instance, with a major difficulty, lived with her family in very poor housing conditions: four weeks before the onset of her depression her sister got engaged not long after returning from 'a good time in Australia', the event perhaps underlining her sister's rosy hopes and her own failure as a homemaker. Another women had suffered from financial hardship for several years and this had got worse after her sister's suicide a year before; her depression began almost on the day of the anniversary of her sister's death. Another woman with major difficulties about money became depressed soon after returning from holiday to find her gas meter burgled (for which she knew she would have to pay). We were able to convince ourselves that about half the twenty-four women with a major difficulty and no severe event had had minor events of this kind not long before onset, although some were less persuasive than these examples. One, for instance, was a widow who said she missed her husband who had died five years before. She was financially responsible for a lodger in poor health who lived with her for many years and we recorded this as a 'major difficulty'. Onset occurred the night she had attended a friend's husband's funeral (which was not rated as an event and thus does not figure in the above results). However, with the results of the statistical analysis, they do suggest that minor incidents (not always included in our measurement of events) can provoke depression by bringing home to a woman the implications of a major disappointment, loss, or failure. Such an effect would explain the raised rate before onset of minor events reported by Cooper and Sylph (1973) who used the London measure of events in a study of thirty women, attending general practitioners, who had developed a new neurotic disorder.

If the presence of an effect is accepted, it follows, of course, that incidents or even simply thoughts, about which we, as investigators, had no awareness, might also have been at work. Given this and the speculativeness of some of our interpretations we will make no attempt at a precise estimate of the size of the effect. Nor do we wish to reject the possibility of some insidious wearing down process resulting from the long-term difficulties. But, on the whole, we believe that a definite point of appraisal leading to a new assessment of the hopelessness of life is likely to play the most important role in translating a major difficulty into depression.

Depressed women without severe event or major difficulty

To complete this discussion of provoking agents it is necessary to consider the twenty-eight patients who were without a severe event or major difficulty. First, there is again evidence for a raised rate of events involving minor threat in the five weeks immediately before onset: 33 per cent (9/32) in weeks 1 to 5 compared with 7 per cent (2/32) in weeks 6 to 10 ($p<.05$), and it therefore seems likely that major reassessments were provoked in some instances.

The second obvious possibility is that some of the women had events and difficulties of a kind that we have already established as sufficient to provoke onset but that, for some reason, our rules had laid down as not severe or long-lasting enough to be classified as provoking agents. There in fact seems little doubt that three patients had been 'misclassified':

1   Fifteen weeks before onset the patient, and her family, had moved to a council flat after waiting four years in overcrowded accommodation. Within two weeks damp appeared and eventually spread to all rooms except the kitchen – 'there was a musty smell everywhere'. The council did not send anyone for six months – and when interviewed she was on the waiting list. (This was not included as an event and since it had only lasted three months, it was not included as a *major* difficulty.)

2   Two weeks before onset the patient had been forced by her landlord to have the dog she had had for ten years put down. 'He was our baby – our whole life was devoted to him.' She was widowed and was living with an elderly mother. The event, according to our 'rules', could not be rated severe, since dogs were not classified as close ties.

3   Her husband had started staying out late at the office for six months before onset and 'had gone off sex'. He had told her that 'he was working too hard'. She said she resented the loneliness. Just before onset, according to the case records (she did not tell us), she found lipstick on his handkerchief. Because she did not tell us of this particular incident we could not rate it an 'event'; the husband's slow change in behaviour in itself could not be seen as an event.

With certain women we could not be so sure: but in several other instances it is not difficult to believe that the event had had important implications:

4   A widow who had had trouble for two months with pains in her hands and feet had been forced to change her work by the swelling in her joints. Just before onset a doctor at the hospital said she had rheumatiod arthritis and it was 'incurable'. She said she had been terribly upset and worried about the future but 'must learn to live with it'.

5   The patient considered that her depression had been due to the recent loss of a family friend whom she and her husband had deliberately avoided because of problems he had. She had also recently moved to another part of London and saw much less of her two 'confidants'. At the same time she had been forced to participate in her husband's busy professional life which she felt she 'couldn't keep up with'. (The friend's death was not rated as an event according to our stringent rules about close ties and the move was not considered severe on the contextual scale.)

6   She had not long left an interesting job to have her first child and was lonely on a new estate away from her friends. (The move was not rated severe on the contextual threat scale.)

7   The patient's mother had recently gone to Newcastle for an unlimited stay with another daughter. She usually spent all day with her mother who was about her only social contact apart from her husband. The marriage was considered poor. Since she did not name her mother as a confidant we erred on the conservative side and rated the change as non-severe.

8   She became depressed not long after she found out that a man at work on whom she had a crush was in fact married. This was not counted as an event.

9   Not long before onset she learnt that her firm was to leave London. She had been there eleven years.

10   Just before onset she had been told she must lose six teeth and that 'she had a mouth full of poison'. She was also involved in important changes at work.

11   Some time before onset her brother got engaged; her own boyfriend was very ambivalent about getting married.

12   Just before onset she learnt that the boy she had been in love with for some time was now living with someone else. She had left home about six months earlier and her living conditions were bad. This was not rated severe since, although

she said she was in love with him, he was no longer her boyfriend – another of our rather stringent rules.

13   Her daughter who had lived at home got married and left to live in Scotland. The patient herself was married and had two other children so by our rules this separation could not be rated as severe. (She told us she had been extremely upset and we rated the event severe on the self-report scale of threat.)

There were other instances – but they become increasingly speculative. The first three, at least, of the thirteen listed events would seem to warrant inclusion as severe threat events but we found it impossible to form a firm judgement on the rest of the twenty-eight. It was, of course, to prevent such difficulties that our approach to measurement was developed. However, some do have a convincing ring, and we can add an overall judgement that among the patients there were only four people who did not seem to have any recent experience that could meaningfully be related in some way to onset of depression in terms of threat, loss, or feelings of hopelessness. Among the thirty-seven onset cases, only four had no provoking agent; in two cases there were marked difficulties which had lasted only eighteen months and so did not quite qualify for the category of major difficulty. In all four there were minor events of the kind we have defined as highlighting the elements of loss and disappointment in the current situation – for example in a context of uncertainty over the continuation of an extra-marital affair she and her husband bought a house, thus highlighting the fact that one day she must choose one and lose the other (and indeed after her depressive onset, her boss did end the affair).

When these examples are read in conjunction with the statistical analysis it seems reasonable to conclude that our estimates of the size of the aetiological effect of the social environment are somewhat conservative. We will return to this point later when we deal with the issue of endogenous depression – depression essentially produced, it is sometimes claimed, without psychosocial factors.

We have now completed our survey of provoking agents but before we go on to present in detail an account of how they provoke depression, we will follow the course of the analysis that led us to this theory, an analysis that tried to relate both the provoking agents and depression to other social variables. In the next two chapters we look first of all at some of the general descriptive variables, such as class and then at factors that more clearly reflect the individual experience of the women.

10 Social class,
provoking agents, and depression

Now we have some notion of how women become depressed we can turn to the question of social class. The circumstances associated with the aetiology of depression might well be expected to occur more commonly among working-class women, and yet there is a widespread belief that it is more common among middle-class women. A sociologist, Pauline Bart, in a recent review asserts that 'Middle-aged, middle-class, married, never divorced housewives, those women who assumed the traditional roles of wife and mother have a higher rate of depression than working women or women who have been divorced' (Bart, 1974: 144). A psychiatrist, Ernest Becker, states that depression is more common among middle-class women: 'high expectations leave a middle-class woman particularly vulnerable to feelings of disappointment with attendant feelings of guilt, low self-esteem and depression. Since she is less able than a working-class woman to explain her disappointment in terms of social deprivation she does so in terms of personal failure' (Becker, 1964). In an equally stimulating discussion of depression Charles Costello, a psychologist, also suggests that upper- and middle-class women have more depression and that this may be due to the expectation that is 'developed that one is individually responsible for one's position in life – that things are under one's control' (Costello, 1976: 71). But although commonly asserted, systematic epidemiological research gives no support. There have been a number of surveys of psychiatric disorder in whole populations: in an earlier chapter we discussed those in Manhattan and Nova Scotia. Barbara and Bruce Dohrenwend in a valuable review note that of eleven studies examining social class and psychiatric disorder in urban communities eight report the highest rate in lower social class groups.[1] This has been confirmed by Michael Rutter and his colleagues at the Institute of Psychiatry using a clinical-type interview in an Inner London Borough and also by Naomi Richman who carried out a psychiatric interview with the mothers of children under five living on a council estate in a working-class district in North London (Rutter *et al.*, 1975; Rutter and Quinton, 1977; Richman 1974). Since most psychiatric disorder among women is likely to be some form of affective condition, these results are indirect evidence, at least, that lower-class groups have a higher rate of depression. Other than our own there have been two recent direct population studies of depressive symptomatology. The first by Warheit, Holzer, and Schwab (1973) used an eighteen-item questionnaire on a random sample of adults in a city of 75,000 in the south-eastern United States. The questionnaire was not validated but had grown out of research with psychiatric patients. Twenty-one per cent of the white women were considered to have a high score (this is double that of white men, the same as black men, and one third less than black women). Using a five-fold measure of social class there was a seven-fold difference between the top and bottom categories, the higher the class the lower the rate. Comstock and Helsing (1976) recently surveyed a large city and a semi-rural area in the United States using a similar questionnaire. The patterns of differences according to socio-economic indicators (income and years of schooling) were comparable but not quite so large.

Our own survey of 458 women in Camberwell, based on clinical-type interviews, also shows large class differences. Psychiatric disorder, and depression in particular, is much more common among working-class women: 23 per cent were considered cases in the three months before interview compared with only 6 per cent of middle-class women (p<.001). Later we will discuss how we defined the class groups – but for the present we can say that it matters remarkably little which of various alternative measures are employed – they give essentially the same result.

In addition to class we have found it important to take into account five 'life-stages' dealing both with the age of the woman and the age of the youngest child at home. Three consist of women with a child at home where the youngest child is: *less than 6, between 6 and 14* and *15 and over*; and two where there is no child at home, consisting of *younger* women of less than thirty-five and *older* women of over thirty-five years of age. Somewhat over a third of the younger group had never been married; those with a child at home were nearly all married and while almost three-quarters of the *older* women were married they contained the majority of the widowed, divorced and separated.[2] Among the working-class women two groups stood out – the highest rate of psychiatric disorder was 31 per cent for women with a child of *less than* 6 and the lowest rate 12 per cent for younger women, the remaining three life-stages each having a rate of about 20 per cent. Middle-class women showed no differences in terms of life stage (see *Figure 1*).[3] The great majority of the cases were depressive and the social class differences remain unchanged when others disorders were excluded.

Figure 1   Prevalence of caseness in Camberwell in the three months before interview by social class and life-stage

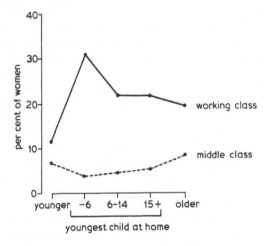

At this stage we are dealing with results descriptively. Interpretation is not straightforward. For example, women with a child under six are more likely to have more than three children under fourteen and it may be this rather than having a young child as such that is crucial. But this is not to conclude that the presence of a child is not of some significance. When a woman has one under six *and* three or more under fourteen living at home, she is particularly vulnerable and roughly twice as likely to be disturbed as other women with three or more under fourteen and four times more likely than the rest of the women with a child at home (p<.001).[4] It is hazardous to jump to conclusions from descriptive material: theory is needed to help make sense of such material. But to anticipate, having three or more children under fourteen at home is directly implicated in increasing risks of depression and finds a place in our causal model.

Two further diagrams are useful as an introduction. The first deals with chronicity. Half the women had been disturbed for less than a year (onset cases) and half for more than a year (chronic cases). All but one of the onset cases were depressed and the one exception had prominent depressive features. Only working-class women with children had a greater risk of an *onset* – a four-fold greater risk than comparable middle-class women (p<.001). *There was no class difference in risk of developing depression among women without children.* The incidence of depression among women without children was less than half that of working-class women with children *(Figure 2A)*.

Figure 2 Proportion of women in Camberwell who were cases in the three months before interview by social class, life-stage, and whether onset or chronic

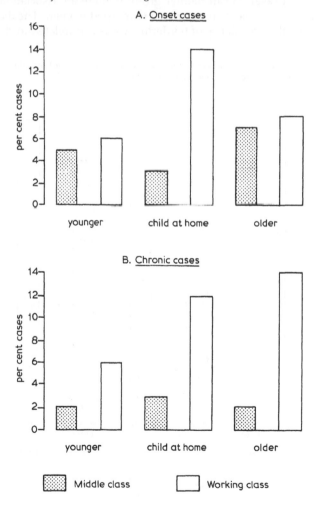

A. <u>Onset cases</u>

B. <u>Chronic cases</u>

Middle class   Working class

Class differences among chronic conditions are also considerable. Chronic disorders were not a major focus of our study, but these differences are striking and sobering. Not only do working-class women have a much higher overall rate of chronic conditions, they do so in *all* life-stages, the class differences being no longer restricted to women with children at home – *Figure 2B*: p<.01.[5]

The final diagram (*Figure 3*) shows that single women have a particularly low rate of psychiatric disorder (one in twenty is a case) and those widowed, divorced, and separated a particularly high rate (one in three is a case), but in neither group is there an association with class. Class differences are restricted to married women. The diagram shows that the prevalence of borderline cases is unrelated to class: 19

Figure 3   Proportion of women in Camberwell who were cases or borderline cases in the three months before interview by marital status

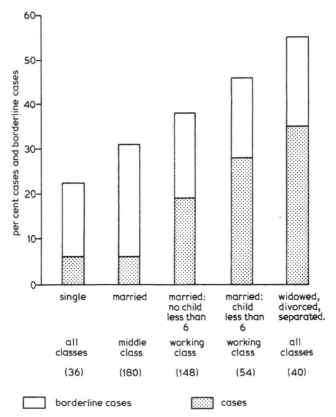

		married: no child less than 6	married: child less than 6	widowed, divorced, separated.
single	married			
all classes	middle class	working class	working class	all classes
(36)	(180)	(148)	(54)	(40)

☐ borderline cases   ▨ cases

per cent of working-class and 17 per cent of middle-class women experienced a borderline disorder in the three months before interview.[6]

Well over a century ago Farr (1859) documented for the whole of France how 'if unmarried people suffer from disease in undue proportion, the have-been-married suffer still more'. Probably more well known are suicide statistics showing that the single and widowed adults of both sexes are in general more vulnerable than the married and that when incidence for the married of either sex is taken as standard, the single and widowed male is relatively more vulnerable than his female counterpart. Durkheim showed this by using what he called a coefficient of preservation.[7] Gove (1973) has recently extended this method to a range of conditions using United States Public Health Statistics. His conclusions on suicide are broadly similar to Durkheim's findings and he obtains similar results for homicide, motor accident deaths, cirrhosis of the liver, lung cancer, tuberculosis, and diabetes. He argues that the results follow from the fact that men find being married more advantageous than do women, and being single, widowed, or divorced more disadvantageous. Briscoe and Smith (1973) supply one of the most recent of many studies demonstrating the high rate of psychiatric disorder among the divorced. What our study appears to add is the importance of studying class *and* 'life-stage'. In Camberwell the single have lower rates of psychiatric disorder than the married only among working-class women and there are no class differences among the widowed, divorced, and separated.

There are, therefore, very large class differences to be explained. But at this point we will interrupt the analysis to consider what we mean by social class.

Measurement of social class

Like almost everyone else who has studied social class we have relied on 'hard' indicators such as occupation and education. We began, in fact, by using the well-known Registrar General's six-fold social class classification of occupations, which claims to be based on 'general standing within the community of the occupations concerned' (OPCS, 1970). But the use of occupation raised the question of what to do about the many women who either do not work or are in part-time jobs; like most others we avoided the problem by using, where possible, the occupation of a-man-as-chief-breadwinner. We classified a woman by the occupation of her husband or her father, if she was living with either of them, and only by her own when she was not. We made one exception. For anyone who was widowed, separated, or divorced we used the husband's usual occupation where her economic circumstances had not apparently changed a great deal – if they had, we took her current, or if she was not working, her last occupation. For example, one woman who did not go to work had been married to the manager of a fish shop who had died twenty years before. She was now quite poor and we placed her in terms of the 'unskilled' cleaning jobs she had had in recent years.[8]

Throughout our analyses of social class we have sought to divide the women in Camberwell into two roughly equal class groups. We wanted to do this in order to facilitate analysis: using such a division gives larger numbers and makes it easier to cross-tabulate class results with other variables.

In the first Camberwell survey of 220 women we took account of education and an index of 'prosperity' in order to do this, since the usual manual/non-manual division gave unequal groups.[9] We refer to this as the *Bedford* measure. At this point Goldthorpe and Hope (1974) published a large scale enquiry to put the Registrar General's use of occupation on a firmer basis and, since this could be used to divide the population into groups of more or less equal size, we have used it in the analysis of both surveys. One hundred and twenty-four occupations were ranked in terms of criteria such as 'standard of living' by people in the general population. A number of the resulting occupational positives make more intuitive sense than the six-fold scheme of the Registrar General: for instance, 'drivers' are no longer placed among 'skilled' workers. For purposes of our research we used thirty-five occupational groups provided by Goldthorpe and Hope, defining a middle-class group by categories 1 to 22. Representative occupations are, starting from those nearest to the 'working class': printer compositor, sheet metal worker (22), accounts clerk, assayer for silversmith (21), warehouse foreman (20), self-employed carpenter (19), maintenance engineer (18), technician in laboratory, builder's foreman (17), car mechanic, television engineer (15), manager of shop (14), and at the upper extreme, managing director (3), university lecturer (2) and doctor (1). Representative occupations for the working-class group are bricklayer, carpenter, gas fitter, plumber (23), hairdresser, chef (25), lathe turner, welder, boiler-man (26), train driver, crane driver (27), shop assistant, cinema projectionist (28), self-employed taxi-driver (29), butcher, machine operator (30), scaffolder (32), driver, bus conductor (33), barman (34), window cleaner (35). The scheme also, of course, allowed us to divide the women up in other ways: a three-fold classification we occasionally use is 'high' (1 to 18), 'intermediate' (19 to 32 excluding 26) and 'low' (33 to 35 including 26).

Class refers to many things, though most sociologists would probably stress its relation to socially valued resources both in terms of access (owning a house) and in terms of motivation (wishing for university education for one's children). It can determine in complex ways what people desire as well as their access to what they want. What justification then is there for using such a crude and arbitrary method of classification? The first and most obvious point is that occupational measures correlate well with overall ratings of social class based on interviews with respondents about their way of life. Equally important they correlate well with a variety of 'dependent' variables such as mortality and educational achievement of children.[10] In this sense current measures demand to be taken seriously. Having said this it is also clear that any particular category of such a class index represents at best some 'average' experience and that within any one category there is bound to be substantial variation in whatever phenomena are of significance. This is inherent in the whole approach and the point has probably been reached when further attempts at refinement of overall measures of class will not be worthwhile. No one measure can hope to deal adequately with the complexity. We therefore take a pragmatic view, following much the same argument as our earlier discussion of 'units' and 'qualities'. Class measures have so far proved sufficiently highly correlated with relevant 'dependent' variables for them to be used to establish that there *are* issues worth investigating; once this is done, as many 'qualities' of the categories as an investigator cares to measure can be used to try to specify what is going on. 'Drivers' can be divided by whether they 'own' a house, and so on. The Camberwell research confirms the value of this approach. The Bedford and Goldthorpe-Hope measures give highly similar results for differences in prevalence of psychiatric disorder in spite of the fact that the two are only modestly correlated. Even the Registrar General's scheme gives similar results.[11] We used the Goldthorpe-Hope scheme because it is simpler and because it could be used to divide the Camberwell population roughly equally.

The use of a husband's occupation to study women can also be criticized.[12] In Camberwell we used it to characterize 83 per cent of the women and for about half the rest, we used that of their father with whom they lived. In practice, taking account of a woman's current or past occupation added practically nothing to the size of the association between social class and prevalence of psychiatric disorder obtained by the use of husband's occupation alone.[13] Nor did a woman's educational level show an association with prevalence of disorder over and above that of the current occupational measure. It also appears that it is measures of the present that are critical. When the social backgrounds of the fathers of the women were considered, the measure representing the current situation showed by far the greatest statistical association with prevalence of disorder, suggesting that it is the on-going situation that plays a dominant aetiological role.[14]

It follows from the view just outlined that we require not better measures of social class but better theory about reasons for results obtained by the use of the measures we have. It is only when we have these reasons that we can hope to be at all sure about what we have measured. In short we argue for an approach that emphasizes the understanding of causal processes rather than the accuracy of the general measure of class. A crude index may be quite enough to generate and test complex and sensitive theoretical ideas about under-lying causal processes. And it is to this we now turn. We start by considering the relation of class to the two provoking agents – severe events and major difficulties.

Social class, life-stage, and events

Life-events, as they have been defined, involve more than the usual everyday ups and downs of life – we have seen, for example, that only a very small part of the spectrum of illness is included. In spite of this 'events' are surprisingly common. Fourteen hundred occurred to the 458 women in Camberwell in the twelve months before our interview, all but 13 per cent of the women having at least one. As many as one in six experienced one judged 'marked' on long-term threat. These were usually major catastrophes: suffering a stroke, learning that a husband had cancer, arrangements for a desperately wanted flat falling through, an unhappily married woman's lover leaving to live abroad. They form part, it will be remembered, of the broader category of *severe* events. Thirty-one per cent of the women had at least one severe event, the additional women having an event of only moderate long-term threat, but again, as with marked events, potentially capable of provoking depression. They were, for example, being forced to give up an enjoyable job in order to look after an ailing mother, a woman confidant returning to Ireland, a break with a regular boyfriend, and a hysterectomy for a youngish woman who already had two children.

With such a broad range of incidents, not unexpectedly, certain types are more likely to be severe. This can be shown when events are classified by groups ranked in terms of the proportion of severe events they contain. At one extreme 'death' and 'illness to subject' contain one in ten of all events but three in ten of the severe events, while at the other 'residence change' and 'role change to others' contain one in six of events and only about one in 100 of those that are severe.

Severe events were not, of course, the only unpleasant events. Each

Table 1 *Events occurring to women in Camberwell ranked by ten categories in terms of the proportion of severe events they contain*[15]

	percent of severe events in category	
1 deaths	62	(28/45)
2 illness and accidents to subject	41	(42/103)
3 interaction changes	24	(37/152)
4 important news, decisions, disappointments	22	(33/150)
5 miscellaneous crises involving loss of pets, burglaries etc.	14	(31/220)
6 illness and accidents to others	14	(29/211)
7 role change to subject	11	(10/92)
8 job changes to subject and others	6	(13/221)
9 residence change	3	(2/63)
10 role changes to others	0	(0/142)
total	16	(225/1400)

woman in Camberwell had on average a further 1.6 containing a lesser degree of either short- or long-term threat. For instance a miscarriage in a newly married woman one week after learning of a pregnancy, a daughter living nearby announcing she was to move with her family to a New Town, learning that a daughter's husband had left her, a brother being admitted to a mental hospital. There was no correlation between experiencing a more minor event of this kind and having a severe event. The women therefore experienced a large number of unpleasant events in the year: 31 per cent had one or more considered severe, 14 per cent had at least three, 34 per cent one or two of lesser threat, and only 21 per cent were without one involving some short- or long-term threat.

There were still other events. It will be remembered that we included incidents such as buying a new house, which women generally reported to have been welcomed. For the most part these involved pregnancy, changes in employment, changes in residence, increased contact with relatives and friends, marriage, engagements to marry, and various kinds of achievement such as passing an examination – although under certain circumstances they could be rated as threatening. Judgments on the contextual scales about lack of threat and a woman's report of her feelings about events usually agreed, but a small number of incidents were rated as threatening – at least in terms of short-term threat – and yet were reported as welcome. These mainly involved births, incidents that served to alleviate a long-term difficulty, and a few reported positive responses to what in general terms were clearly negative events – such as hearing that one is to have a major operation.

Of the total 1400 events, 463 (or one-third) were said by the women to have been welcome. As just indicated, a number of these 463 were considered by us to involve some degree of threat. Excluding these leaves 23 per cent of the total 1400 events as unambiguously welcomed. But this conclusion, of course, concerns only incidents that we had defined as 'events'. We therefore asked women a direct question about other incidents they experienced as positive and these were also recorded separately from events. However, even the possibility of including these incidents cannot overcome the basic crudity of the approach to positive experience and we are not convinced, as we are with negative occurrences, that the measure necessarily gives a reasonable estimate of positive experience. Our research devoted most of its time to developing measures of unpleasant experience and a good deal more work will be required to deal with the more pleasant side of life. We have at most made a start.

In Camberwell the frequency of events declines steeply and steadily with life-stage, *older* women having less than half that of the *younger* group (*Figure 4*); this includes those said by the women to be welcome. However *the rate of severe events remains at much the same in all life-stages*. Moreover when social class is considered *it is only severe events that show a class difference and then only among women with children*. The most straightforward way to present class differences is therefore in terms of the number of women with at least one severe event. Almost exactly one in three of those without children in both working- and middle-class groups had at least one in the year; among working-class women with children the proportion was still one in three but was only one in five among middle-class women with children (*Table 2*). Middle-class women, therefore, once they have children are surprisingly protected. But it is only when type of event is considered that a full picture emerges. Almost half of the severe events occurring to the younger women are of a *socio-sexual* nature – that is concerning boyfriends, confidants, and sexual crises of one kind or another (e.g. a close confidant leaving London, an illegitimate pregnancy). The overall rate of these events then falls markedly in the next four life-stages (*Figure 5*). Severe events involving *miscellaneous* crises (e.g. job losses) are rare but also tend to decline. By contrast, events concerning illness (including death) greatly increase with life-stage. Most significant are *household* events concerning finance, the home itself, and husband or child (excluding anything to do with health). These reach their peak, not surprisingly, among women with children. But while they form as

Figure 4   The experience of life-events in Camberwell by life-stage and severity

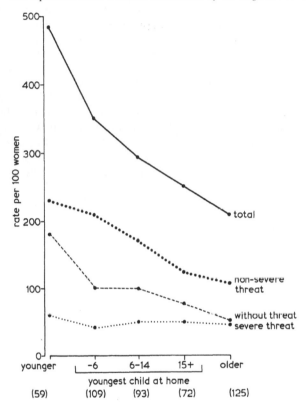

Table 2   *Percentage of women in Camberwell with at least one severe event in the year by life-stage and social class[16] (chronic and onset cases included)*

	middle class %	working class %
without children at home	34 (33/98)	34 (29/86) n.s.
with children at home	22 (26/120)	34 (52/154) p < .05
	p < .02	n.s.

little as a third of the total of severe events, *it is only among them that there is a class difference*. We have therefore managed to specify remarkably precisely the class difference in events: working-class women have a three times greater chance of having at least one severe household event, other severe events not differing by class (*Table 3*).

A simple listing of household events occurring to those with children, even when omitting details of the context that gives them significance, is enough to suggest their class-linked nature. For working-class women they were: subject given a month's notice at a job she had had in a laundry for many years, husband losing his job, son in trouble with the police, son killed while at play, husband sent to prison, husband from whom she had been estranged coming home to live after being away for many years at sea, house-move to escape from difficult neighbours, leaving a job in order to look after her son, left alone after

Figure 5   The experience of severe events in Camberwell by life-stage and type

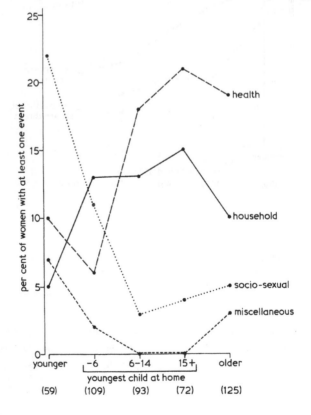

Table 3 *Proportion of women in Camberwell with at least one severe event by type, social class, and presence of a child at home**

		with child %		without child %		total %	
Household event	middle class	7	(8/120)	5	(5/98)	6	(13/218)
	working class	19	(29/154)	13	(11/86)	17	(40/240)
		p < .01		n.s.		p < .01	
Health	middle class	13	(16/120)	16	(16/98)	15	(32/218)
	working class	15	(23/154)	16	(14/86)	15	(37/240)
		n.s.		n.s.		n.s.	
Other	middle class	7	(8/120)	18	(18/98)	12	(26/218)
	working class	8	(12/154)	10	(9/86)	9	(21/240)
		n.s.		n.s.		n.s.	

* A woman with at least one household and at least one non-household severe event will have been counted twice, etc.

move of daughter, arrangement about a new flat falling through, notice to quit flat, threatened with eviction by landlord, husband released from prison, court appearance for not paying rent (husband out of work), overdose taken by step-daughter who was living with them, being forced to have an unwanted abortion because of housing conditions, forced to leave aunt's house where she lived, disabled son's row with father and his leaving to live alone, overdose taken by school-age daughter (for two different women), told by mother to leave home, house taken off redevelopment list which meant she probably would not be rehoused, husband had row at work and lost job, husband left job with no job to go to, crisis when divorced husband sent children to live with her, divorced woman forced to move from parents' house, husband stayed away over night unannounced (and later left her). All were severely threatening – for instance the family who moved to avoid their neighbours could not affort the rent of the new flat; they acted in desperation. 'Household' events occurring to middle-class women with children were: lover leaving for abroad (forcing the woman to place her children and husband before the relationship), finding her husband had got involved with a woman at work, learning that their landlord intended to sell the land on which their rented house stood, builders working on their house leaving owing them money, husband 'walking out' and staying away a week, discovering husband having an affair, husband discovering her affair, and a son having to go to a special school because he was 'backward'.

We have already noted that events of lesser severity do *not* show an overall class difference – there are on average 156 and 170 per 100 for working- and middle-class women respectively. *Household* events, which form a fifth of these lesser events show, at best, a slight class difference – 38 per 100 for working- and 32 per 100 for middle-class women.

Difficulties and social class

Ongoing difficulties present broadly the same social class differences. The total number was quite close to that of events (1481, excluding 134 resulting from an event in the year, compared with 1400 events) and a similar proportion of the women had at least one difficulty (93 compared with 87 per cent for events). In what follows, in order to avoid duplication, we will exclude difficulties resulting from an event in the year except for a few instances where the difficulty turned out to be clearly more threatening than the event. Most difficulties had gone on for a number of years. Only 18 per cent had lasted less than a year. (This proportion is only increased to a quarter by the inclusion of those arising from events in the year.) A further 16 per cent lasted under two years, 26 per cent between two and five years, 20 per cent between five and ten years, and 21 per cent over ten years. The severity of difficulties was unrelated to the length of time they had lasted.

In presenting results we had a choice of dealing in detail with those we have called *major* difficulties known to be capable of provoking depression or *marked* difficulties, which include all rated 1 to 3 of any duration. We have taken the latter as there is a strong possibility that it is not just difficulties of two years or more that play an aetiological role and there is in any case no denying the unpleasantness of marked difficulties irrespective of their length. This means dealing with 148 women with at least one marked non-health difficulty instead of the ninety-nine with a major difficulty. A further sixty-eight women had a marked health difficulty, giving a total of 216 with a marked difficulty of any type or length.

A quarter of the total difficulties were *marked* either in terms of a non-health or a health problem and, as just noted almost half of the women in Camberwell had at least one such difficulty.[17] The thirty-four difficulties rated on the top severity point can only be described as harrowing and the 121 on the second and the 198 on the third were anything but trivial. We placed, for example, on the third point a woman with diabetes who had to cook her own meals and live within easy access of her work. Her husband wanted a child but she had been told that if she became pregnant she would have to enter hospital ten weeks early, which would have meant leaving her husband, who also had a serious health problem, alone at home. Also on the third point was a woman worried about her husband who went out drinking every night. He regularly came home the 'worse for drink' and then 'fidgetted in his sleep all night long' and 'ranted, raved and cursed on'. She said she tried to ignore him and they had periods of not saying a word for three to four days at a time.

In addition to the 47 per cent with a marked difficulty, 24 per cent had at least one moderate difficulty (scale point 4), and a further 22 per cent one of lesser severity.

So far results for difficulties broadly follow those for events. However, unlike events, their frequency does not differ with life-stage at any level of severity.[18] (It will be remembered that life-events decrease in frequency with life-stage except for severe events). However, not surprisingly they have lasted a shorter time in the first two life-stages – of those with a marked difficulty the proportion with one lasting over five years is 27 per cent for the first two and 55 per cent for the last three life-stages.[19]

However, differences do emerge with life-stage when *type* of difficulty is considered. In much the same way as with severe events, marked *health* difficulties increase with life-stage; *household* difficulties are more common among women with children at home, with the remaining difficulties, particularly involving socio-sexual issues, decreasing after the first stage (*Figure 6*).

As would be expected, there are again social class differences. Sixty-one per cent of the working- compared with 38 per cent of the middle-class women had at least one marked difficulty. When type is considered there is one clear departure from the pattern for severe events. It is not only *household* but also *health* difficulties that show large class differences. Nineteen per cent of middle- and 34 per cent of working-class women have at least one marked *household* difficulty and 19 and 31 per cent respectively one concerning *health* ($p<.01$). Only the remaining types of difficulties involving 7 per cent of the women show no class difference. That concerning health is reminiscent of the findings of the psychiatric survey itself where, although among women without children, the occurrence of *new* cases did not differ by class, working-class women with and without children had far more chronic conditions. *Table 4* gives details.

As with events, it is the most unpleasant that occur more commonly among working-class women. Social class differences in rates of difficulties of lesser severity are very much smaller: overall, working-class women had only 9 per cent more health and 18 per cent more non-health difficulties. But probably the most important finding is that

Figure 6 The experience of marked difficulties in Camberwell by life-stage and type

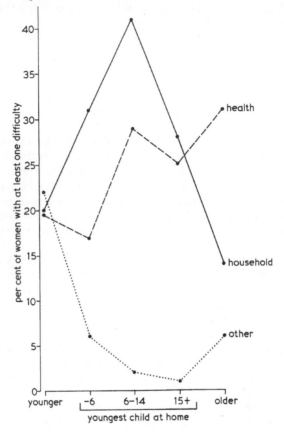

difficulties last longer for working-class women. One of the most straight-forward ways of showing this is to compare severe events with difficulties lasting more than two years. It is clear that if difficulties last comparable periods of time in the two classes, the ratio of severe events to marked difficulties lasting more than two years would be much the same in the two classes. They are not. Severe events, as we know, are more common among working-class women: 28 per cent more than middle-class women had at least one in the year. And yet as many as three-quarters more had a marked difficulty lasting more than two years. Since almost by definition severe events lead, for at least a time, to a marked difficulty, the explanation for this difference must be that difficulties occurring to working-class women take much longer to

Table 4 *Proportion of women in Camberwell with at least one marked difficulty by type, social class, and presence of child at home – those deriving from an event in year excluded*

		with child %		without child %		total %	
Household	middle	24	(29/120)	12	(12/98)	19	(41/218)
	working	41	(63/154)	21	(18/86)	34	(81/240)
		p < .001		n.s.		p < .001	
Health	middle	15	(18/120)	23	(23/98)	19	(41/218)
	working	29	(45/154)	34	(29/86)	31	(74/240)
		p < .001		n.s.		p < .001	
Other	middle	3	(3/120)	13	(13/98)	7	(16/218)
	working	4	(6/154)	12	(10/86)	7	(16/240)
		n.s.		n.s.		n.s.	
Total	middle	36	(43/120)	41	(40/98)	38	(83/218)
	working	59	(91/154)	48	(41/86)	61	(132/240)
		p < .001		n.s.		p < .001	

resolve. Consistent with this is the fact that marked difficulties lasting *less* than two years, but not resulting from a severe event in the year, show no class difference. Comparable results emerge when events and difficulties are considered by type – household, health, and other – and by whether or not a woman had a child at home.[20]

In order to complete this descriptive account we give in *Table 5* the proportion of women within various life-stage and class groups who had a provoking agent in the year. Some of the more interesting points we have made are masked but the table makes the class differences

Table 5 *Proportion of women having at least one severe event or major difficulty (lasting two years, non-health) by class and life-stage*

	younger %	−6 %	6–14 %	15 + %	older %	total %
middle class	40 (17/42)	29 (15/51)	42 (16/38)	39 (12/31)	45 (25/56)	39 (85/218)
working class	76 (13/17)	59 (34/58)	58 (32/55)	54 (22/41)	52 (36/69)	57 (137/240)
	p < .01	p < .001	n.s.	n.s.	n.s.	p < .001

p < .001 (spanning −6 through 15+)

clear. It also shows some convergence, a narrowing of the class difference with life-stage.

Provoking agents, class, and depression

We are now ready for the most important question of this chapter. We have seen that risk of depression (that is incidence of onset cases), is related to class only among women with children. We have also seen that it is only women with children who show a class difference in the rate of severe events and major difficulties. Does this class difference in the occurrence of the provoking agents explain the class differences in risk of depression? Surprisingly only a modest part of the risk of working-class women is explained in this way. When women with children who have had a severe event or major difficulty are considered, 31 per cent of the working- compared with 8 per cent of middle-class women developed depression. *Working-class women with children at home therefore have a four times greater chance of developing depression even when only those with a provoking agent are considered.* But the greater risk is restricted to women with children. The risk for working-class women without a child at home but with a severe event of major difficulty was, if anything, less than that for middle-class women. Finally, it concerns only those with a provoking agent. For

Table 6 *Percent of women developing a psychiatric disorder (i.e. onset caseness) in the year by whether they have children at home, social class, and whether they had a provoking agent (always before any onset). Chronic cases are excluded.*

	severe event/ major difficulty		no severe event major difficulty		total	
	%		%		%	
Women with child at home						
working class	31	(21/67)	1	(1/68)	16	(22/135)
middle class	8	(3/36)	1	(1/80)	3	(4/116)
Women without children at home						
working class	10	(3/30)	2	(1/44)	5	(4/74)
middle class	19	(6/31)	1	(1/63)	7	(7/94)
All women						
working class	25	(24/97)	2	(2/112)	12	(26/209)
middle class	13	(9/67)	1	(2/143)	5	(11/210)
total	20	(33/164)	2	(4/255)	9	(37/419)

those without there is again no class difference, risk being about one in sixty in each social class group (see *Table 6*).

Differences in rate of events and difficulties cannot therefore explain the greater vulnerability of working-class women to depression. In arithmetical terms, making allowance (i.e. standardizing) for class differences in events and difficulties reduces the overall class difference in risk by one quarter. This clear-cut and largely negative result provided a fulcrum around which our investigation turned. It indicated that further factors must intervene to modify the impact of severe events and major difficulties and that these had to be discovered if class differences in depression were to be explained. We turn, therefore, to consider whether there were other circumstances affecting the lives of the women in Camberwell, which increased risk of depression once an event or difficulty had occurred.

Part III
Vulnerability factors

11 Vulnerability

The last chapter gave a hint that psychosocial factors might play a role in creating vulnerability to depression as well as provoking it. To summarize: while almost all the women in Camberwell who developed depression in the year of the survey had a severe event or major difficulty, only a fifth of those with such provoking agents broke down. What about the exceptions? Why in general are some far less vulnerable and, in particular, why are middle-class women so protected? Since one in three working-class women with a provoking agent and only one in twelve middle-class women were onset cases, any explanation of this class difference would go a long way to explain the general question of vulnerability (*Table 6*, chapter 10).

Intimacy and vulnerability

If social factors act to protect and to make vulnerable, the most obvious point at which to begin the investigation was with the social ties of the women. For each event and difficulty we had asked about emotional and practical support received from friends and relatives. Mrs Smith, whom we discussed at length in chapter 5, received 'some' support during the trouble with her daughter – her father had kept her in touch with what was going on and a number of friends gave support. This kind of assistance was associated in the total sample with a somewhat reduced risk of depression.[1] The size of the effect is modest but enough to encourage a closer look at the protective role of more enduring relationships. Lowenthal and Haven (1968) have noted the paucity of references in the social sciences to the quality and depth of personal relationships. Sociologists have traditionally made assumptions about categories of relationships (e.g. kin, neighbours, close friends) and concentrated on the frequency of contact and the provision of practical help. Some qualitative studies have done more but in a rather unsystematic way. The anthropological literature has similarly tended to neglect the emotional qualtiy of relationships although there are many valuable insights. In their own study of people over sixty in San Francisco, Lowenthal and Haven asked 'Is there anyone in particular you confide in or talk to about yourself or your problems?'. Miriam Komarovksy's important study, *Blue-Collar Marriage*, asked about emotionally significant events in the week or two before interview and then with whom they were discussed – if at all. In addition when the interviewer was told of some experience of apparent significance she was asked whether the husband or anyone else knew about it (Komarovsky, 1962: 134).

In the interviews in Camberwell each woman was asked to name people to whom she could talk about things that were troubling her, and our rating of the quality of relationships depended mainly on replies to these questions.[2] The woman was encouraged to mention more than one person. We have used 'a', 'b', 'c', and 'd' to label the four points of the scale. Women on the high point, 'a', were considered likely to have a close, intimate, and confiding relationship with a husband or boyfriend, those on 'b' and 'c' other confidants and those on 'd' none. In order to obtain an 'a' rating, a woman had to name her husband or boyfriend in answering the standard questions, but there were three exceptions to this rule. What they said was occasionally ignored in the light of the wider discussion of the marriage (or relationship with boyfriend) and of other things that came up in the course of the interview. First, women mentioning their husbands as confidants when their answers were clearly contradicted by their description of the marriage were not rated as 'a'. Second, we rated women as 'a' when, from the general discussion of their marriage, it was clear they had a close tie with their husband although he had not been named as a confidant. But on most occasions we rated strictly according to what was said in response to the direct questions. Third, in a few instances we included as 'a' a close relationship with a woman when it had some of the characteristicts of a marital tie – particularly a common domicile. In placing emphasis on ties with men we were influenced by Robert Weiss's stimulating discussion of the apparent failure of various types of friendship and social relationships to substitute for each other. In a study of divorced men and women in Boston he conjectured that relationships tend to be relatively specialized. 'Attachment' is provided by ties from which participants gain a sense of security and place and where individuals

'can express their feelings freely and without self-con-
sciousness . . . For a relationship to provide intimacy there must be
trust, effective understanding and ready access. Marriage can provide such a relationship and so, often, does dating, at least for a
time. Occasionally a women may establish a relationship of this
kind with a close friend, her mother, or a sister.'   (Weiss, 1969: 38)

This comes close to our general notion of an 'a' relationship. But this
does not mean that a sexual relationship is necessary. One woman in
Camberwell (a single working-class woman), for instance, had seen a
married man almost daily for twenty years and named him as a confidant. They met only away from home, usually in the same pub
during the day – and did not share their close friendship with anyone.
Indeed, when he died suddenly in the year, she only learnt about it
indirectly a week or so after he had not turned up for a meeting.
    The importance of the measure for us is not in its ability to describe
life in Camberwell but the insight it affords about the origin of depressive disorders. It is a crude measure. Communication between husband and wife is difficult to assess and our questioning was limited. If
we were in doubt we made a practice of erring in rating an 'a' relationship as present.[3] We did so as long as the woman mentioned her
husband as confidant and there was no positive evidence that things
were held back from each other. We sometimes felt that we could make
the rating only because the tie had not been tested in the year by an
urgent issue; and that had there been a crisis it might well have been
clear that the relationship was not close. This might seem a threat to the
validity of the whole enterprise. If many couples with an 'a' rating
should have been given a 'non-a' rating, our results might appear to
have little meaning. However, this is less threatening than it might at
first appear. For our purpose the crucial women were just those who
had had to weather a crisis in the year – that is had had a provoking
agent; and it was for these women that we felt most confidence in the
validity of the rating. A test for the protective role of intimacy only
requires an examination of those with a severe event or major difficulty, comparing the risks of depression among those with and those
without an intimate relationship; the intimacy levels of those without a
provoking agent are not important. Mrs Black provides an example.
Her young daughter was killed in an accident one evening six months
before we saw her. She said that her relationship with her husband
'had been bad for years' and that they had a serious row about his
betting on horses at least once a month – but she conveyed that she
expected this and that it did not really bother her. They had sexual
intercourse about once every four months; went to a pub once a week

and occasionally to a dance. She did not 'hanker for more'. She said she did not confide in him. At the time she was told of her daughter's death he was out at a pub and she coped alone with the help of neighbours. Her husband was unable to talk to her about it, even though he did make a change in his routine, going out rather less often for a couple of weeks. She said she found no emotional support from this change and developed a curious way of deriving comfort; she would retire to bed early and concentrate inwardly on the image of the wounds and physical damage to her dead child; she could rely on this to send her to sleep within a short time. After a few months she took an evening job.

The second point 'b' was kept for women without an intimate tie with a husband or boyfriend (or very occasionally a woman in the same household) but who nevertheless reported a confiding relationship with someone else such as a mother, father, sister, or friend whom she saw at least weekly. The third point 'c' covered all other women reporting a confidant who was seen less than weekly, and the final point 'd' those who mentioned no-one. Of the 458 women in Camberwell 63 per cent were rated 'a', 22 per cent 'b', 8 per cent 'c', and 6 per cent 'd'.

Intimacy acts as a powerful mediator between the provoking agents and onset. Women were far more likely to develop depression if they had a 'non-a' relationship. In the presence of a provoking agent one in ten of 'a', one in four of 'b', and one in every 2.5 of 'c' or 'd' developed depression. Moreover, low intimacy *without* a provoking agent was rarely associated with depression: only two of the sixty-two women with a 'non-a' relationship and with no provoking agent developed depression (*Table 1*). The importance of an 'a' relationship is clear. It is of interest that there is some suggestion that a 'b' relationship also provides some protection when compared with relationships in the two lowest categories.

These findings concerning confidants hold for all women; but it is important to note that women without children at home were much less affected by the absence of an 'a' relationship, – the proportion of those with children at home who became cases was almost twice as high. However, if a woman had an 'a' relationship, the presence of children at home made no difference to her risk of depression.[4]

We also established in some detail the frequency of contacts with relatives and friends; but once the intimacy context was allowed for there was no association between frequency of such contacts and risk of depression. It is of interest here that in the San Francisco study, 'social contacts' bore no relationship to 'adjustment' as long as the person had a confidant.

Table 1 *Percentage of women in Camberwell who experienced onset of caseness in year by whether they had a severe event or major difficulty and intimacy context (chronic cases excluded)**

	intimacy					
	'a' (high)		'b'		'c' or 'd' (low)	
	%		%		%	
severe event or major difficulty	10	(9/88)	26	(12/47)	41	(12/29)
no severe event or major difficulty	1	(2/193)	3	(1/39)	4	(1/23)

*The figures in this table (and the rest of this chapter) are based on the whole year before interview, not just the 38-week-period used in chapter 7 in order to be comparable with the patient data.

What about bias? Since the rating of intimacy is based on the situation existing *subsequent* to any event occurring before onset, a few women were rated 'non-a' as the result of a crisis. One woman had, for example, married quite late in life and moved to live in London with her husband, her whole life 'revolving about him'. When he suddenly died of a heart attack she was left with no close tie and was rated 'd' on intimacy. Thirteen of the 164 women who experienced a severe event or major difficulty changed from a high rating in this way as a direct result of an incident in the year; but when these women are excluded, results remain substantially the same. (We do not wish to suggest that the reasoning involved in rating these thirteen women as 'non-a' is circular in terms of an aetiological effect – simply that this cannot be ruled out.) There is also a possibility that the women who were depressed might give a more jaundiced view of their close ties. We were, of course, aware of this possibility and did our best to make a 'non-a' rating only when there was good evidence that failure of communication had occurred well before onset of any psychiatric disorder. In order to give the reader some idea of the ratings we reproduce two further examples from the first Camberwell series. The material is typical, although we have deliberately included an instance where we felt there was particular difficulty in making the rating.

Mrs Murdoch was twenty-six and had been married four years and was rated 'a'. She and her husband finished their education in their early twenties and came from middle-class backgrounds. In the year Mrs Murdoch's mother came to stay in order to come to a decision about divorcing her husband. She stayed three to four weeks but at the time it seemed she would remain much longer. Mrs Murdoch had known that her father was seeing another woman but she had not felt that it would lead to divorce. She was upset by the situation, especially by the way that she was forced to act as confidant to each parent. (In addition she was pregnant and living in very cramped accommodation with an outside lavatory.) She spoke very warmly and enthusiastically about her husband and talked of him as a protective figure. They had many interests in common. While she mentioned him as her main confidant she also named a girl friend whom she saw once or twice a week. In general her contacts were high: she saw two sisters once a week, her parents and her parents-in-law a few times a month, and fifteen friends at least once a week. (She named each friend.) On two occasions in the year friends in serious trouble came to talk things over with her (and stayed the night). She and her husband went to the cinema about once in two months and they did a lot of browsing together in shops and galleries. She was particularly articulate and there was no doubt about her enthusiasm for these activities.

Mrs Drew was also middle class and was also pregnant, having been married just over a year. In the year she telephoned a close friend and confidant after learning of a crisis her friend had had with her husband. We judged as a severe event an incident in which she was quite unexpectedly given 'the brush off' by the friend. She said that this was a great shock as she thought they were extremely close. She was very hurt and, although she tried to contact her again after this, she did not persist as she felt she did not want to be humiliated by seeking her friendship. She also told us that she had some difficulty in her marriage. Before becoming pregnant she had been on the pill and for some time had lost all sexual interest. This had worried both her and her husband and they had had long and tense discussions. She said she felt her husband did not understand it and *she* could not understand *how* he could not understand it. When she came off the pill things improved and she became pregnant. Her husband was not mentioned as a confidant – she mentioned her mother with whom she got on very well and a friend. However, we rated her 'a' on the evidence that it was basically a good marriage with a great deal of communication. She spoke warmly of her husband and the things they enjoyed doing together. The fact that she did not mention her husband as a confidant may well suggest something adverse about the marriage; on the other hand, it seemed to us more likely that she did confide in him and she had simply not understood that the question intended her to include her husband as a potential confidant. (Our ratings, particularly in the first Camberwell series, did at times involve more interpretation than we would have liked.)

Sidney Cobb (1976) has recently undertaken a broad review of the socio-medical literature for any suggestion that social support acts to prevent ill health. The studies are a mixed bag and evidence rather poor but his review is enough to suggest that support may play a role in mediating between stress and other forms of disorder. Two studies with a longitudinal design are particularly interesting: that by Nuckolls, Cassel, and Kaplan (1972) showed that women without social support stood more chance of complications in pregnancy, following life crises; and one by Gove (1973) that arthritic symptoms were more common after loss of job in men who had previously been rated low on social support. An important task in the next decade will be to develop more sensitive measures of 'support' that can be used in fairly large-scale social enquiries. Meanwhile the Camberwell results are no more than suggestions. It is clearly impossible to rule out the possibility of bias: since other respondents cannot be used to check on the validity of replies, longitudinal research is now required. In our own analysis we therefore looked for 'harder' measures that might show the same kind of effect.

Further factors affecting vulnerability

Three further factors proved to play a similar role. For two the effect can again be seen by looking simply at women who experienced a provoking agent and who were not already suffering from a chronic psychiatric disorder. The first concerns loss of mother before eleven: 47 per cent of women who had lost a mother compared with only 17 per cent of remaining women developed depression in the year – p<.01. None of those who had lost a mother but were *without* a severe event or major difficulty did so (*Table 2A*). This also illustrates exactly the characteristics of a vulnerability factor – that it contributes to depression only in the presence of a provoking agent. Only loss of mother before eleven is important. Loss of mother after eleven is not associated in any way with depression, nor is the loss of father at any age.[5]

A second factor, having three or more children under fourteen living at home, acts in much the same way as early loss of mother; but the effect of a third, lack of employment outside the home, can only be seen when considered in relation to the other factors.[6] When analysed together, the three 'hard' measures approach much the same order of effect as intimacy alone.

In order to make clear the role of employment we will consider all four factors together. *Table 3* does this. Although somewhat complicated it deserves fairly close study. Women in Camberwell are first classified by whether they had a provoking agent and then in terms of three categories of increasing vulnerability based on the measures of 'intimacy', three or more children under fourteen, and loss of mother before eleven. Group A contains those with an 'a' on intimacy context *regardless* of the presence of three or more children or loss of mother; B, those who are 'non-a' but without the other two factors; and C, those with a 'non-a' relationship but with at least one of these two. Finally the role of the fourth factor, employment, is considered within each of the groups.

Table 2   *Percentage of women in Camberwell who suffered onset of depression in the year by whether they had a severe event or major difficulty and the loss of a parent before 11 (chronic cases excluded)*

	A loss of mother before 11		B loss of father before 11 (excluding 30 women with a loss of mother before 11)	
	Yes	No	Yes	No
severe event or major difficulty	47 (7/15)	17* (26/149)	20 (3/15)	17 (23/135)
none	0 (0/15)	2 (4/240)	0 (0/17)	2 (3/222)

* p < .01.

In the presence of a provoking agent, one in ten of women in group A developed depression. This is much lower than the risk of depression in groups B and C and, furthermore, it remains much the same whether or not the women were employed; indeed, although not shown in the table, it remained similar irrespective of whether they had three or more children under fourteen at home or had lost a mother before eleven. In other words, high intimacy afforded the same degree of protection irrespective of the presence of the other vulnerability factors.

In group B when there had been a provoking agent, women had double the risk of depression of group A. But now going out to work halved the chance of becoming depressed. Finally, there is group C, in which, it will be remembered, in addition to a 'non-a' on intimacy, there had to be either loss of mother or three or more children under fourteen. While there are only twenty-three women in this group, as many as three-quarters of those with a provoking agent developed depression. Chances of developing depression were so high that a third of the women with an onset of depression belonged to this group. But even in this very high risk group going out to work reduced chances of becoming depressed.

Although there is a marked increase in risk of depression in the presence of a provoking agent, as one moves from group A to group C, without a provoking agent risk of depression does *not* increase. Particularly notable are the nine women in the highest risk group, who did not have a severe event or major difficulty. None developed depression, although almost all would have been expected to do so if there had been a provoking agent. While the numbers are small the difference is statistically significant and it does underline the point that vulnerability factors increase risk of depression only in the presence of a provoking agent.

To summarize, groups A and C provide the extremes of protection and vulnerability. 'A's have a husband or boyfriend as confidant and this appears enough to neutralize the effect of the three other vulnerability factors – early loss of mother, three or more children under fourteen, and lack of employment. Risk is progressively increased in groups B and C and it is only in these that work outside the home serves a protective function. It halves risk of depression in the presence of a provoking agent.

Table 3   *Proportion of women developing psychiatric disorder in the year among women who experienced a severe event or major difficulty by vulnerability factors (intimacy, employment status, early loss of mother and 3+ children under 14 at home)*

		with event or difficulty		without event or difficulty	
		%	%	%	%
A 'a' intimacy regardless	employed	9 (4/53)	} 10 (9/88)	1 (1/117)	} 1 (2/193)
	not employed	11 (5/45)		1 (1/76)	
B 'non-a' intimacy excluding early loss of mother or 3+ children under 14 living at home	employed	15 (6/39)		0 (0/34)	
	not employed	30 (7/23)		11 (2/19)	
C 'non-a' intimacy relationship with early loss of mother and/or 3+ children under 14 living at home	employed	63 (5/8)		0 (0/7)	
	not employed	100 (6/6)		0 (0/2)	
		20 (33/164)		2 (4/255)	

Social class and vulnerability

We have dealt with differential vulnerability in general and now turn to the second issue – the class difference in risk of depression.

The same four factors are significant. Intimacy not only explains vulnerability in general but forms an important part of the overall greater vulnerability of working-class women. *Figure 1* shows the percentage of women in Camberwell who had ever been married and were rated high on intimacy (i.e. 'a') by social class and life-stage. (Widows have been excluded.) Three class groups are used, since on this occasion the difference between the 'intermediate' and the 'low' group is of particular interest. The 'high' group shows no decline in intimacy by life-stage, the 'intermediate' a steady decline, and the 'lowest' a dramatic change when there are children – in this lowest group only four in ten of those with a child under six at home were considered to be high on intimacy. However, level of intimacy improves with successive life-stages and in the final stage the lowest-class group comes close to the high-class group in the proportion having an 'a' relationship. Of course, a series of cross-sectional surveys on different groups can be misleading if seen in the same light as longitudinal data on the same group. (By the time they reach the last life stage the present 'young' group might be relatively low on intimacy.) But the very low level of intimacy among the lowest status women when they have children is enough to suggest one of the reasons why working-class women and women in that life-stage are at greater risk.

But in addition to having a husband less often as a confidant, working-class women are also more likely to have lost a mother – 11 per cent (26/240) versus 6 per cent (14/218) – and to have three or more children under fourteen at home – 13 per cent (32/240) versus 7 per cent (15/218). They are not, however, more likely to be without work.

When all vulnerability factors are considered, a third of working-class women fall into category B and 9 per cent into category C, compared with 21 per cent and 2 per cent of middle-class women.[7] Since working-class women with children also have a higher rate of severe events and major difficulties, they have a greater chance of experiencing *both* a provoking agent and a vulnerability factor. *And this is enough to explain the entire class difference in risk of depression among women with children* – at least in statistical terms.[8]

We will leave until a later chapter *why* these factors serve to protect or make a woman vulnerable to depression and continue to develop a causal model of depression in terms of the measures as we have so far presented them.

Figure 1 The experience of high intimacy with husband/boyfriend among ever-married women in Camberwell by life-stage and class (excluding widows)

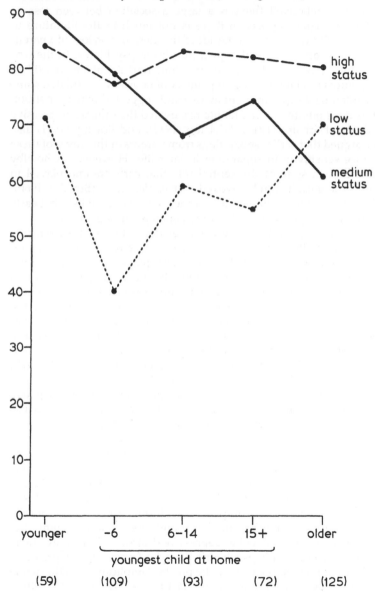

Early loss of parents and depression

While in Camberwell there is a large association between loss of mother and later depression there is not much in the literature to support such a clear-cut result. Indeed the literature on loss of a parent and depression is one of the great puzzles in psychiatry. In the first paper by a psychoanalyst on depression, Karl Abraham in 1911 in conformity with Freud's two-step theory of neurosis, postulated some early infantile disappointment in love and suggested that a repetition of this disappointment in later life reactivated the primary depressive condition. Fairbairn (1941), Edelston (1943), and Bowlby (1951) also have argued that earlier separations from parents or the threat of these enhance sensitivity to separation in later life. However, as Bowlby points out, in spite of the central role that early trauma played in Freud's theories, he rarely invoked such explanations (Bowlby, 1960). This omission foreshadowed the curious failure to establish that early loss of parents plays any role in the aetiology of depression.

In spite of a great deal of research, evidence for an effect remains elusive. Granville-Grossman's conclusion in 1968, that there was no unambiguous evidence that loss of parents plays an aetiological role, was undoubtedly a fair one. Since then Birtchnell has carried out two large-scale studies with essentially negative results. The first failed to find any relationship between parental death and depression; the second, involving much larger numbers, did find a statistically significant relationship between loss of a parent by death before ten and later depression, but the size of the association was so miniscule that the result can hardly be judged positive evidence (Birtchnell, 1970, a, b, and c, 1972). And yet the persistence of the research effort over so many years in the face of so many ambiguous and outright negative results undoubtedly reflects a widespread belief among psychiatrists that early loss of a parent is in some way important.

In Camberwell, loss of mother before eleven by death or other means was linked to a greatly increased risk of depression in adulthood. Such a loss made women more vulnerable to the effects of a provoking agent, but this result only refers to onset cases. When considered together with chronic cases, 22 per cent of the total cases had lost a mother before eleven in comparison with only 6 per cent of normal women. Loss of father before eleven and loss of either parent after eleven was again unrelated to depressive disorder.[9] Since only one in five of all women with psychiatric disorder (most often depression) had lost a mother before eleven, the practical implications of this result should not be exaggerated. But the fact that 43 per cent of the forty women with loss of mother before eleven were psychiatric cases (all depressed), compared with 14 per cent of the remaining 418 women, is impressive evidence for an aetiological effect (p<.001).

We did, in fact, look in all at four forms of past loss:

(i) loss of a mother or father before the age of seventeen because of (a) death, (b) separation *of* parents or separation *from* a parent lasting at least one year;

(ii) loss of a sibling by death while the subject was between one and seventeen;

(iii) loss of a child at any age through death or adoption;

(iv) loss of a husband by death.

They are called *past* losses to distinguish them from events in the year. Loss of husband by separation and divorce was excluded, as in drawing up the list we bore in mind the need to exclude losses that might themselves have been the result of a psychiatric episode. Furthermore, in order to avoid muddling the question with that of the impact of recent crises, we ignored losses within two years of the date of interview. In almost all instances, as far as we could tell, the past loss preceded the first episode of clinical depression in a woman's life. The various ages and time periods were chosen very much by hunch, but subsequently loss of parents and siblings *after* the age of seventeen was examined and found to be unrelated to any of the processes investigated by us.

Past loss is common: 37 per cent of the women in Camberwell had had at least one of the losses just listed. The experience was related to class, and, as would be expected, to age. Women of forty-one and over had more than those under forty, and working-class more than middle-class women.[10] Results are quite clear cut. We have already seen that loss of father does not increase risk of depression among women in Camberwell; it can now be added that no other kind of past loss does so.[11] It is only loss of mother before eleven that matters.

How different are provoking agents and vulnerability factors?

It will have struck the reader that some of the provoking agents (a marked marital problem) are not dissimilar from some of the vulnerability factors (lack of intimacy with husband). Leaving aside the question of theoretical support for a sharp distinction between the two, how far is it justified in terms of our results? First, we do not claim that the two sets of factors are uncorrelated. There is bound to be an association, if only in the obvious sense that a woman with a major marital problem is hardly likely to be rated high on intimacy. (In fact, the association is much lower than might be expected: only 12 per cent of the women with a 'non-a' relationship had a *major* marital difficulty –

i.e. a provoking agent). The two sets of factors will also be correlated to the degree that vulnerability factors increase chance of occurrence of events and difficulties. Women with large families, for instance, are more likely to have a crisis involving a child simply because there are more children to whom untoward things can happen. Not surprisingly, therefore, provoking agents and vulnerability factors are quite highly associated.[12] The key question however remains: how far can we claim that they behave differently?

The most obvious way to examine this question is to deal with the two factors in the same way in analysis and compare results. We did this in two ways. We first took women with either a provoking agent or a vulnerability factor but not both. Eleven per cent (4/35) of those with a provoking agent but no vulnerability factor developed depression compared with only 1 per cent (2/151) of those with a vulnerability factor but no provoking agent. While numbers are admittedly small there is nothing here to suggest that provoking agent and vulnerability factor are interchangeable in terms of the production of depression. In the second exercise, women with a provoking agent and *one* vulnerability factor were compared with those with two or more vulnerability factors but *no* provoking agent. Twelve per cent (10/83) of the first group developed depression compared with only 3 per cent (1/39) of the second and there is, therefore, again nothing to suggest that provoking agents and vulnerability factors have comparable effects. If they had, women with two vulnerability factors would have had as high a risk of depression as those with one vulnerability factor and a provoking agent.

It is not our wish to claim that we have settled this question. A great deal more remains to be done. However, a reasonable case has, we believe, been made that the two sets of measures reflect distinct aetiological processes. When we later elaborate the theory behind these connections, the distinction will also be seen to fit quite well the emotional processes we postulate to underlie the development of depression.

Patients and vulnerability

So far, in discussing vulnerability factors, we have dealt with the general Camberwell population. We now turn to patients. Results for early loss of a parent are much what would be expected from previous research on early loss. There is little difference to be found in the rate of loss of mother before eleven among patients and the Camberwell sample – 10.5 per cent compared with 8.7 per cent. While this form of comparison is the one that has been used in previous research, it is

misleading because the general population group also contains depressed women who have a high rate of early loss of mother. When
these women are excluded a greater difference emerges – 10.5 per cent
and 6.0 per cent respectively – but one still not reaching statistical significance and in any case falling far short of the order of difference found
in the Camberwell survey itself. Loss of father shows no association.

One clear difference involving loss does emerge. If loss of mother
before eleven is ignored, 49 per cent of patients and 28 per cent of
normal women had a past loss (p<.01). However, for a number of
reasons we believe that this does not indicate that past loss in general
increases risk of onset of depression. In other words the general
population and patient results do not in fact differ in terms of the effect
of past loss. Since the argument is lengthy we have relegated it to a
footnote.[13] We believe the evidence is convincing enough for us to
assume that past loss plays at best a minor role in increasing risk of
depression once loss of mother before eleven is taken into account. We
should add that it would not jeopardize in any way our general argument about the aetiology of depression if past loss *did increase risk of
depression*. We take our position on strictly empirical grounds: the
evidence reviewed in the footnote does, we believe, make such a
general effect unlikely.

So far we have shown that, for patients, loss of mother before eleven
has not the same importance as for women developing depression in
the Camberwell sample. There is a second important difference. While
the patients are much the same on the intimacy measure as onset cases,
they do not differ from normal women in the proportion having three
or more children under fourteen living at home.[14] How are we then to
explain these two inconsistencies? Does it mean that our original set of
conclusions about the four vulnerability factors is misleading? We
believe not. We suggest that a young and relatively densely spaced
family does increase chances of depression in the presence of provoking agents, and that the patient result is explained by the fact that
once a woman is depressed, contact with a psychiatrist is made *less*
likely by the presence of young children. They work in one way to
influence risk of depression and in the opposite way to influence
contact with a psychiatrist. If this argument is extended to early loss of
mother, it has the added attraction of explaining the inconsistent and
often negative results of previous research. One reason why it can be
extended is easy to see. Early loss of mother is correlated with the
presence of three or more children under fourteen at home. (It is also
correlated with low intimacy.)[15] Therefore, since three or more young
children decrease chances of a mother seeing a psychiatrist, early loss
of mother will also be associated with a reduced chance of seeing one.

Selection of this kind might well be sufficient to explain the results of previous research, all of which has been based on psychiatric patients. We conclude therefore, that the four vulnerability factors *are* likely to be important in the aetiology of all forms of depression; but that this will not always be apparent in women treated by psychiatrists, as two of the factors at least appear not only to increase risk of depression but, once it has developed, to *decrease* chances of seeing a psychiatrist. This argument is corroborated by the special group of thirty-four women attending their general practitioner with a depressive disorder. The proportions with the various vulnerability factors are almost identical with the main patient series, suggesting the same factors may also act to inhibit contact with a general practitioner (see note 14).

In the general community sample we could examine this last possibility more directly, as at each interview we asked women about whether they had seen a doctor about their psychiatric symptoms and what he had done about them. For onset cases there was a large association between number of children and employment and whether the woman had seen a general practitioner about her condition. Of those with fewer than three children under fourteen at home, 83 per cent (10/12) of those not employed and 50 per cent (8/16) of those employed had seen their general practitioners. Of those with three or more children under fourteen at home, only 11 per cent (1/9) had done so, irrespective of whether they were employed (p<.01). This, of course, is just what one would expect in terms of 'effort barriers' to care. Cartwright and Jefferys (1958) report a lower than average rate of *all* contacts with general practitioners with increasing number of children for women under forty-five. Hare and Shaw (1965a) in their Croydon study found that, although there was no overall relationship with family size, the average number of consultations per child decreased with size of family. Andersen and Kasper (1973) suggest much the same occurs in the United States. It is of interest, however, that in Camberwell the effect was not present among chronic cases – 72 per cent received some form of care for their condition from a general practitioner, compared with half the onset cases.[16]

One further result is relevant at this point. The class difference in prevalence of depression in Camberwell is not found among the 114 patients who have much the same class distribution as if they had been drawn at random from the total Camberwell population.[17] This, of course, is further evidence that those receiving psychiatric treatment are not representative of the total population of women suffering from depression in Camberwell. This lack of a class difference among the patients also suggests that the reasons we have so far given for differential selection into psychiatric care are probably far too simple. Many processes could underlie such a class result – for instance working-class women with young children may less often receive treatment because they are more likely than other women to blame their conditions on the quality of their lives and see medical attention as irrelevant. It would be pointless to discuss such possibilities without more data and, in any case, we only wish to make a case that the vulnerability factors can also serve to make psychiatric treatment less likely. This is not only important in its own right but, as already noted, would explain much of the puzzling inconsistency of previous research on early loss of parents. While the argument can be no more than plausible until further research is done, it should be noted that whatever the details of the links, the existence of factors determining selection into treatment is more than merely hypothetical. One has only to consider the very large differences in the referral rates to psychiatrists by individual general practitioners to make clear that a great deal of selection does occur (Shepherd *et al.*, 1966). The question is not whether it takes place but the particular reasons for it.

Social class and suffering

In the social sciences there has been some uncertainty about the significance of adversity. Keith Thomas's imaginative use of statistics in *Religion and the Decline of Magic* documents the seventeenth-century Englishman's liability to pain, sickness, premature death, and many other threatening events. He then notes

> 'Poverty, sickness and sudden disaster were thus familiar features of the social environment of this period. But we must not make the anachronistic mistake of assuming that contemporaries were as daunted by them as we should be, were we suddenly pitchforked backwards in time. In Tudor and Stuart England men were fully accustomed to disease and a low expectation of life. Parents were slower to recognise the individuality of their children, for they well knew they might lose them in their infancy. Husbands and wives were better adjusted to the idea of the surviving partner marrying after the other's death. The attitude of the poor to their lot seems to have been one of careless stoicism. Many middle-class observers commented on their insensibility in the face of the dangers of the plague, and were shocked by the general reluctance to obey regulations designed for their own safety.' (Thomas, 1973: 20).

Such doubt about the suffering of the less privileged is common. Philippe Aries dealing with much the same period writes: 'it may be that the child that had died soon in life was buried almost anywhere, much as we would bury a domestic pet, a cat or dog' (1962: 37).

Durkheim, in discussing rates of suicide, notes the very high rate for those with independent means which

> 'sufficiently shows that the possessors of most comfort suffer most. Everything that enforces subordination attenuates the effects of this state. At least the horizon of the lower classes is limited by those above them, and for this same reason their desires are more modest. Those who have only empty space above them are almost inevitably lost in it, if no force restrains them.'
>
> (Durkheim, 1952: 257).

At this point it is tempting to take Barrington Moore's view in his *Reflections on the Causes of Human Misery:*

> 'Presumably it requires no laboriously accumulated proof to demonstrate that human beings have hardly every really enjoyed 1) being tortured or slaughtered by a cruel enemy; 2) starvation or illness; 3) the exactions of ruthless authorites that carry off the fruits of prolonged labour; 4) the loss of beloved persons through the acts of others over which one has little or no control; . . .'
>
> (Moore, 1972: 2).

But this unquestioning mood falters. He continues: 'On this score too there are of course variations. Due to cultural and social conditioning some groups of people are better able to withstand suffering than others, and culturally sanctioned attitudes towards suffering vary considerably' (1972: 2).

Thomas and Aries also show uncertainty – but now about how far in fact suffering was lessened with familiarity. Thomas notes: 'Alchohol was thus an essential narcotic which anaesthetized men against the strains of contemporary life. Drunkenness broke down social distinctions, and brought a temporary mood of optimism to the desperate' (Thomas, 1973: 222). And Aries is puzzled that signs of increased solicitude and involvement in young children occurred *before* a significant drop in their death rates (Aries, 1962: 39).

On the assumption that severe events and major difficulties are comparable in the two classes there is nothing so far to suggest that there is *any* difference in the appraisal of adversity in the different classes in Camberwell – working-class women simply have more. There is certainly enough to check any assumption about class differences in capacity for suffering. But it may be asked how equatable are the provoking agents and vulnerability factors in the two classes? It would be foolish to deny class differences in response to them. Indeed the contextual scales were designed to take account of some of them; the birth of a third child will clearly differ in meaning if it occurs to a working-class woman in bad housing and low income than to a middle-class woman in good housing with domestic help, and it is just this kind of obvious difference in circumstance that the contextual scales take into account. They are less able to deal with more subtle differences in value and attitude but even here something could be done – they take into account, for instance, a birth's unplanned inter-ruption of a busy professional career. But too much should not be claimed for the contextual scales. We cannot claim without more research that the events and difficulties included as provoking agents are equatable for the two classes and the same clearly holds for the vulnerability factors. Conclusions about class response to adversity would depend on the direction of bias. If, as seems most likely, we have tended to underestimate the impact of events and difficulties for middle-class women or to over-estimate their impact for working-class women, a correction would be needed to increase the rate of provoking agents occurring to the middle class. If this were done it would mean that an even smaller proportion of middle-class women would break down in response to them and that we have underestimated the relative vulnerability of working-class women. But it can be argued that we have exaggerated the significance of the vulnerability factors for middle-class women; having three or more children under fourteen for instance, might well be less of a 'liability' for them. There is no way of settling the matter at present, although, if there has been bias, it is curious that when provoking agents and vulnerability factors are con-trolled for, there is no class difference in risk of depression (see note 8). If Ernest Becker and others were correct about the greater sensitivity of middle-class women to depression a class difference would have been expected here. Whatever position is taken it is difficult to see the result reported in this chapter as being compatible with the notion that working-class women suffer less because they have less – indeed, the opposing, equally plausible view, is as likely: that because they have less (and the promise of less) they suffer more in response to loss or disappointment. It will be time enough to worry more about these somewhat academic possibilities when more has been done to equate risk of the obvious adversities in our society.

12 Borderline and chronic conditions

We have so far dealt with the onset of definite depressive disorders among women in Camberwell during a twelve-month period. It is also possible to consider two further types of affective disorder: definite psychiatric conditions that had lasted continuously for more than one year (i.e. chronic cases) and borderline case conditions which, although involving psychiatric symptoms, were not judged to be severe enough to be classified as cases. It must, however, be borne in mind that it was not part of our central purpose to study them and our conclusions are inevitably less secure.

Onset of borderline case conditions

Borderline case conditions are probably seen in large numbers by general practitioners. A third of those in the Camberwell sample had consulted their general practitioner about their symptoms. There has now been a good deal of research on psychiatric disorder in general practice – much of it from the General Practice Research Unit at the Institute of Psychiatry (e.g. Kessel, 1960; Shepherd *et al.*, 1966; Goldberg and Blackwell, 1970). In a review of the work, Cooper, Fry and Kalton (1969) suggest that in any one year at least one in ten of a general practitioner's registered patients will consult him with frank psychiatric symptoms. In one London suburban practice they surveyed, where continuous records had been kept by the general practitioner, 6 per cent of men and 17 per cent of women in the practice were given a psychiatric diagnosis in any one year. Recently Johnstone and Goldberg (1976) screened 1093 consecutive attenders at a general practice surgery in Manchester for minor psychiatric disorder – 32 per cent were considered to have 'conspicuous psychiatric disorder' that was recognized by the general practitioner taking part in the study and a further 11 per cent 'hidden psychiatric disorder' in the sense that it was only picked up by the use of a psychiatric screening schedule developed for use in general practice (Goldberg, 1972). The bulk of such disorders are affective and 'depression is ubiquitous' (Goldberg and Blackwell, 1970). In the Camberwell survey this morbidity has, of course, not been approached by means of a treatment setting. It is impossible to say just where categories of disorder overlap (they undoubtedly vary somewhat from study to study in any case); but from knowledge of the prevalence of case and borderline case conditions in Camberwell and the proportions among them seeking help from general practitioners, it seems that a good number of those classified as borderline cases in our Camberwell sample would be classed as 'conspicuous psychiatric disorder' in these studies.

We collected evidence about the onset of thirty-one borderline case conditions. Although this is bound to be an underestimate of the annual prevalence of such episodes, as reporting tends to fall off with distance from interview, thirty-one is a substantial enough number with which to consider the aetiological role of severe events and major difficulties.[1] *Table 1* shows that onset is again linked to the presence of a provoking agent; but it also shows that rather more of the borderline cases than the cases are without a provoking agent. But this is only so for middle-class women; almost all of the borderline cases *without* an event or difficulty are middle-class – eleven of fifteen compared with only three of sixteen of the working-class women were without a provoking agent. In fact most of the women did have an upsetting event which, for one reason or another had not been rated 'severe' on long-term threat – for example, a wedding of a woman who had sexual

Table 1   *Onset of caseness and borderline caseness in the year by whether there was a severe event or major difficulty*

	onset cases (excluding chronic cases)	onset borderline cases (excluding cases and chronic borderlines)	total: onset cases or borderline case (excluding chronic cases)
	%	%	%
no severe event or major difficulty	2 (4/255)	6 (14/226)	7 (18/255)
severe event or major difficulty	20 (33/164)	17 (17/100)	30 (50/164)
	p < .01	p < .01	p < .01

problems, death of a mother-in-law who lived nearby, buying a house to share with a sister (this highlighting the fact that now she 'probably would never get married'), and an examination. However, we have not been able to find a convincing explanation for the puzzling class difference. Two obvious possibilities are, one, that borderline case conditions at times develop in response to less threatening events than full case conditions, and second, that the long-term threat of some of the events occurring to middle-class women has in some way been underestimated.

A clear answer can be given to a second question. We know that women in Camberwell are far less likely to develop a definite depressive disorder in the presence of a provoking agent if they have an intimate 'a' relationship with husband or boyfriend and are more likely to do so to the extent they have a 'non-a' relationship and one or more of the other vulnerability factors. We can now add that the less vulnerable a woman the more chance she has of developing a borderline case rather than a case condition. It is those least at risk in terms of the four vulnerability factors that are most likely to develop borderline conditions. This can be seen by considering the ratio of onset cases to

Table 2 *Overall vulnerability by onset caseness and onset borderline caseness*

	onset cases		onset borderline cases		remaining women excluding borderline and case conditions	
	%	(n)	%	(n)	%	(n)
A all with 'a' intimacy relationships regardless	30	(11)	45	(14)	77	(226)
B 'non-a' intimacy, regardless of employment, excl. those with early loss of mother or 3+ children under 14 at home	40	(15)	55	(17)	20	(60)
C 'non-a' intimacy with early loss of mother and/or 3+ children under 14 living at home	30	(11)	0	(0)	3	(9)
	100	(37)	100	(31)	100	(295)

Columns 1 and 2, p < .001; 2 and 3, p < .001; 1 and 3, p < .001.

onset borderline cases for three groups of women characterized by increasing liability to depression. The three groups are:– (i) those without a provoking agent; (ii) those with a provoking agent but 'low' on vulnerability; and (iii) those with a provoking agent and 'high' on vulnerability.[2] The ratios of cases to borderline cases are 4:14 in the first and lowest risk group, 16:14 in the second, and 17:3 in the third and highest risk group (p<.01).

An alternative way of considering this effect is to compare onset cases, onset borderline cases, and women without a psychiatric condition in terms of the three overall vulnerability groups described in the last chapter. In line with the results just presented, onset cases contain the greatest proportion of the most vulnerable, borderline cases the next, and women with no case or borderline conditions the least (*Table 2*).

The causal model established for onset of clinical depression, therefore, can now be enlarged to take account of borderline conditions. Women may develop these in response to a provoking agent rather than a definite disorder and they are more likely to do so to the extent they are 'protected' by the absence of the four vulnerability factors.

Chronic conditions

While 8 per cent of the women in Camberwell developed a psychiatric disorder in the year, a similar proportion suffered from a chronic condition of comparable severity that had lasted continuously for at least a year. There is again a large class difference. Prevalence of chronic case conditions in the three months before interview was five times greater among working- than among middle-class women (12.5 and 2.3 per cent – p<.001). The less severe chronic borderline conditions did not differ by class (14 and 16 per cent), although when cases are excluded from the total used in this calculation, a small difference does emerge (12 and 18 per cent). Arguably these are the most disturbing of our findings and we felt bound to do what we could to understand them. The provoking agents are the most obvious starting point. Is it possible that they can perpetuate as well as begin a depressive disorder? Major difficulties and severe events were certainly common among women with chronic case or borderline case conditions. When compared with the women without a psychiatric condition they have twice the proportion with a severe event and three times the proportion with a major difficulty. Also notable is the large number with a major physical health difficulty lasting at least two years – a quarter had one compared with a tenth of the remaining women, including those with onset conditions (18 per cent of the chronic conditions had a health difficulty concerning themselves and 16 per cent one concerning a close relative). The results are presented in full in *Table 3*: in whatever way they are considered, those with chronic psychiatric conditions have a large number of severe events and major health and other difficulties.

Table 3   *Women in Camberwell with at least one severe event or major difficulty (lasting at least two years) in the year by psychiatric condition*[3]

psychiatric condition in the year	A severe event	B major difficulty	C marked health difficulty lasting at least 2 years	D any difficulty — B or C	E total — A, B, or C
	%	%	%	%	%
onset cases (37)	73	49	11	59	89
onset borderline case (31)	42	26	10	32	55
all onset conditions (68)	59	38	10	47	74
chronic case (39)	44	41	28	67	69
chronic border-line case (56)	36	34	23	57	66
all chronic conditions (95)	39	37	25	61	67
other women (295)	21	13	10	23	35

Note: these figures refer to the 12 months before interview and not to the 38 week period as used in chapter 6, which was both shorter and, for onset cases, always preceded the disorder.

Unfortunately it is difficult at present to relate these results in any kind of convincing way to causal processes. The high rate of events and difficulties among chronic conditions could be explained in a number of ways:

(i) Current events and difficulties could be the direct result of those that brought about the psychiatric condition in the first place, with the further complication that they may or may not have then served to perpetuate the condition.

(ii) They may have occurred quite independently of the original provoking agents and have served to perpetuate the condition under way.

(iii) Finally, they may have arisen as a direct result of the disorder itself – for example, severe debt because of unemployment. The association of chronic neurotic conditions with both social problems and physical illness of the patient has already been noted (Eastwood, 1972 and 1975; Cooper, 1972). Unfortunately the causal processes involved remain quite obscure. While, as just suggested, social and physical problems may be the direct result of the psychiatric disorder, there is no reason why they should not then in turn serve to perpetuate the psychiatric condition that gave rise to them. The chances of a psychiatric disorder starting such circular processes may be quite high. Indeed, a good deal of the effectiveness of current psychiatric care (including physical treatment) may lie in the way it serves to break up such negative 'feedback loops'. But, leaving this aside, it is clear that issues of the complexity we have outlined cannot be taken too far with the Camberwell material; at best there can be pointers to what may be going on.

With this in mind, we first looked at those major difficulties that appeared to be the least likely to be the result of the psychiatric disorder, applying for this purpose the same criteria of 'independence' developed for life-events: a difficulty was 'independent' if it seemed on *logical* grounds unlikely to have been brought about by the woman's disorder. While there are bound to be errors in such judgments we are convinced that women with an 'independent' difficulty could not on the whole have done much more to help themselves. Most concerned financial hardship and housing, about which, as far as we could see, the woman could not do anything. We describe three occurring to women who were chronic cases which give an idea of the kinds of problem considered 'independent':

(1) The subject and husband share two rooms and a tiny 'cubicle kitchen with son and daughter-in-law and three children (ranging from fourteen to a small baby). There is no bath or basin and one leaking lavatory for the whole house. The house is in a demolition district of the local authority and most of the street is deserted and derelict with rats and mice in the surrounding area. The rooms are incurably damp. The family has a low income. The subject's husband is a bad 'coper' and she is left to try to get new housing. The local authority bought the house eighteen months ago but they have been given no date for rehousing despite her visits to the Housing Department, taking medical certificates with her. There is a good deal of tension between her and her husband, and also between him and his

daughter. Her husband appears to be chronically depressed and irritable, the baby getting on his nerves constantly. (Rated '1' on both the contextual and the general difficulty scale.)

(2) The subject is a young woman whose husband left her. She lives alone with a small baby. She cannot afford a baby-minder (she has tried) and has therefore not worked since the baby was born; she manages on Social Security. Her flat is damp and smells musty all the time: even the clothes in the wardrobe have to be redried before they can be used. Caring for the baby in these conditions is difficult: he has bronchitis and catarrh constantly. She is a private tenant and has tried to get the landlady to do repairs but she always procrastinates. The upstairs flat has overflowing and smelly drains that also bother her. She has no proper kitchen and has to cross a yard to the only lavatory in the house. Her brother has helped her to try to damp-proof the walls internally but it has not helped. The new paper they put on together is very damp again and mildew grows everywhere. She has tried to get both the council and 'Gingerbread' (a voluntary society) to rehouse her, but in both instances she was told her priority was low because she was not actually homeless. (Rated '3' on the contextual scale and '2' on the general difficulty scale.)

(3) The subject is a married woman with two small children whose marriage is breaking up. Poor housing has been a contributing factor to the tensions. Originally private tenants in their old terrace house, they tried constantly to get the landlord to damp-proof and to put in a water-heater and renew the wiring. He refused, knowing the house was scheduled for demolition. The house has a very small 'kitchenette', no bathroom or hot water and dangerous electric wiring; two rooms are too damp to use. The area itself is very decayed with many houses boarded up. There is no open space at all for the children and she says they are constantly in trouble for climbing into deserted property. The council are now buying up the area but she has no idea when they might move – she has been very persistent with the council and has twice managed to get a visit from a housing official but was told she was not top priority and she had plenty of space.

Just over a quarter of women in Camberwell had a major 'independent' difficulty – that is, excluding health. Substantially more of those who had such a difficulty suffered from a *chronic* psychiatric condition – 35 per cent did so compared with 17 per cent of women without such a difficulty (*Table 4*). Half the women with such a difficulty had one concerning housing, and this was again related to chronicity: 28 per cent of the chronic cases had a major housing problem, 13 per cent of chronic borderlines, 1 per cent of onset case or borderline case conditions, and 6 per cent of the remaining women – p<.001.[4]

Table 4 *Percentage of chronic and onset psychiatric conditions among women with and without a major 'independent' difficulty*

	women with an 'independent' major difficulty		women with no 'independent' major difficulty	
	%	N	%	N
chronic cases	17 ⎫	17	6 ⎫	22
	⎬ 35		⎬ 17	
chronic borderline case	18 ⎭	18	11 ⎭	38
onset case or onset borderline case	25	25	12	43
remaining women	39	39	71	256
		99		359

p < .001

Major housing problems are therefore highly associated with chronic psychiatric conditions and particularly with case rather than borderline case conditions. Twenty-eight per cent of chronic cases had a major housing difficulty and a further 15 per cent a major difficulty of another kind, compared with 13 per cent and 20 per cent respectively of chronic borderline case conditions. Housing difficulties are about the 'hardest' set of difficulties that were available to us. Visits were made to everyone's home and the interviewer therefore had some direct experience of the difficulty; and, since we applied our own standards of 'severity' they are probably the least likely of the difficulty ratings to be subject to reporting effects. All involved either severe overcrowding, extreme physical shortcomings, or major problems involving noise or security of tenure – in other words, probably they contributed to the perpetuation of the psychiatric conditions, leaving aside any role they might also have played in the original onset. Of course, this clear-cut result concerning housing makes it easier to accept that other kinds of major difficulty could play a similar role. In any case it would be erroneous to conclude from these results that housing problems were in all instances (or even most) a direct cause of the chronicity of the psychiatric disorder. Poor housing is often linked with marital and other problems in a way that makes any simple interpretation of causal processes hazardous. The most likely way in which major difficulties influence psychiatric state would seem to be by perpetuating feelings of hopelessness, which well might have dissipated if the woman's self-esteem and ability to cope had been greater. Difficulties with money, husband, and children, often associated with bad housing, can obviously be as significant as the housing itself in eroding a woman's sense of success in her roles of homemaker, mother, and wife. But the point should not be taken too far: poor housing, even without financial hardship and problems with husband or children, may well make it less likely that a woman can refurbish her sense of self-worth, especially if some of her contemporaries have already been rehoused, thus underlining her sense of deprivation.[5] The higher rate of marked health difficulties among women with chronic psychiatric conditions has already been discussed in chapter 9. In the absence of material about provoking agents preceding their chronic conditions, it is impossible to decide between a number of possible interpretations – that the health problem results from an earlier health crisis which also provoked the depression, that the physical state is a long-term consequence of the chronic psychiatric disorder, and so on.

Another characteristic of chronic conditions is their association with a high rate of severe events (*Table 3*). Four in ten of chronic conditions as against only one in five of the rest of the women (excluding onset cases and onset borderline cases) had a severe event in the year (p<.001). Most of the severe events appeared to originate from the long-term major difficulties that are so common among these women – for example, a young daughter's suicide attempt arising in the background of a tense home and poor marriage or a move to a new house falling through in the context of poor and overcrowded housing. When this kind of severe event is excluded the proportion of chronic conditions with a severe event does not differ from that of normal women.[6] Such crises may obviously also serve to perpetuate both the difficulty itself and feelings of hopelessness and thus perhaps, as we have speculated, the woman's depression.

So far we have discussed unpleasant experience. It follows logically from our argument that events decreasing feelings of hopelessness should be capable of favourably influencing the course of disorder. Most obviously this would be the reversal of the problem provoking the depression. Sadly this probably occurs very rarely among women entering psychiatric treatment. By the time a woman has seen a psychiatrist, very little can probably be done about the loss and disappointment provoking or perpetuating the depression. Improvement of the situation produced by the provoking crises reasonably soon after onset of depression is not likely to be all that common in any case, but when it does occur, the woman in question would probably be less likely to see a psychiatrist. Among the thirty-nine chronic cases in Camberwell, five showed a definite improvement in the year – enough at least for the women to be considered no more than a borderline case at interview. One woman said she had begun to improve about six months before we saw her, after she had won £200 on the football pool. Another woman when first seen was considered to be suffering from a long-lasting depressive disorder and had lived in bad housing for even longer. When she was seen by the research psychiatrist some three to four weeks later, she was very much improved (although he considered she had earlier been a case of depression). Between the dates of the two interviews she had received a letter from the local housing authority offering her alternative accommodation. The other three women whose symptoms improved apparently had no such events but our measure of 'positive' events was too crude and the alleviation of long-term difficulties probably too infrequent for much to be expected from such an analysis. There was one other hint of the existence of such an effect. The association between major housing difficulties and chronic psychiatric disorder was stronger in the first series of 220 women seen in 1969 than in the second seen five years later. Twelve per cent of the first sample and 8 per cent of the second had a major difficulty: furthermore, of those with such a difficulty, 46 per cent of the first series and 32 per cent of the second had a chronic psychiatric condition. In summary, 5.5 per cent of the first series had a chronic condition *and* a major housing difficulty and 2.5 per cent of the second. While this difference does not reach statistical significance, there had been between the dates of the two surveys a large local authority housing programme – albeit one that has not escaped severe criticism for its reliance on massive 'high-rise' flats. While the possibility of a direct link between improved housing and lower prevalence of psychiatric disorder should not be ruled out, there is unfortunately a second interpretation. By the time of our second survey there had been an influx of West Indian families into Camberwell from neighbouring Brixton. Since we did not interview these women, it is possible that we underestimated the overall numbers in bad housing in Camberwell and that the changes are, in part at least, the result of an artefact. Nonetheless we are disposed to believe they reflect some hope for change and improvement: if we argue that social factors are important in influencing the onset and course of depression, it follows that the improvement of social problems can have a real impact on the prevalence of disorder.

Part IV
Symptom-formation factors

13 Severity of depression

Hitherto we have simply talked of 'depression' and ignored characteristics of the condition itself. The fact that provoking agents play the same role for onset cases in the general population and for the more severe in-patient cases suggests that they do not directly influence severity of depression. But we have also shown that vulnerability factors play a role in the presence of a provoking agent in determining whether a woman develops a case or borderline case condition and here vulnerability factors could be said in some sense to play a role in determining severity. But these points have been thrown up in the course of other analyses. We need to consider the question directly. Are there *symptom-formation* factors that influence the form and severity of depressive conditions? Are these distinct from the aetiological factors so far established?

The number and variety of symptom patterns subsumed under the diagnosis of depression are so many that there were a number of routes we could take to tackle the question of severity. We could concentrate only on the intensity and frequency of a symptom or, in addition, take into account the disorder's effect on a woman's functioning, her performance at work, and her running of the home. We could also give certain symptoms greater weight than others in assessing overall severity. Is loss of weight a more 'severe' symptom than disturbance of sleep? Is loss of energy somehow more severe in terms of the depression than irritability, tension, and restlessness? The very term 'depression' seems to imply a giving up of hope, where a person sinks back into herself; unlike desperation where she may continue to struggle helplessly, often violently, and with agitation. Yet judged clinically, both can be part of depression. Agitated depressions are still 'depression'. And in terms of the intensity of the symptoms and their interference with the person's normal functioning, the acting out of despair in a dramatic suicidal gesture may well be more 'severe' than a so-called 'mild endogenous depression' where sufferers lose interest, energy, appetite for food and sex, and sense of meaning and purpose but somehow carry on the essentials of their lives. Yet paradoxically the loss of hope and of a sense of meaning may be greater in the latter.

One way we tried to come to terms with this complexity was by rating severity of a number of symptom areas – of anxiety, of socially unacceptable behaviour, of appetite disturbance, of depressed mood, of pre-occupational thinking, and so on – as well as the severity of interference with employment and routine. But even within these categories we still found ourselves comparing rather different things: a 'severe depressed mood' might include both those who cried almost continuously and those who felt so depressed that they were unable to cry; 'severe impact on relationships' might include both people who withdrew from contact and those who became constantly irritable, plangent, and perhaps violent. It seemed, prima facie, impossible to rate either of such alternatives as more, or less, severe than the other.

Although, as this suggests, we were not completely comfortable with our measure of severity, we felt it important to have an overall assessment – first, because standard psychiatric commentaries talk in such terms, and second, because we felt that the topic might be so complex that an overall measure would be essential before we could move on to further subcategories which might prove to relate to our social variables. In a parallel way, when dealing with events, we had started from a global concept of overall severity of threat rather than the various dimensions of each event. Furthermore despite our discomfort the reliability of the overall rating of severity was high. (We have already given examples in chapter 2 and Appendix 2.)

The second major aspect of depression that we considered was the classic psychotic-neurotic distinction. Our perspective here is not original. We believe that the distinction is closely linked with the severity of the depression itself (Lewis, 1934). To anticipate: we have come to see the psychotic-neurotic division in terms of severity of hope-lessness, or the degree to which a person has given up, in the way described by Engel (1967). A retarded psychotic has given up more radically than a restless neurotic. While severity of hopelessness would correlate with overall severity, there would not be complete correspondence. Whereas the most psychotic patients would be expected to have the highest scores on overall severity, among neuro-tics there might well be a discrepancy: those with a dramatic suicide attempt and other flamboyant symptoms might rate high on severity, but, in terms of hopelessness and 'giving up', might seem less severe than others with mild endogenous depressions. (It is interesting how the terminological switch from 'psychotic' to 'endogenous' makes it possible to avoid using a phrase that might otherwise appear self-contradictory, that is 'mild psychotic depression'.)

These ideas about the psychotic-neurotic distinction developed as we gained experience and as we analysed the clinical material. Fortunately, in terms of measurement, the ratings of overall severity and those of psychotic-neurotic were kept distinct, and they proved to be independent of each other. The judgments of psychotic and neurotic depression were made for us by our psychiatric colleague, John Copeland, who followed the traditional ideas of this distinction. They were not influenced by the notion that the crucial feature underlying the dimension might be the degree of hopelessness. This was an idea that came to us much later. We therefore set out to explain both severity and diagnosis. We start in this chapter with severity.

In-patients and out-patients

In-patients are on the whole more depressed than out-patients and we have found it useful to deal with severity of depression in terms of these treatment groups. Indeed, understanding severity proves to be very largely a question of the reasons for the differences between in-patients and out-patients. At the time of 'admission' 90 per cent of the former and 44 per cent of the latter fell in the top two points of the five-point scale of overall severity of depression (p<.001). In spite of this there was no difference in severity between the two groups *at onset*. Why should they diverge only some time after initial onset?

We described in some detail in chapter 2 how we established points of marked change ('change-points') after the disorder was under way. Since these were dated, it was possible to look at the role of events in bringing them about. Only one in seven of the onset cases in Camberwell had a change-point and we will therefore deal with the patient series where change-points were both common and important. Forty-two of the patients had a second and ten a third 'change-point', involving an unmistakable worsening of their depression. We have described the changes in Mrs Gray's condition in detail in chapter 2, but a quick summary may be useful. About sixteen weeks before her admission she had an 'onset', becoming depressed, tired, and irritable, crying and shouting at the children. For about a month she became gradually worse and then stayed much the same for about two months. The second 'change-point' occurred three weeks before her first visit to the psychiatrist. Within a period of a few days she got much worse, crying a good deal more than before and finding she could not go on a bus or into a shop. She felt she could not swallow; her appetite waned and she lost weight. She could not be bothered to talk to anyone and could not bring herself to go out. Household chores became even more of a burden, though she forced herself to do them perfunctorily. She also had great difficulty in getting off to sleep.

The answer is made simpler by the fact that the difference in severity is almost entirely accounted for by deterioration occurring at the points of maximum change, that is at the change-points. In-patients were more disturbed first, because they more often had a change-point after onset (44 per cent as against 24 per cent); and second, because they tended to deteriorate further than out-patients if they had one. In terms of the scale of severity, in-patients deteriorated on average practically a full scale point while out-patients moved only a third of a point.[1] When looked at as a whole the differences between the two groups is due to discrete rather than gradual changes.[2] Since the two treatment groups do not differ in severity at onset, the question becomes twofold: why do in-patients have more change-points after onset and why do they deteriorate more than out-patients between change-points? We will consider first the role of provoking agents. Since these are capable of bringing about depression, is it possible that they can lead to a worsening of the disorder when they occur *after* onset?

Severe events and worsening of depression

The role of severe events in the worsening of a depressive disorder after onset can be seen as part of the issue of additivity. We have seen that the occurrence of more than one severe event can increase risk of developing depression, although at most one in five who became depressed had had onset influenced in this way. In general our results so far support Lear's:

> 'But where the greater malady is fixed,
> The lesser is scarce felt.'

But in spite of this, once a depressive disorder is established a severe loss or disappointment can lead to a marked deterioration in the sense of an increasing depth of depression – at least in the patient group.

In order to test for the aetiological role of severe events, we could not follow exactly the same procedure used with onset: we needed to control for the possibility that an increased rate of events was not due to a causal effect but to the fact that either the depression itself had increased the number of events (e.g. giving up a job) or that severe events occurring before onset had led to others after onset (e.g. learn-

ing that a husband had been arrested might be followed by his impris-
onment). Either could produce a raised rate of severe events before
change-points that had no aetiological significance. Fortunately both
possibilities could be controlled. The first could be met by excluding
altogether 'illness-related' events such as giving up a job or a suicide
attempt. The second could be met by using for comparison not the rate
of severe events in the general population but that for short time-
periods after those onsets that had *not* been followed by a change-
point. Since these would be equally subject to any higher rate of events
resulting from severe events before onset, any difference in the rate of
severe events was likely to be due to the fact that they had played a
causal role.[3]

Since 47 per cent of the change-points had been preceded by a severe
event compared with an expected proportion of 16.3 per cent, severe
events are apparently capable of bringing about a marked worsening of
an established depression.[4] Details are given in *Table 1*. (The expected
proportion is an adjusted figure that allows for the fact that the comparison periods were somewhat shorter than those between onset and
change-point.)

Table 1 *Severe events occurring before second (C2) and third change-points (C3)
with expected number of severe events*

length of periods in weeks	severe events before change-points (onset to C2 and C2 to C3)**			expected number of severe events based on actual numbers in periods (onset to 'admission' and C2 to 'admission')		
	severe event	no severe event	% severe event	severe event	no severe event	% severe event
4 to 10	8	13	38	2	43	4
11 to 20	8	9	47	3	16	16
21 and over	7	4	64	4	7	36
all	23	26	47	9	66	12*

*standardizing for length of periods at risk 16.3
**only one severe event was taken for each patient in each period

Only a third (7/23) of the severe events occurring before a change-
point were 'related' to a severe event before onset (in the sense we have
defined in chapter 6); and even if those 'related' to a major difficulty
are considered, the proportion is still only about one half (12/23). Much
the same process appears to be involved here as with onset itself, major

losses and disappointments producing further 'onsets' in an established depression. Surprisingly there is again little to suggest that more minor events play a role.[5] Only severe events appear to be important. It is as though new loss and disappointment increase the depth of a woman's hopelessness and this leads to a worsening of her depression: that a woman depressed after the emigration of her son to Australia might not have got worse if her father had not died ten weeks after the start of her depression.

This effect is strictly no more than an extension of work already presented. Severe events still seem best conceived as acting as provoking agents producing change-points (or as it were further 'onsets') within an established depressive disorder. This is confirmed by the fact that severe events influence severity only in this indirect fashion. The presence of a provoking agent *before* onset is not related to severity of depression either at onset or at any later change-point. Nor is the degree of threat of particular events or difficulties, nor the number of events and difficulties, related to severity of depression. If the role of events in influencing severity of depression at 'admission' is therefore a special case, are there still other factors that, while not increasing risk of depression, more directly influence its severity?

Past loss and severity

A major loss in the past, particularly in childhood and adolescence, is much the most significant factor influencing severity of depression. The measure of past loss was described in chapter 11 where it was concluded that only loss of a mother before eleven increased risk of onset of depression in adulthood. Loss of mother between eleven and seventeen had no influence. Now it must be added that *past loss* as a whole, defined as loss of mother or father before seventeen, loss of a sibling between one and seventeen, loss of a child at any age, and loss of a husband by death, related to severity of depression at *admission* (gamma = .47). Most of the loss had occurred in childhood and adolescence.

The only other factor found to be associated with severity was a previous depressive episode (gamma = .58) We have already shown that the presence of a severe event after onset also relates to severity (gamma = .28). When all three factors are taken into account, a simple additive score ranging from 0 (all absent) to 3 (all present) relates quite highly to severity – gamma .65.[6]

The association is sufficiently large to explain almost the entire difference in severity between out-patients and in-patients. The argument is as follows.

Since in-patients and out-patients did not differ in severity at onset, we only need to explain the *change* in severity after onset. Since no woman rated '2' on severity at *onset* moved to point '1' by admission, those rated '1' and '2' at onset can be disregarded. For the remaining sixty-five women the simple index just described is highly related to severity: 18 per cent with 0 points, 52 per cent with 1, 82 per cent with 2, and 100 per cent with 3 were rated in the top two scale points of severity. This entirely explains the association between type of treatment and overall severity – at least in statistical terms.[7]

The role of events in these results is obvious and in later chapters we will argue that past loss acts through some cognitive process. The mode of action of previous episodes is unclear. Is it related to some general 'constitutional' vulnerability which leads to both the earlier and the present episode, or to the fact that an earlier episode subsequently increases a person's 'physiological' vulnerability? Or should the effect be seen as cognitive? (To anticipate the discussion in Chapter 15, a person who has had a previous painful depressive episode might, for instance, be more likely to 'deny' important aspects of a subsequent loss thereby increasing risk of a severe depression.) There is one result that may be of some relevance. The three factors will in general have occurred largely in the time order – first, past loss; then, previous episode; and last, severe event after onset. Where there has been a past loss, a previous episode does not relate to severity; the latter only relates in the absence of past loss. In the same way the presence of a severe event after onset is associated with severity only in the absence of past loss or previous episode.[8] It is almost as if the first cut were the deepest: once someone has had an important past loss, the role of a previous episode in contributing to severity is relatively less important. Similarly, once a person has experienced a past loss or a previous episode, the role of an event after onset is relatively less important.

One question remains to be answered at this stage. Do these symptom-formation factors overlap with the other factors in our model? Severe events have already been dealt with; only in a very special sense can they be said to act as symptom-formation factors. Their presence before onset does not serve in any way to increase severity. Provoking agents and symptom-formation factors in general do not appear to overlap. We have already seen in chapter 11 that except for loss of mother before eleven, past loss does not act as a vulnerability factor and it is therefore only necessary to consider whether a previous episode can act as a vulnerability factor. For the patients there is no suggestion of this:[9] previous episodes do *not* increase vulnerability, although, unfortunately, we did not collect this information systematically for women in the general community. We conclude, therefore, that at least among patients the three symptom-formation factors that serve to increase severity of depression do not by and large relate to the measures we have used so far in our model. Indeed a clear-cut case begins to emerge for a three-factor model of depression – provoking agents, vulnerability factors, and symptom-formation factors – with only early loss of mother before eleven capable of acting in more than one way. We now turn to complicate the model for the last time by considering the psychotic-neurotic distinction.

14 Psychotic and neurotic depression and the existence of endogenous depression

In this chapter we continue with the issue of symptom-formation factors and particularly their relation to the classic distinction between psychotic and neurotic depression. In collecting material for this chapter we used a traditional psychiatric diagnosis of psychotic and neurotic depression, relying on the clinical judgment of a psychiatric colleague at the Institute of Psychiatry who took into account criteria such as the presence of early morning waking and retardation, which are fairly generally accepted as distinguishing features of the two forms of depression. Since 'psychotic' and 'neurotic' symptoms can occur in both types of depression, a judgment has to be made on the basis of the total clinical picture rather than the presence of particular symptoms. For example, just over half the patients considered psychotic and just over a fifth of the neurotic patients had early morning waking. Using such an overall judgment, sixty-three patients were classified as psychotic and forty-nine as neurotic. (Two with some manic symptoms were excluded from this part of the analysis.)

The psychotic-neurotic distinction was only modestly associated with our measure of overall severity.[1] It was therefore necessary to explain both features of clinical depression. We should, however, remind the reader that this refers only to severity as defined by our measure, in the choice of which we had had to face certain complex issues already discussed in the last chapter. As the analysis proceeded, in fact, we began to feel that, had we concentrated more on the severity of the patient's hopeless resignation rather than on the intensity and number of the total symptoms, a different picture would have emerged: that there would have been a substantial association between such severity and a psychotic type of depression and that to a large extent this was what underlay the traditional distinction between the two forms of depression.[2]

The two-fold diagnostic division was subjected to a number of statistical analyses. One of the most important was a discriminant function analysis. This took account of all the clinical material but excluded consideration of factors such as age, provoking agents, or previous episodes in order to avoid the kind of circularity of argument we earlier outlined in the discussion of unit and quality. We used only clinical material collected about the current episode. The discriminant function analysis derived weights for each symptom according to its association with the psychotic and neurotic groups, those items which were the most important in the distinction having the highest loadings, either positively if they were associated with the psychotic group, or negatively if they were associated with the neurotic group. An overall score was obtained for each woman by adding the weights of her symptoms. Various scores can be allotted in this way according to the level of significance at which one is prepared to accept the initial association of the symptoms with the diagnostic distinction and thus the number of items summated for the score. We elected to use scores based on the seventeen clinical items that differed between the two groups at the 20 per cent level of significance. On the basis of the distribution of the patients' scores using these seventeen items a particular score was chosen to represent the best cut-off point between psychotic and neurotic patients. This gave an overall misclassification rate of 23 per cent; that is, the original psychotic and neurotic groups could be successfully reconstructed on the basis of these scores with only a little more than a fifth of the patients being wrongly allocated. The items and their weights are much what would be expected from the literature. In general, the psychotic patients tend to be more retarded in movement, thought, and emotion and the neurotic group to be more active and to show more emotion.

This seventeen-item discriminant function analysis was used to differentiate the extreme and the less extreme halves of each of the two original groups. The extreme psychotic group was the 'most psychotic' and the less extreme the 'least psychotic'; and the extreme neurotic group the 'most neurotic' and the less extreme neurotic the 'least neurotic' (and nearest the psychotic).[3]

We will start by dealing with the most obvious question – the relation of the two provoking agents to the psychotic-neurotic division.

Endogenous versus reactive depression?

The concept of reactivity has a long history in the development of psychiatric theory and has not always been clearly distinguished from the concepts 'psychogenic' and 'exogenous'. Brian Cooper (1976) traces the use of the term from Sommer (1894) and Breuer and Freud (1895) where 'reaction' referred to the psychological correlates or antecedents of neurosis rather than to the clinical phenomena themselves; through the idea that the manic phase of a circular psychosis might be a reaction to the depressive phase (Ziehen 1894); to Edward Reiss's monograph on affective illness (1910), which he sees as the first clear definition of a group of reactive disorders, laying the trail along which Karl Jaspers and later Schneider were to follow. But in Schneider's classification all psychoses were assumed to have a somatic pathology and thus by definition were not reactive, a notion in marked contrast to the Scandinavian psychiatric tradition where a distinct group of psychogenic, or reactive, psychoses is recognized (Stromgren, 1968). The greater attention paid to the concept of reactivity by the Scandinavians is also apparent in the Norwegian distinction between neuroses and neurotic reactions. The international differences in this area are highlighted by the fact that the Canadian system, cited by Stengel (1959), differs from the system of the American Psychiatric Association (1965) in classing neurotic disorders as reactions but not the psychoses; the American system, influenced by Adolf Meyer, lists schizophrenia, manic-depressive psychosis, and psychoneuroses as reactions. As Cooper concludes 'after more than eighty years the psychiatric concept of reactivity remains nebulous, and its value for classification uncertain'.

Within the area of depression, there has been a belief linking psychotic with endogenous and neurotic with reactive depression, and we felt it important to examine these notions despite the existing conceptual confusion. The topic is generally formulated in terms of two contrasting viewpoints: on the one hand there is a tradition in psychiatry that maintains psychotic and neurotic depression are two quite separate entities, with symptoms clustering bimodally along a dimension of symptom scores – neurotic depression arising in response to precipitating events and psychotic depression in their absence. Much of the statistical and empirical work supporting this view has come from Martin Roth and his colleagues in Newcastle (Kay et al., 1969; Carney, Roth, and Garside, 1965; Garside et al., 1971). On the other hand is what may be called the dimensional viewpoint, which sees depression as a continuum of varying symptom patterns with no clear boundary between psychotic and neurotic types. This view is associated with the name of Aubrey Lewis (1938) and has most recently been given support by the work of Kendell (1968 and 1976). While there are other classifications which have been developed around this distinction (e.g. Foulds, 1973; Overall et al., 1966; Paykel, 1971) these two have traditionally been the focus of the debate. The second approach does not logically involve any definite commitment to a belief about the presence or absence of precipitating events, although in practice there is usually the assumption that the presence of these will be associated with depressions at the more neurotic end of the continuum; (in fact the assumption is often built into the research design by the use of 'precipitating event' as one of the items among the symptoms in just the way we have criticized). It is clear, however, that there are two distinct issues involved in the debate in the sense that different sorts of evidence are required to confirm each one. The first requires evidence to show whether depressive symptoms regularly tend to form separate clusters, rather than most symptoms combining with most others. The second issue requires evidence to show whether events regularly precede any of these clusters or any depressions classified in accordance with traditional criteria, but in the absence of knowledge about precipitation by the diagnostician.

In our patient series the psychotic and neurotic groups were defined by the research psychiatrist without knowledge of the patient's experience of provoking agents. The two groups showed no difference in the proportions having a severe event or a major difficulty: 71 per cent of the psychotics have one or the other and 80 per cent of the neurotics.[4] It is possible that this negative result is due to the unreliability of the diagnostic assignment, but fortunately this can be checked. Since the discriminant function gives weights that maximize clinical differences between the diagnostic groups, patients can be reassigned according to their score so the most 'psychotic' of the neurotic group are placed with the psychotic group, and vice versa. When as many as a fifth of each group are reallocated in this way significant differences between

Table 1 *The halves of the psychotic and neurotic groups by whether they have a severe event or major difficulty*

	severe event		major difficulty without severe event		severe event or major difficulty	
	%		%		%	
Psychotics						
extreme half	48	(15/31)	16	(5/31)	65	(20/31)
less extreme	68	(21/31)	10	(3/31)	77	(24/31)
Neurotics						
less extreme	68	(17/25)	12	(3/25)	80	(20/25)
extreme half	63	(15/24)	17	(4/24)	79	(19/24)

the groups in the proportions with a provoking agent still do not emerge.[5]

A second way of considering the existence of an 'endogenous' depression is to look at the relation of provoking agents to the position of patients on the discriminant function score *within* the original psychotic and neurotic groups. Psychotics located toward the upper extreme of the discriminant function score distribution are less similar to the neurotic group as a whole than less extreme psychotics, and the most extreme neurotics are less similar to the psychotic group as a whole than the less extreme neurotic patients. The extreme psychotic group when compared with the rest of the patients do have fewer with a provoking agent: 65 per cent have experienced a severe event or major difficulty before onset compared with 77 per cent of the less extreme psychotics, 80 per cent of the less extreme half of the neurotic group, and 79 per cent of the extreme neurotic group. Although not statistically significant, this does hint that the extreme psychotic patients may be somewhat less 'reactive' (*Table 1*).

We employed a third approach. This time we started with the provoking agents and used them to form a 'reactive' depressed group who had a severe event or major difficulty and an 'endogenous' group without either. It should be emphasized that this approach is using the terms 'endogenous' and 'reactive' in an unusual way to describe the presence or absence of provoking agents and not particular symptom patterns in order to avoid the circularity found in so many medical concepts where aetiology and symptom pictures are confused. Of course, if there is a truly 'endogenous' group, clinical differences will emerge between groups defined by the presence or absence of a provoking agent. But conclusions were much as before. Clinical differences between the 'endogenous' and 'reactive' groups were few indeed. At admission they differed significantly on only four of the seventy-four clinical items and at onset again on only four – differences that are very little more than would be expected if the associations were a purely haphazard matter. Despite this, it is of interest that the four items on which the two groups differ at admission relate in the direction predicted by traditional psychiatric teaching. The two items, significantly more common in the 'endogenous' group, were loss of appetite and early morning waking and the two more common in the 'reactive' group suicide attempts and feelings of hopelessness about the future (*Table 2*).[6]

Therefore while we cannot claim the 'reactive' and 'endogenous' depressives are completely clinically indistinguishable, the analyses considered together suggest that the psychiatric tradition has been misleading in its claim that there are, in any sense, two *clearly* distinct forms of depression and that the psychotic type is in general not 'reactive'.

These findings are not the only challenge to the tradition. Paykel, Prusoff and Klerman (1971) carried out a principle components analysis on twenty-eight symptoms and concluded that their second factor provided 'strong evidence that symptoms characteristic of endogenous and neurotic depression tended to cluster together so as to form two contrasting patterns'. They then examined the association between factor scores and two alternative stress scores, total stress score and maximal event score. There was a significant but very low correlation between total stress score and this second factor but this fell to a level below significance when the effect of age was partialled out.

Table 2   *The incidences of a selection of symptoms in the 'endogenous' and 'reactive' groups. Percentages of each group positive on each item at onset and admission*

items associated with the diagnostic dichotomy at admission or onset	onset			admission		
	'endogenous'	'reactive'	p	'endogenous'	'reactive'	p
	(n = 28) %	(n = 83) %		(n = 28) %	(n = 83) %	
loss of appetite	71	53	n.s.	89	67	<.05
loss of libido	43	22	<.05	46	29	n.s.
early morning waking	50	29	<.05	61	35	<.05
suicide attempt	4	11	n.s.	0	16	<0.05
feelings of hopelessness about the future	32	60	<.01	57	78	<.05
feeling tired; no energy	57	77	<.05	75	87	n.s.
a sample of items not associated with the 'endogenous'/'reactive' dichotomy at admission or onset						
retardation	43	39		61	52	
slowness of thinking/speech	29	19		43	30	
diurnal variation, worse morning	18	33		32	41	
irritability	75	66		82	75	
verbal attacks	18	30		25	39	
specific worry	61	55		57	59	
preoccupational thinking	43	54		46	64	
auditory hallucinations	0	8		4	8	
panic attacks	14	19		29	23	

Garmany (1958) found precipitants common among depressives diagnosed as endogenous. Unfortunately, he counted physical illness such as influenza among his stresses so that it is not possible to quote an exact percentage for his psychosocial stresses. However as many as 80 per cent of his endogenous cases had stress factors and only 17 per cent of them had physical stress precipitants, some of which were combined with psychosocial factors. Thus, a rough estimate of two thirds of his endogenous patients with a psychosocial stress factor gives a figure close to our own. Similarly Thomson and Hendrie (1972) found using the SRE measure of life-events that patients with reactive depressions did not have significantly higher life-change scores than patients with endogenous depressions. Leff and his colleagues (1970) found the incidence and type of stressful event occurring in their thirteen endogenous patients (as defined by the presence of five of six classical symptoms) similar to those occurring in their twenty-seven non-endogenous patients.

The distinctions made between provoking agents, vulnerability factors, and symptom-formation factors have therefore again held up remarkably well – provoking agents are not in an important way related to the form of the depression. Let us therefore turn finally to consider, as with severity, whether there are special symptom-formation factors associated with the psychotic-neurotic distinction.

The psychotic-neurotic distinction and past loss

While we have seen that past loss is related to severity, it has an even greater association with diagnosis. Two-thirds of psychotic patients had a past loss compared with 39 per cent of neurotic patients and if the extreme and less extreme halves of the psychotic group are distinguished, this association is increased. Seventy-four per cent and 58 per cent respectively had a past loss and 39 per cent of the neurotics. (See dotted line in *Figure 1* (p<.01).)

But this ignored *type* of past loss and, indeed, no one has taken up the hint by Freud in *Mourning and Melancholia* that this might be significant:

'In melancholia, the occasions that give rise to the illness extend for the most part beyond the clear case of loss by death and include all those situations of being slighted, neglected and disappointed which can impart opposed feelings of love and hate into a relationship or reinforce an already existing ambivalence.,

(Freud, 1971: 161).

When past loss due to *death* is distinguished from loss by *separation* (i.e. absence of parents, adoption of child) the differences are increased still further. In order to distinguish women with a death from those with a separation, in the few instances where both kinds of loss occurred, the *earliest* has been taken (4 per cent of patients and 3 per cent of women in the general population had both). Loss through *death* and through *separation* are both strongly related to diagnosis, but related in opposite ways: 74 per cent of the extreme psychotic, 45 per cent of the less extreme psychotic, and 16 per cent of the neurotic group had had a past loss through death (p<.01). By contrast none of the extreme psychotic, 13 per cent of the less extreme psychotic, and 22 per cent of the neurotic group had had a past loss by separation (p<.01). (The two halves of the neurotic group are not distinguished by type of past loss.) In other words, although past loss is not a potent aetiological factor, it may well be a most powerful influence on symptom pattern when women *do* get depressed: loss by death predisposing to psychotic depression and loss by separation to neurotic depression.[7]

These differences were so remarkable that we looked for a way of checking them. Fortunately, Robert Kendell had examined a series of consecutive female in-patients in the Maudsley Hospital suffering

Figure 1   Per cent with past loss by death and by separation among depressed patients by whether 'psychotic' or 'neurotic'

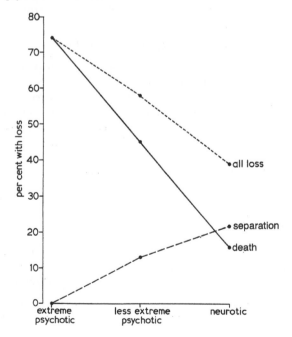

Table 3 Per cent of patients by type of past loss and degree of psychotic/neurotic depressive features according to discriminant function score in the present series (N = 111) and Kendell's series (N = 70)

	Present series		Kendell		Both series	
	% loss by death	%separation	%loss by death	% separation	% loss by death	% separation
1st quartile (most psychotic)	71 (20/28)	0 (0/28)	50 (9/18)	0 (0/18)	63 (29/46)	0 (0/46)
2nd quartile (least psychotic)	50 (14/28)	7 (2/28)	37 (7/17)	12 (2/17)	47 (21/45)	9 (4/45)
3rd quartile (least neurotic)	25 (7/28)	25 (7/28)	29 (5/17)	12 (2/17)	27 (12/45)	20 (9/45)
4th quartile (most neurotic)	15 (4/27)	22 (6/27)	17 (3/18)	39 (7/18)	16 (7/45)	27 (12/45)
	41 (45/111)	14 (15/111)	34 (24/70)	16 (11/70)	38 (69/181)	14 (26/18)
	p < .01	p < .05	p < .05	p < .01	p < .01	p < .01

Note: In order to ensure greater comparability with Kendell's series we have divided our series differently here from our three-fold classification in Figure 1.

221

from depression and also had a diagnostic index score based on his clinical judgment of psychotic and neurotic depressive states (Kendell, 1968). He was kind enough to allow us to use this material. We also consulted the hospital case notes to obtain details of past loss.[8] The results for the two samples are very close when their respective discriminant function scores were divided into four more or less equal groups (*Table 3*). Therefore, leaving aside the interpretation, the result itself seems secure. There is also a methodological point: the results confirm that we are not dealing with idiosyncratic clinical judgements on the part of the psychiatrist.

Since a good deal of the significance of this result depends on the distinction of type of loss, the question arises whether type of loss has an influence on severity as well as on diagnostic group. In order to look

Figure 2 Per cent with past loss by death and by separation among depressed patients by severity and whether 'psychotic' or 'neurotic'

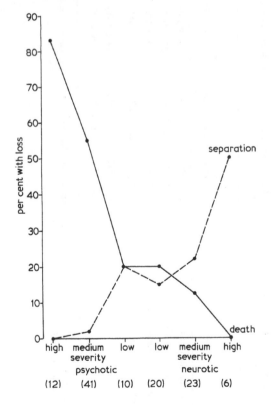

at this, since death has little or no relation to the neurotic group and separation to the psychotic group, the term *effective loss* has been used for death for psychotic and separation for neurotic patients (remembering that in the small number of instances where both have occurred the earliest has been taken). When effective loss is considered, the association of past loss with severity is increased from a gamma of 0.47 to one of 0.68.[9] This raises the further question: does past loss have an effect on severity independent of its effect on diagnosis? A number of ways of looking at this all indicated that type of past loss has an independent effect on both severity and on diagnosis. One of the most interesting is shown in *Figure 2*: type of past loss is related to severity *within* the psychotic and *within* the neurotic groups but in a different way. Loss by death is related to severity for the psychotic group and loss by separation is directly associated with overall severity in the neurotic group. Although numbers are small the general trends are impressive.[10]

There are two final results concerning loss: the choice of loss of parent or sibling before the age of seventeen had been decided at the level of a hunch. We therefore also examined loss of a parent or sibling after the age of seventeen but they played no part either in increasing vulnerability or in symptom formation. Nor did the inclusion of marital separation and divorce influence the results: there were only two patients who had experienced a divorce or separation who had not also experienced a still earlier loss.

Other background factors

Having dealt with past loss, what about other factors? In the last chapter we showed that the presence of a previous episode was associated with greater severity. It is therefore not surprising that psychotic patients also more often had a previous episode (52 per cent compared with 33 per cent of the neurotic group). Again a division into subgroups reflecting the degree of psychotic and neurotic symptoms reinforces differences found for the two diagnostic groups as a whole: 71 per cent of the extreme psychotic group had a previous episode as against 39 per cent of the less extreme psychotic group. The two halves of the neurotic groups are again, as with type of past loss, similar (32 and 33 per cent respectively).

Before considering what might be involved we must consider a factor generally recognized to be associated with psychotic depression – age. Many have shown that those with psychotic depression are older (e.g. Spicer, Hare, and Slater 1973). There is also a striking age difference in our series: psychotic patients had a mean age of forty-five as against 29.5 for neurotic patients (p<.001). The extreme psychotic group are older – on average they are 45.5 as against 39.1 in the less extreme half. Again the neurotic group are not distinguished: in this instance the less extreme neurotic group nearest the psychotic is just a little older – 31.4 and 29.2 respectively.

Further analysis makes it fairly clear what appears to be happening. The association between previous episode and diagnosis is much reduced when age is taken into account but that between age and diagnosis remains when previous episode is controlled. Those results taken together mean that the interpretation represented in *Figure 3a* can be rejected in favour of that in *Figure 3b*.

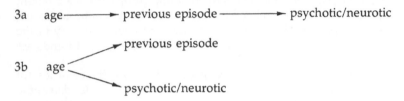

If, as in *3a*, age brought about previous episode and this in turn the diagnostic distinction, the relationship between the latter and age would disappear (or be greatly reduced) when previous episode was controlled. This does not occur.[11] On the contrary, control for age suggests that the relationship of previous episode to diagnosis is largely a result of the age of those who have had a previous episode. Most likely this is because the older the women the greater time she has had to have a previous episode. It is therefore *the relationship of age rather than previous episode to diagnosis that needs explanation*.

One possible explanation might be an increasing severity of depression with age. But this is not supported. Age is not associated with overall severity.[12]

Let us then turn to consider the relation of age to past loss in more detail. Although older women are more likely to have experienced a past loss there is little to suggest that age has any influence on the association of past loss and diagnosis. This holds within each of the age groups 18 – 25, 26 – 40, and 41 – 65 and with almost exactly similar results being obtained for Kendell's series (*Table 4*). Moreover, if age at which the first onset of psychiatric disturbance occurred is controlled, the differences remain as marked.[13]

Whether the loss occurred before or after the age of ten is irrelevant (*Table 5*) and again a similar result was obtained for the Kendell series. Since results hold for those who experienced a loss before eighteen, the effect is not to be explained by losses occurring in adulthood. It is worth noting, however, that a third of the losses by death occurring to the psychotic group happened after eighteen, while losses by separation during adulthood are rare.

Age is therefore significantly related to the psychotic-neurotic distinction, independently of other factors we have considered. We leave discussion of the reasons for this until the next chapter.

Table 4 *Age of patients by proportion with a past loss by death and by separation by whether psychotic or neurotic compared with women in the general population*

	18—25	26—41	41—65	Total
Death	%	%	%	%
psychotic	33 (3/9)	56 (5/9)	66 (29/44)	60 (37/62)
neurotic	5 (1/22)	25 (4/16)	27 (3/11)	16 (8/49)
general population	13 (9/72)	23 (34/145)	39 (94/241)	30 (137/458)
Separation	%	%	%	%
psychotic	0 (0/9)	11 (1/9)	7 (3/44)	6 (4/62)
neurotic	32 (7/22)	13 (2/16)	18 (2/11)	22 (11/49)
general population	7 (5/72)	10 (14/125)	5 (12/241)	7 (31/458)

Further subclassifications of depression

We have concentrated upon the psychotic-neurotic classification of depression because that has been widely acknowledged to be related to the presence of precipitating events. Other typologies of depression have also been found useful. The distinction between unipolar and bipolar depressive illness is well known. We aimed to focus on patients currently exhibiting depressed rather than manic symptoms and only two of the patients had any manic features. Six of the others had been given a diagnosis of manic-depressive psychosis but only one of these had any evidence of previous manic symptoms; the diagnosis seemed to have been based on the degree of agitation rather than on previous hypomanic features. Under these circumstances there was no way of examining the relationship of social background factors to the unipolar-bipolar distinction.

(i)   *Early vs. late onset*

A two-fold division according to the age of the patient at first onset of depression has been subject to an increasing number of investigations

Table 5   *Per cent of patients with a past loss by death or by separation by age loss occurred and whether psychotic or neurotic*

	−10		11–17		18+	
	death	*separation*	*death*	*separation*	*death*	*separation*
	%	%	%	%	%	%
psychotic	27 (17/62)	2 (1/62)	11 (7/62)	3 (2/62)	21 (13/62)	2 (1/62)
neurotic	6 (3/49)	12 (6/49)	6 (3/49)	8 (4/49)	4 (2/49)	2 (1/49)

(Winokur, 1972; Woodruff, Guze and Clayton, 1971; Baker, *et al.*, 1971; and Perris, 1966). These authors have distinguished what they call depressive spectrum disease, the prototype of which is onset of the condition before the age of forty among females, from pure depressive illness, the prototype being in late-onset male patients. When this dichotomy is described it is usually coupled with the dimension of family history of mental illness: female patients with an early first onset, before the age of forty, are described as tending to have a history of alcoholism or sociopathic disorder in their first degree male relatives. Unfortunately, although we had data on family history, we became increasingly dissatisfied with it as the work progressed; since it had not been a main focus of the study, we had not put enough effort into eliminating the sort of biases we have discussed at length in connection with measurement of life-events. Only very detailed interviewing with systematic checking of medical records for all relatives could really meet the criteria we came to see as minimal for proper family history data, criteria which are expensive and all too rarely met. For this reason we analysed our information in terms of age at first onset only. This proved to be of little significance.

Sixty-eight per cent of the patients had had their first onset before the age of forty. In this early onset group exactly half had had at least one episode prior to the one we studied compared with two-thirds of the late-onset group but this difference was not significant. Twenty per cent of the early onset group had no provoking agent with the current episode whereas 36 per cent of the late onset group had no current provoking agent, a difference that was not significant. More of those currently diagnosed neurotic rather than psychotic fell in the early onset group: 16 per cent of neurotics and 45 per cent of the psychotics had a first onset after forty (p. <,01). The direction of this trend was not however maintained within the psychotic group.

We have already mentioned that past loss did not relate to age at first onset; and no other factor emerged as associated with age at first onset either among the provoking agents, the vulnerability factors, or the symptom-formation factors.

The absence of significant associations between late onset and other factors may be a feature of our concentration upon women: the prototype in the literature of 'pure depressive disease' is the late onset male rather than female. Although there is this ambiguity, it seems safest at present to treat the spectrum-illness dichotomy with as much circumspection as the neurotic-psychotic one.

(ii)   *Anxiety and depression*

A final diagnostic classification dealing with anxiety and described in Chapter 2 did show interesting associations, although it should be emphasized that it is a relatively crude categorization developed after our experience in the Outer Hebrides.[15] On North Uist we found anxiety, both with and without concurrent depression, to relate to certain background demographic factors, which could be seen as indices of integration into the community. The highest proportion of cases and borderline cases with anxiety features were found among the most integrated women, that is those who lived on a croft, who had been brought up on the island, and who attended church regularly (Brown *et al.*, 1977). Living on a croft obviously could not be examined in Camberwell and neither of the other factors seemed to relate to degree of anxiety, something hardly surprising in view of the very different meaning they must have in the two communities.

Although degree of anxiety showed some relation to the psychotic-neurotic distinction and to overall severity, its relationship with past loss was less clear.[16] The proportion of patients with a past loss by separation was similar in the three diagnostic groups – (i) case anxiety/case depression; (ii) case depression/borderline case anxiety; and (iii) case depression. Past deaths, however, were associated with a somewhat lesser degree of anxiety – 33 per cent of those with case anxiety/case depression and 28 per cent of the case depression/borderline anxiety had a past death compared with 48 per cent of the case depression group. Overall the results suggest that the association of type of past loss with the psychotic-neurotic dimension is not mediated by anxiety.[17]

While the presence or absence of provoking agents and vulnerability factors did not relate to anxiety, there is some suggestion that the type of provoking agent might be associated with the degree of anxiety accompanying the depression. Among the patients the case anxiety/case depression group was only 18 per cent of the total but it had as many as 31 per cent of the severe events that had no loss component. Put another way 24 per cent of those with a case anxiety/case depression diagnosis had such an event compared with 12 per cent of the other two groups. Conversely only 24 per cent of the case anxiety/case depression group had a loss event compared with 53 per cent of the other two.

There is therefore some suggestion that events can act as symptom-formation factors and that the link is much what would be expected from everyday emotional responses to events. In general, feelings of depression will follow something that has happened and about which little or nothing can be done, while anxiety accompanies a situation of uncertainty. In the context of a loss, anxiety would be expected where something can still be done to restore the situation. In these terms a severe event may give rise to a number of emotions: disappointment on learning of a husband's unfaithfulness may go with concern that he may leave home.

Further evidence for this sort of effect is seen when the nature of health difficulties is considered. Although health difficulties did not increase risk of depression, they were much more common among chronic cases and chronic borderline cases. Furthermore, among these chronic conditions they tended to be more often illnesses of the woman herself, whereas among onset cases they tended somewhat more often to concern close relatives. When the threefold depression-anxiety typology is considered those with anxiety at either a case or a borderline case level tend to have more health difficulties concerning others and those with only depressive symptoms have more concerning their own health. The results occur among patients, cases, and borderline cases and are especially marked among the chronic conditions; the trends hold both for marked and for moderate health difficulties.[18] At first the fact that anxiety is associated with health difficulties concerning others may seem paradoxical; in the last paragraph we suggested a connection between anxiety and severe non-loss events, many of which were disorders concerning the woman herself. But this is no longer a contradiction if the contrast made in chapter 9 between a discrete health crisis and a long-term health difficulty is remembered. It would be explained if the health difficulties in contrast to crises tended to be associated with an actual *loss* of activity or role. This would be expected first, if the disorders had been going on for some time and thus were difficulties rather than events, and second, if they concerned the woman herself rather than another person. This was confirmed by looking at the loss of role and loss of activities consequent upon the differing physical illnesses among those with health difficulties.[19] Again these results make sense in terms of the general notion that actual loss is associated with depression and uncertainty with anxiety. Alternative explanations cannot however be ruled out. Chronic mild depressions, with their non-specific symptoms of exhaustion, tension, and distress may well be part of the illness itself, a sort of physical exhaustion syndrome as well as an emotional result of the illness. Moreover the association of anxiety with bearing the burden of sick relatives might be spurious, particular personality types being more likely to have married invalids or not to have left their aged parents' neighbourhood. Another, more psychoanalytic explanation might invoke the repression of the inevitable frustration caused by sick relatives as the cause of the anxiety. But before these alternatives are explored, the basic result will need to be replicated. More generally while there is support for the possibility that events may give rise to 'mixed' clinical pictures according to their emotional implications, the basic research remains to be done.

These results suggest from yet another viewpoint that the crucial aetiological link is between a loss and the experience of hopelessness rather than through upset in general; and that the more complete the loss (actual rather than threatened, death rather than separation) the more depressed, less anxious, the reaction will tend to be. It is this connection between loss and hopelessness that we turn to in the next chapter where we discuss a theory to explain the various causal connections we have detailed in the last eight chapters.

Part V
Interpretation and conclusions

15 Depression and loss

The time has now come to draw together the various factors we have identified as significant in producing and shaping depression. The main task of this book has been to develop a causal model of clinical depression: this has been done and, we believe, it is sufficiently well based for some attention to be paid to the theory that we have developed to make sense of it. But the two must be kept distinct: claims that we make for the causal model cannot be made as yet for the more speculative theory.

We have identified three broad groups of factors; the provoking agents, the vulnerability factors, and the symptom-formation factors. These we believe relate in differing ways to a central experience of hopelessness which develops out of the appraisal of particular circumstances, usually involving loss.

Hopelessness and depression

Recognition that loss plays an important role in depression has, of course, been widespread. While a good deal of the extensive research literature has dealt with death, Freud made the point in *Mourning and Melancholia* that the object need not necessarily have died but simply have been lost as an object of love. The way in which we have categorized events follows a similar line of thought. Basically we have seen loss events as the deprivation of sources of value or reward. We now go further to suggest that what is important about such loss for the genesis of depression is that it leads to an inability to hold good thoughts about ourselves, our lives, and those close to us. Particularly important, as Melges and Bowlby (1969) have argued, is the loss of faith in one's ability to attain an important and valued goal. But this must not simply be equated with disappointment and adversity. Most of us (we will not bother with rare exceptions) strive to hold ourselves and those close to us in high esteem – as a good mother, or father, wife or husband, housewife, worker, friend, home decorator, and tennis player, although each of us differs in the relative importance we give to such activities and roles. Sources of value can come from a person, a role, or an idea; but it would also be misleading to see such rewards as mutually exclusive. A mother can value a child for his presence, obtain a sense of identity from her maternal role, and gain reward from fantasy about what he will become. A further point is that it is possible to hold good thoughts about them even when all is far from well with our world. The fact that we are beset by difficulties will not *necessarily* detract from our ability to feel all right about things; indeed, if we can believe we have stood up well to adversity, feelings of pride and self-worth may increase. The point is not obscure: the ability to feel good about things is not a straightforward function of the amount of 'difficulty' and 'failure' in our lives.

The fact that reward can be got simply from ideas means that the past, the present, or the future are involved; it follows also that scope for suffering is increased. Ideas about the future may have had only a tenuous link with reality and yet still be experienced as great loss if they can no longer be believed. This independence of ideas from place and time is important for an understanding of loss. The worth of a person or a role does not necessarily disappear with the loss of the person or the role – a widow can continue to have good thoughts about her marriage. In the same way, good thoughts will not necessarily be possible even if person or role remain unchanged. A woman deprived of a lover will not always lose good thoughts about herself or lose hope of gaining another. She may retain the warmest memories and remain confident of her attractiveness and capacity to love. Alternatively, the parting may cast doubt on what she had seen as a successful relationship and lead her to question her ability to rebuild any worthwhile relationship with a man. In other words, the implications of loss usually stretch far beyond the fact of the loss itself. Like Melges and Bowlby we believe hoplessness is the key factor in the genesis of clinical depression and loss is probably the most likely cause of profound hopelessness. But it is not just loss of a particular 'object' that has to be dealt with, so much as its implications for our ability to find satisfactory alternatives. The process of loss can be likened to a series of Russian dolls one within the other – but in a Lewis Carroll world where each succeeding doll may prove to be larger than the last. In loss it is not always just the current situation that is involved (although, we believe, the significance of this is often underestimated). The present is

bound to some degree to awaken our past. This has long been recognized: that crises will often awaken 'unresolved conflicts',
memories, and emotions. Some emphasise the potential for growth
and adjustment here – stressing that the crises give us another chance
of dealing with the past. Clinical experience abounds with examples of
individuals and families who 'rise to the occasion' when confronted
with crises, thereby not only successfully mastering the exigencies of
the current situation, but also dealing more adequately with long-
standing conflicts that have been suppressed or repressed (Parad and
Caplan, 1965: 57).

The immediate response to loss of an important source of positive
value is likely to be a sense of hoplessness, accompanied by a gamut of
feelings, ranging from distress, depression, and shame to anger. Feelings of hopelessness will not always be restricted to the provoking
incident – large or small. It may lead to thoughts about the hopelessness of one's life in general. It is such *generalization* of hopelessness
that we believe forms the central core of a depressive disorder. It is this
that sets the rest of the syndrome in train. We are not the first to believe
this (or at least something like it). Aaron Beck has focussed upon a
similar cognitive component of clinical depression. While we do not
rule out that at times physical factors may be largely responsible for
clinical depression, we believe that in most instances a cognitive
appraisal of one's world is primary – and it is from this that the
characteristic bodily and psychological symptoms of depression arise.
This is not to deny the importance of research on the physical basis of
depression. Clinical depression involves profound bodily changes.
What we assert is that until such work is extended to take account of
bodily processes *before* the onset of depressive symptoms, it has no
strict aetiological relevance in the sense used in this book; for the bodily
changes may well form part of the dependent rather than the independent variable.

Our argument so far is incomplete. Why do relatively so few people
develop such hopelessness? A less familiar component of our theory is
that a person's ongoing self-esteem is crucial in determining whether
generalized hopelessness develops – that is, response to loss and
disappointment is mediated by a sense of one's ability to control the
world and thus to repair damage, a confidence that in the end alternative sources of value will become available. If self-esteem and feelings of mastery are low *before* a major loss and disappointment a
woman is less likely to be able to imagine herself emerging from her
privation. It is this, we believe, that explains the action of the vulnerability factors in bringing about depression in the presence of
severe events and major difficulties. They are an odd assortment: loss

of mother before eleven, presence at home of three or more children under fourteen, absence of a confiding relationship, particularly with a husband, and lack of a full- or part-time job. (Reversal, of course, will express them as protective factors – *not* losing a mother before eleven and so on.) We suggest that low self-esteem is the common feature behind all four and it is this that makes sense of them. There are several terms other than self-esteem that could be used almost interchangeably – self-worth, mastery, and so on. In the end we chose it because it was a term sometimes used by the women themselves (although they more often talked of lacking confidence). We were particularly interested in a few of the women who took up employment a few weeks *after* the occurrence of a severe event, none of whom developed depression. One working-class woman who had previously not worked for six years commented that 'the money was not much' but it 'gave me a great boost' and 'greater self-esteem'. The relevance for the women of the three vulnerability factors occurring in the present would probably lie in generating a sense of failure and dissatisfaction in meeting their own aspirations about themselves, particularly those concerning being a good mother and wife – this giving them chronically low self-esteem.

When discussing Henry VIII's reaction to the possibility of Katheryn's adultery we related the idea of meaning to plans of action – the King was unprepared in the sense he had 'formed neither a plan nor a preference' for another liaison. McCall and Simmons in *Identities and Interactions* (1966) made the point that the major source of our plans are *role identities*, the imaginative view an individual has of himself as an occupant of a particular social position. While these are usually socially based, quite idiosyncratic ideas of oneself can be incorporated. We believe it is these role identities that are usually involved in the hopelessness that precedes clinical depression. McCall and Simmons see the identities as woven into various more or less cohesive patterns.

> 'The basis for this clustering is ordinarily that several role-identities involve similar skills, have the same persons "built into" their contents, or pertain to the same institutional context or period of one's life. These clusters may themselves be linked more or less closely with other clusters or may be quite rigidly "compartmentalized" or "dissociated" from others.'
>
> (McCall and Simmons, 1966: 76–7)

The more a woman has committed herself to a given identity or cluster of identities the more her 'assumptive world', in Parkes's sense, will be caught up in it and the greater the severity of a crisis that deprives her of an essential part of it. Our concepts of general and specific appraisal were based on the way women respond to 'external' events and difficulties – the way they put them together in their mind. In general appraisal there is a simple addition of distress as if the thought 'oh yet another thing' is the final cause of breakdown. In specific appraisal, additivity of events rests on the particular implications of the first event for the second. It is not, however, easy to move from these ideas to the impact of provoking agents on role identities. It is possible to imagine the general appraisal of a number of 'unrelated' severe events influencing just one role identity – learning that one's child is in trouble with the police and that another has failed an important examination may be quite unrelated in an 'exteranal' sense but jointly have a devastating impact on a woman's notion of herself as an effective mother. It is also possible to conceive of a specific appraisal of 'one' event influencing several identities – and even more complex possibilities. Since little is known about the organization of these identities, we can only speculate. In our various discussions of the 'additivity' of provoking agents we have suggested that it is hopelessness about restoring a particular source of value that is usually crucial. This may be something that was once had (a husband's love) or something which was only wished for (a new place to live). It is now clear that this must not be taken too literally; although the hopelessness usually starts from a particular focus, just what is involved in terms of 'psychic additivity' will depend on the underlying role identities. A general appraisal may relate to a specific identity and a specific appraisal to a number of quite disparate identities. However, on the whole, some broad comparability between the two would be expected. It is possible that what is *left* of a role identity or identities after a provoking agent will determine vulnerability. If important role identities are left, a woman will have more on which to build for the future; and one way of viewing vulnerability is in terms of the hope a woman can bring to her situation.

It is not difficult to see how three of the factors we have identified as enhancing vulnerability may relate to role identities or how their reversal (having a full or part-time job, a close relationship with husband, not having three or more children under fourteen at home) can be protective. In the case of employment, not only does the role identity of worker become available to a woman but her extra social contacts will often provide her with new interpersonal identities. The existence of an intimate relationship most probably acts by providing not only a role identity but also one that is likely to be appraised as successful, and thus a source of self-esteem. In a similar way it is probably usually easier to perform successfully in the role of mother when there are fewer than three children under fourteen, and it is easier for a woman to spend time outside the house building new role identities if she has fewer children who can be left with neighbours or relatives, or even accompany her more easily.

We therefore suggest that the vulnerability factors play an important role because they limit a woman's ability to develop an optimistic view about controlling the world in order to restore some souce of value. Of course, an appraisal of hopelessness is often entirely realistic: the future for many women *is* bleak. But given a particular loss or disappointment, ongoing low self-esteem will increase the chance of a general appraisal of hopelessness:

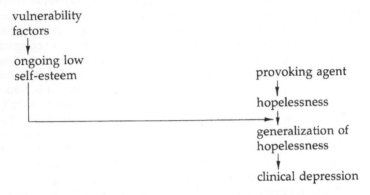

In this view loss itself is less important in producing depression than feelings of profound hopelessness, which may or may not stem from loss. The fact that major loss *is* often present before onset of depression means no more than that it is the most common way in which sources of value can be placed in jeopardy.[1] But hopelessness may occur simply in response to thoughts about a possible loss. The hopelessness of the divorced women who became depressed when her young daughter returned from holiday apparently stemmed from her pessimism about her future loneliness and this was triggered by her dwelling on the time when her daughter would finally leave home.

Loss of someone much loved will not necessarily lead to hopelessness. Even with great grief and distress there may be awareness of new possibilities and an underlying sense of hope. In our research we have been forced to neglect 'personality' factors as it was impossible to collect them accurately enough when dealing with women already depressed. If they play a role, it is probably substantially related to such a dimension of optimism-pessimism.

So far we have speculated that the common feature of three of the vulnerability factors is their association with feelings of low self-esteem and lack of mastery. Since they all concern the present, it follows that it is the current environment that is the most important influence. Intensive studies of the life of women in London are now needed to move beyond this. Recent studies of housework and attitudes of women with young children towards employment outside the home begin to do this (Gavron 1966; Oakley 1974; Ginsberg 1976).

For example, Susannah Ginsberg argues that work outside the home becomes a source of self-esteem for many women within a society where status accrues to economic gain. A woman may have spent years caring for her children but still not be considered qualified for any job – child-care or other – on the basis of this experience. The relatively low status attributed to the work of child-care can sometimes be internalized by the women in terms of feelings of low self-esteem. Although work outside the home may share the monotony and bore-dom that, as Ann Oakley describes, many women find in child-care and housework, it at least gains recognition in terms of economic reward. This may be one reason for the protection provided by paid employment. Of course, this does not rule out the more obvious assets of a job outside the home – social contacts and respite from the demands of small children.

The presence of loss of mother before eleven among the four vul-nerability factors is more difficult to explain. It may lead to enduring changes in personality of the woman herself or, given that such a loss is correlated with low intimacy and three or more children under four-teen, it may impart a greater risk of undergoing certain adverse experi-ences, it being these that leave her more vulnerable. Both, of course, may be at work and indeed may be so in the same woman. The women may have greater dependency needs as suggested by Birtchnell (1975); and these may make them more likely to marry the 'wrong' man, if only because they are more likely to settle with the first man willing to live with them. While we have no means at present of a direct test of these possibilities there are some clues.

We have already noted that loss of mother before eleven is related to low intimacy with husband and to having three or more children under fourteen. Table 1 goes further by showing that even when one or other of these factors is present, loss of mother is still associated with a greater risk of depression for women with a provoking agent: two-thirds of the women with low intimacy or three or more children under fourteen became depressed if they had lost a mother before eleven compared with only a quarter of those without such a loss (p<.05). This suggests that early loss of a mother leads not only to certain adverse experiences (e.g. low intimacy and three or more children under fourteen) but also to changes in the personality of the woman herself. It is certainly not unlikely that loss of mother before eleven may have an enduring influence on a woman's sense of self-esteem, giving her an ongoing sense of insecurity and feelings of incompetence in controlling the good things of the world.

But although depression among women with loss of mother before eleven is extremely common, we do not suggest that the experience is inevitably linked with psychiatric disorder and unhappiness. With luck (or wisdom), especially in choice of a husband, such women may do particularly well.[2]

Table 1   *Women in Camberwell developing depression by whether they had (i) low intimacy with husband/boyfriend or 3 or more children under 14 (ii) lost a mother before 11 and (iii) a severe event or major difficulty*

severe event or major difficulty	low intimacy with husband or three or more children under 14			high intimacy with husband and less than three children under 14		
	loss of mother before 11			loss of mother before 11		
	Yes	No		Yes	No	
	%	%		%	%	
yes	64 (7/11)	23 (18/78)	p < .05	0 (0/4)	11 (8/71)	n.s.
no	0 (0/6)	3 (2/71)	n.s.	0 (0/9)	1 (2/169)	n.s.

If this general view of loss of mother as a vulnerability factor is accepted, it is still necessary to explain its two special features. First, that the loss of any other close *relative* does not increase risk of depression and second, that loss of mother *after* the age of eleven plays no part. The first can possibly be explained by the fact that the mother will usually be the largest source of appreciation and support. A father's or sibling's disappearance is likely to be a less painful experience for a child. The second point might be explained by the fact that until a child is about eleven the main means of controlling the world is likely to be the mother. Thereafter the child is more likely to exert control directly and independently. The earlier the mother is lost, the more the child is likely to be set back in his or her learning of mastery of the environment; and a sense of mastery is probably an essential component of optimism. Thus, loss of mother before eleven may well permanently lower a woman's feeling of mastery and self-esteem and hence act as a vulnerability factor by interfering with the way she deals with loss in adulthood.[3]

The writings of John Bowlby on the infant's reaction to separation lend support to this view. In his two volumes *Attachment and Loss* he has built an impressive theoretical edifice reshaping classical psychoanalytic instinct theories in the light of the studies of ethologists, particularly Lorenz and Hinde, and of child development psychologists, such as Ainsworth, who have studied mother and infant in the first years of life. He elaborates a dimension of the security-insecurity of the child's attachment to a principal figure (usually, but not necessarily, the natural mother), which he sees as the basis for the growth of self-reliance as an enduring personality characteristic. Following Ainsworth's data he argues that closeness and 'relatively much physical contact in the earlier months . . . does not make [an infant] into a clingy and dependent one year old; on the contrary it facilitates the gradual growth of independence' (Bowlby, 1973: 405). It follows that the converse, abrupt severing of an attachment, can interfere with the growth of self-reliance. This idea has many echoes in the writings of psychoanalysts. Bowlby's 'security of attachment' seems clearly to refer to the same feature of infancy that Benedek (1938) refers to as 'relationship of confidence', that Klein (1948) refers to as 'introjection of the good object', and that Erikson (1950) refers to as 'basic trust' (Vol 1: 339). Bowlby also cites the object-relations theories of Fairbairn (1952) and the works of Winnicott (1958): 'maturity and the capacity to be alone implies that the individual has had the chance through good-enough mothering to build up a belief in a benign environment' (Bowlby, 1973: 409). But what Bowlby has done is to transfer these maxims developed through clinical experience to the centre of a carefully thought out theory of human attachment which can be, and to some extent has been, subjected to the criterion of confirmation and falsification so necessary to any scientific idea.

In his two volumes so far, Bowlby has devoted less attention to the role of separation from principal attachment figure in childhood in leading to depression in adult life and more to its effects in childhood itself and its relationship with later agoraphobia. He does, however, argue plausibly for a depressive component in certain types of agoraphobia (1973: 352–4). The weight of the evidence he presents supports his contention that 'separations, threats of separation and losses . . . divert development from an optimum pathway (for personality development) to a suboptimum one'. Although the separations upon which he focusses are mainly before the child's third birthday, there is nothing in his model to rule out a similar role for separations between the ages of three and ten.

It is clear that our notion of a sense of mastery and self-esteem is very close to Bowlby's concept of self-reliance. Indeed when he discusses the conditions that contribute to the development of secure attachment he cites work not only by Ainsworth but by David and Appell (1969), Sander (1962, 1964), and Bettelheim (1967) which suggests that one important aspect of self-reliance is an environment so regulated that an infant can derive a sense of the consequences of his own actions – a feature clearly related to the development of a cognitive set involving a feeling of being able to control things, that is of not being helpless.

Bowlby's two volumes represent the most concerted theoretical presentation of this viewpoint, but the work of Birtchnell among psychiatric patients, on the loss of parents in childhood, has also collected important data. Although, as we have earlier discussed, his results on early loss of parents are at best conflicting, there is one study which bears directly on the issue of vulnerability (Birtchnell 1975). Using a scale developed by Navran (1954) to measure dependence from a personality measure (MMPI) he found that women who had lost their mothers before the age of ten were significantly more dependent than women who had not. Later examination of the profiles of women who had lost their mothers between the ages of ten and nineteen revealed a degree of dependence intermediate between the other two groups.[4]

The role of the dependent personality in the onset, and especially the perpetuation, of depressive conditions in women has been highlighted by Weissman and Paykel's study of depressed women (1974). But they conclude that 'dependency' is a result rather than a cause of the depression since it 'disappears' when the depression clears up. It is difficult to assess the importance of this finding, since it is unclear from their measurement whether the dependency completely disappears or is merely reduced. Nor do they give information about loss of attachment figures in childhood, which leaves this issue unexplored.

Another important account of how early experience can crucially determine later reactions to stress is Seligman's comparison of depression with 'learned helplessness'. Using animal experiments he has shown that uncontrollable and unpredictable trauma tends to lead to passive resignation – what he calls learned helplessness. He sees this as primarily a cognitive disposition which, once established, increases the chance of an animal passively undergoing a traumatic situation (such as receiving electric shocks) rather than seeking a solution. 'Absence of mother, stimulus deprivation, and non-responsive mothering all contribute to the learning of uncontrollability . . . Since, however, helplessness in an infant is the foundational motivational attitude which later motivational learning must crystallize, its debilitating consequences will be more catastrophic' (Seligman, 1975: 150–1). The argument has obvious relevance for the study of depression, but we do not believe (as Seligman argues) that loss of mother before eleven is specifically related to so-called 'reactive' or 'neurotic' depression. We have seen that loss of mother before eleven, like the other vulnerability factors, raises chances of *any* form or severity of depression. Further we do not view learned helplessness essentially as depression. We see it as a factor predisposing a person to a depressive reaction along the lines of vulnerability factors. But like Seligman we believe that this helpless predisposition, which is the obverse of Bowlby's concept of self-reliance, can be the result of trauma in early life.

At this point we have said nothing about the most obvious aspect of a major loss – that is grief. It is not, of course, a single 'emotion'. Tennyson's *In Memoriam* and Patmore's *Odes on Bereavement* vividly document the psychological and emotional complexity of the painful search for meaning and acceptance of the loss. Costello (1976) has argued that in evolutionary terms the function of the emotions of depression and anxiety is to force us to think about our lives. Certainly these poems, and grief itself, are as much about thoughts, meaning, and purpose as about feelings. In terms of our previous discussion they explore at length other losses entailed by the primary loss.

There are many fine literary accounts of grief – for instance C. S. Lewis' *A Grief Observed* and Susan Hill's *In the Springtime of the Year*. Work by psychiatrists and social scientists is impressively consistent with such accounts. Lindemann in a classic paper published in 1944 described a syndrome of symptoms found in acute grief; since then Bowlby (1961) and Parkes (1970) at the Tavistock Institute have done much to confirm and amplify his scheme. Colin Parkes described the most characteristic feature of grief not as prolonged depression but acute and episodic 'pangs' – episodes of severe anxiety and psychological pain (1972). They are particularly common soon after loss in what Bowlby has called the phase of yearning and protest (1961). Parkes views such pining as the emotional component of an urge to search for a lost object and believes that in bereavement there is the same impulse to search as shown by many species of animal. With it there is also commonly preoccupation with memories of the lost person. Irritability and anger are also common at an early stage. As primary grief diminishes there seems to follow a period of uncertainty, aimlessness, and apathy which Bowlby (1961) has called the phase of disorganization and despair. The characteristic emotion now is depression. Bowlby and Parkes make it clear that there are in reality no clear-cut phases – that elements of each phase (Bowlby adds a third, reorganization) persist into and alternate with elements of other phases. Although such basic patterns of response to bereavement can be discerned, grief may be delayed, exaggerated, or apparently absent and there is some evidence that these 'distorted' reactions are associated with increased rates of physical illness.[5]

Peter Marris in *Loss and Change* (1974) has related grief reactions to a variety of changes other than death. He describes in situations such as enforced rehousing and the rise of educational elites in East Africa the characteristic need to deny the change and also to accept it, outlined by Bowlby and Parkes; what has happened has to be accepted and some meaningful continuity recognized between past, present, and future. Adjustment to a major loss is therefore likely to be both painful and erratic.

> 'It provokes a conflict between contradictory impulses – to return to the past, and to forget it altogether. Each, in itself, would be ultimately self-destructive, either by denying the reality of present circumstances, or by denying the experience on which the sense of self rests. But their interaction forces the bereaved to search to and fro, until they are reconciled by reformulating and reintegrating past attachments.'   (Marris, 1974: 151–2)

Marris argues that whenever people suffer loss their reaction reflects a conflict that is essentially similar to that seen in the grief processes experienced when an individual loses a person close to him. Parkes (1973; 1975) has also taken this view in a detailed study of reactions to a loss of a limb as has Fried (1965) in a study of a large-scale enforced rehousing programme in Boston.

It is essential at this point to emphasize that the need for meaning and a sense of continuity in our lives is not the same as the need for routine. Major change in routine and interpersonal contacts as such do *not* increase risk of depression. It may indeed be welcomed as long as there is continuity of purpose. (Many seek 'eustress' in dangerous sports and the like as a way of bringing variety and a sense of achievement into their lives – see Bernard, 1968.)

As already argued, it is loss of important sources of value, not change, that is crucial (although it is possible to envisage persons so sensitive to loss that almost any change is resisted). What then is the role of grief in depression, bearing in mind its 'distorted' forms? Since only 11 per cent of patients and 14 per cent of onset cases had experienced a death of someone close in the nine months before onset compared with an expected rate of 4 per cent, bereavement is not a great help in explaining depression as a whole.[6] If grief is significant it must be because it is a common response to severe events and major difficulties – not just to bereavement.

How then does this grief relate to the model we have just outlined in terms of hopelessness and low self-esteem? In chapter 2 we claimed that particularly intense grief reactions might develop features that were additional to the central mourning experience and that corresponded to the symptoms described by Feighner (1972) and his colleagues in St Louis as characteristic of clinical depression. We based this conclusion partly on the results of the surveys of widowing by Clayton and her colleagues (1972), although their conclusions about what was and what was not 'real depression' differ from ours. (It may be remembered that they found that one month after the bereavement one third of the widows manifested enough symptoms to be definitely or probably depressed and a year later the figure was 16 per cent.) Following a parallel line of reasoning to the one developed earlier in this chapter we believe that particularly intense mourning reactions can lead to a generalization of the hopelessness that follows the loss. 'Working through' of grief usually forestalls such a generalization: as mourning proceeds the bereaved usually find hope that they can carry on without the lost person, but occasionally the process is so intense or so prolonged that it can no longer be viewed as 'normal' in the sense of within the range of the average reaction. At this point, we would maintain, grief may quite fairly be called clinical depression.

The concept of 'working through' grief is central; it is the process by which alternative sources of value can be found and accepted, and by which hope can be revived. It is however painful – the extent of pain relating, of course, to the importance of who, or what, has been lost. It will also depend, we now argue, on how 'vulnerable' a woman is, that is how easy it is for her to find alternative value sources. Sachar and his colleagues (1968) have suggested that many symptoms of depression may be regarded as helping a patient avoid this pain, by denying the loss or its significance. This idea will be familiar to those trained in psychotherapeutic techniques designed to assist patients to face losses which they have hitherto 'denied'. While it may not at first seem applicable to those patients who are tearful and sleepless, continually preoccupied by their loss, it can plausibly be applied to those patients who say they are unable to cry, who sit withdrawn and retarded, as if cocooned against too much emotion. Consider Tennyson:

> Home they brought her warrior dead:
> She nor swoon'd, not utter'd cry:
> All her maidens, watching, said,
> 'She must weep, or she will die.'

Then they praised him, soft and low,
Called him worthy to be loved,
Truest friend and noblest foe;
Yet she neither spoke nor moved.

Stole a maiden from her place,
Lightly to the warrior stepp'd,
Took the face-cloth from the face,
Yet she neither moved nor wept.

Rose a nurse of ninety years,
Set his child upon her knee;
Like summer tempest came her tears –
'Sweet, my child, I live for thee.'
(*The Princess*, Book VI)

The last verse suggests the conditions under which 'working through' grief becomes possible; crucial is the presence of hope and the child, with his future stretching before him, continuing his father's line, restores some meaning to his mother's future. There is something of the warrior that has not been lost and can become an alternative source of value. (Perhaps the poem also alludes to vulnerability factors in the role of the aged nurse as a person to whom emotion can be safely shown, recalling features of the measure of intimacy.) We therefore suggest a *second* putative process involving vulnerability and low self-esteem:

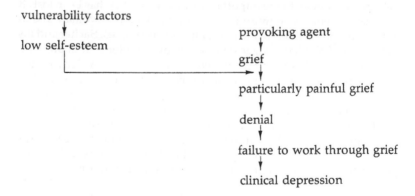

This model relates the response to present loss; but the importance of successful working through of grief perhaps receives indirect support from the material on early loss of mother. There is some evidence that until children are about ten years old they do not readily mourn although they can be taught how to do so (Furman, 1974). If we hypothesize that the way a person will react to later losses will be influenced by their earlier experiences of loss, it seems plausible that a woman with loss of mother before eleven will be more likely to fail to work through her later grief in the way we have suggested. Thus early loss of mother may raise the risk of depression in a second way, by impeding the successful working through of grief, in addition to imparting enduring feelings of low self-esteem and mastery.

At this point we have outlined a theory that we believe accounts for the evidence we presented in earlier chapters about the types of event and difficulty acting as provoking agents and the background factors that make women vulnerable to these provoking agents.

These ideas are sufficient to explain the aetiological role of recent loss and disappointment in the form of severe events and major difficulties and also the way apparently quite minor events can 'bring home' to a woman the hopelessness of her position. They also deal with vulnerability factors that act to increase risk of breakdown in the presence of a provoking agent.

Loss of self-esteem has been given prominence before as a critical intervening variable in the aetiology of depression by a psychoanalyst, Bibring (1953). Although it had been foreshadowed in the writings of Otto Fenichel (1945), Bibring's argument was a radical reshaping of previous psychoanalytical ideas. Such psychoanalytic discussions are apt to focus attention upon a person's internal psychological resources but consideration of the issue in terms of role identities relates it to the social structure, which is where we think it belongs. For it is in the perception of oneself successfully performing a role that inner and outer worlds meet, and internal and external resources come together. Ernest Becker (1964: 111), in commenting on Bibring's views, has suggested that 'nothing less than the full sweep of cultural activity is brought into consideration in the single case of depression'. We agree: our results have pinpointed the importance of class and lifestage in making women not only open to severe events and major difficulties but more vulnerable to their impact. Nevertheless our discussion of vulnerability has so far tended to stress particular factors rather than the 'full sweep of cultural resources' implied by categories such as social class and life-stage. This emphasis has been partly dictated by the evidence itself: there was, for instance, no relationship between the educational level of either the woman herself, or that of her husband, and risk of depression once we had taken account of social class. But there were many 'cultural' factors of which we have not taken account. One is 'intelligence' itself, although it may be objected that this is an internal rather than an external resource. But more important than any such omission was our failure to rate what can be crudely summed up as 'savoir-faire'. Knowing a lawyer, holding an insurance policy, being on good enough terms with a bank manager to be permitted an overdraft, indeed having a bank account in the first place, are external resources in the sense that they can be helpful in certain crises and are obviously closely related to one's class position. Softer, though related measures, would include the network of contacts a person could mobilize, that is, the ease with which they could approach someone with expertise to help them such as a local councillor, a doctor, dentist, accountant, or builder. Here, once again, we face the overlap between outer and inner resources; the ability to mobilize such support will depend not only on the availability of the network of contacts but also on the confidence of the person to approach these contacts, and their ability to build such a network in the first place. Yet again we are faced with the fact that mastery, with which such a network will be associated, is a factor where social and psychological influences are inextricably intermingled. Clearly some of our results are relevant: we have noted how difficulties associated with housing, money, marriage, and children take longer to be resolved when occuring to a working-class woman. We also noted that women usually had little chance of controlling the untoward consequences of the majority of severe events – this indeed is fairly clear from the simple listing of some of them in chapter 10. However, it is important not to go beyond our material.

One glaring inadequacy is our treatment of 'positive' events. We took account of all events to which women had reported a positive emotional response, combined with the number of incidents mentioned in reply to a direct question about pleasant experiences. Although we went beyond our basic life-events schedule, the measure showed only a small association with class position and even less with risk of onset of depression.[7] This result would suggest that positive experiences before onset are not themselves protective. There are various possible explanations of this; one is that only positive experiences *after* provoking agents and before onset of any symptoms can act protectively; another more probable explanation is that not all positive experiences relate to self-esteem or hope, just as we found not all severely threatening events were loss events. Yet another explanation is that most of the positive events we measured were only short-term in their effects and a measure of long-term positive effect would indeed have produced a result associating such events with protection. Finally, again, we would be faced with the same issue we confronted with severe threat: the possibility of a discrepancy between the contextual and the subjective positive rating. If a woman reports as positive the fact that her husband has already survived two months after a dangerous operation, does it mean that it is the event, rated as a positive experience, which is important or is it only because her internal resources of hope are so great that she picks this out as a positive incident to report in the first place? Since in our view hopelessness is crucial to depression it is difficult for us to believe that events that bring hope and a sense of achievement play no role in preventing onset or in improving the course of depression. Like the issue of coping in general the question remains to be explored adequately.

The wider cultural context of self-esteem: a rural study

One of the most intriguing insights that we were able to gain about the role of the 'full sweep of cultural activity' derives from a study of psychiatric symptoms in women in a different cultural setting on the island of North Uist.

In an earlier chapter we suggested that other research supports the conclusion that there is a high rate of depression among working-class women in cities. While there is a general agreement in the literature that rates of psychiatric disorder are lower in rural areas, few have carried out surveys in different areas using the same methods of measuring prevalence of disorder. As an exploratory study, preparatory to a full replication of the Camberwell research in a rural area, in 1975 we carried out a survey of psychiatric disorder in a random sample of 154 women in North Uist in the Outer Hebrides, using exactly the same methods of measurement as in Camberwell.

The most obvious difference between the island and Camberwell is that many island families are still economically productive units, though few depend any longer solely on land or sea for a living. The women were between eighteen and sixty-five years old and almost two-thirds lived in a crofting or fishing household and therefore came into close daily contact with these activities. Over a third of the women had a full or part-time job away from home; just over a third were neither employed nor made any significant contribution to farm work. Men often had other jobs in addition to crofting and fishing.[8]

Psychiatric disorder certainly was not lacking. During the three months before interview 10 per cent of the women in North Uist were considered to be cases (compared with 15 per cent in Camberwell) and a further 14 per cent to be borderline cases (18 per cent in Camberwell), giving a total prevalence of 24 per cent of women suffering from at least a borderline psychiatric condition (33 per cent in Camberwell). However, it is only when further comparisons are made that these figures become meaningful. On North Uist there was no association between social class and psychiatric disorder. Of course, social class must have inevitably different connotations in the two population – most crofters, for instance, would think of themselves as independent farmers although few can support themselves by farming alone. In almost a third of the crofting/fishing households the husband, or brother of the woman had another job. We therefore considered the women in North Uist in two ways. First, according to whether they lived in a crofting/fishing household (62 per cent); and second, by whether the occupation we used to classify them was (i) professional/managerial/ clerical (25 per cent), (ii) skilled manual (12 per cent), (iii) unskilled (18 per cent), or (iv) solely crofting/fishing (44 per cent). In whatever ways the categories were considered, there was no suggestion that 'social class' in North Uist was related to the prevalence of psychiatric disorder. Nor did the presence of a child at home relate to the prevalence of psychiatric disorder. For the women with children at home the rate of overall caseness in the three months before interview on North Uist was quite close to that of middle-class women in Camberwell and very much less than the rate for working-class women in Camberwell. For women without children at home the difference between the classes in Camberwell was somewhat less and the rate on North Uist again approached the middle-class rate in Camberwell (see *Figure 1*).

Certain psychiatrists, writing of the North of Scotland, have had the impression of a high prevalence of depression among Highland women and some general practitioners have suggested that depressive symptoms are more noticeable among the women of the more northerly, predominantly Calvinist islands (Whittet, 1963). These beliefs were not supported by these results. Overall the prevalence of depressive cases on North Uist was about half that in Camberwell (5.8 per cent and 13.3 per cent respectively – p<.02). However, there was an unexpected predominance of other diagnoses on North Uist. If anxiety cases and obsessional cases are combined in a single category the three-month prevalence of such cases was 5.2 per cent on North Uist and 2.4 per cent in Camberwell – the difference does not, however, reach statistical significance. In summary, there was more depression in London and probably more anxiety and obsessional conditions without depressive components on North Uist.[9]

Since data on life-events and difficulties were not collected we were unable to look for vulnerability factors – that is by relating them to provoking agents and onset of caseness. But our data on the relationship of the prevalence of caseness and children at home had already suggested that on the island there might be different factors that were crucial for self-esteem. When we came to look at other broad

Figure 1 Proportion who were cases in the three months before interview among women in Camberwell and North Uist by whether they suffered from depression at the level of caseness or not

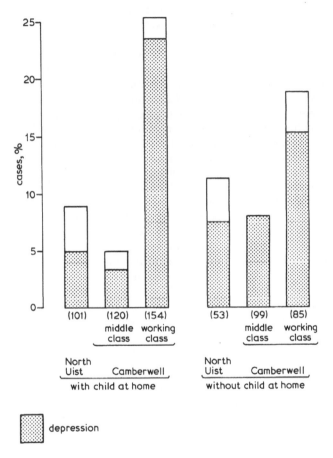

demographic variables we were able to obtain some clues as to what they might be.

Figure 2 suggests that, while the *overall* rate of caseness and borderline caseness may not be crucially affected by them, there are three broad demographic variables which, when combined in an index, relate to the rate of depressive and non-depressive symptomatology. This index, reminiscent of Durkheim's concept of 'integration', includes three factors related to the extent to which a person is part of, or integrated into, the island community: (i) whether or not the woman was brought up on the island; (ii) whether or not she was living in a crofting or fishing family; and (iii) whether or not she attended Church regularly. The rate of depression in the year for combined cases and borderline cases decreased with integration; and the rate of anxiety-other conditions increased, at the extreme the conditions being predominantly ones of depression or anxiety-other.

While more research is needed to draw firm conclusions about this – particularly the high rate of anxiety among the most integrated – a preliminary conclusion about the low rate of depression among the most integrated seems warranted in terms of the views we have outlined about the protective value of the successful performance of roles. A crofting housewife has more opportunity than an urban housewife to perform a range of tasks, which, barring metereological disasters, are limited and successful. Being brought up upon the island will have given a woman from her earliest years a wider range of contacts and thus interpersonal role identities. Regular church attendance offers not only a range of these identities every Sunday but also the higher self-esteem consequent upon the virtuous fulfilment of religious duty. If these are some of the factors that may account for the lower rate of depression on North Uist, there are other explanations. One emphasizes the different kinds of events and difficulties occurring in cities and particularly to the working-class in the 'inner areas'. This is just what we have documented in chapter 10.

In recent years there has been much discussion of an 'urban crisis' involving inner city areas like Camberwell. But although there are undeniably major and specific problems of recent origin, the present situation seems best viewed as the persistence of a problem. David Eversley argues that urban crisis is a

> 'catch phrase used to draw attention to conditions which have always existed and which, if anything, are now less acute than they once were, but which have come into prominence again because of the slowing down, or even reversal, of that long process of economic growth to which we all once looked to dispose of the remnants of squalor and suffering. The "crisis" is nothing but a point in time when familiar conditions suddenly present themselves as being beyond the capacity of our present system to remedy, or at least ameliorate.'   (Eversley, 1977: 18)

One of the most obvious recent problems is the loss of employment opportunities. In the seven-year period 1966–72, firms in the London area shed 217,400 people and these redundancies were mainly in the manufacturing sector. Something like 22 per cent of the total number of jobs in manufacturing industry in London disappeared in this time

Figure 2 Proportion of women on North Uist suffering from depressive or anxiety-other conditions of a case or borderline case severity in the year

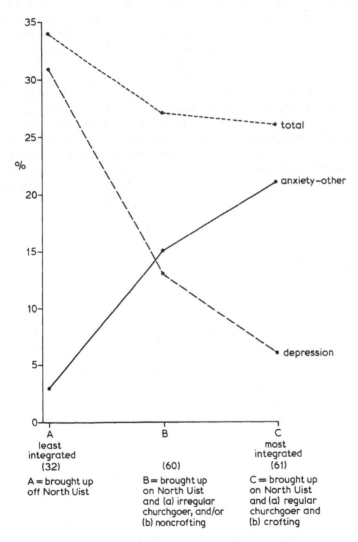

A = least integrated (32)
A = brought up off North Uist

B (60)
B = brought up on North Uist and (a) irregular churchgoer, and/or (b) noncrofting

C = most integrated (61)
C = brought up on North Uist and (a) regular churchgoer and (b) crofting

(Lomas, 1975). This has been, at least in part, the result of successive governments' planning policies. For many years emphasis was placed on building new industrial areas outside the main cities at the expense of the opportunities in the inner city (Field, 1977). There is also in

London, in spite of a good deal of redevelopment, a widely recognized 'crisis in low-income housing' (Eversley and Donnison, 1973). There is simply not enough of it. Often to get council housing (assuming it is desirable) a family has to subject itself to a lengthy period of unpleasant living in barely adequate conditions (Berthoud, 1976). The existence of these problems is not in dispute and they are reflected in our material. One in six of working-class women in Camberwell had at least one 'severe' event or 'major' difficulty involving *housing* and one in fourteen middle-class women. These are disturbing figures bearing in mind the severity of the problems involved. There was also evidence of the movement of industry – 3 per cent of the married women had had a husband who had lost a job through redundancy in the year. (There was, however, no class difference here.) While we now have made a start on the epidemiology of troubles in inner city areas much more needs to be done to establish links with broader economic, political, and cultural structures. For our present purpose, it is enough to say that such links can be made.

It remains to interpret the symptom-formation factors.

Past loss and depression

There is a very large association between past loss and severity and type of depressive symptoms. This only emerges when (i) severity of the depression at admission, (ii) the predominance of neurotic and psychotic features, (iii) four kinds of loss (of siblings, child, and husband and not just of parents), and (iv) whether loss was due to death or other reasons, are distinguished. This has not been done before; but five studies have looked at loss of parent during childhood and adolescence and severity of depression. Most offer some general support for the Camberwell findings. Since they ignore the other three distinctions just listed, only a modest association between loss and severity could be expected. Birtchnell (1970c) provides results for women with a loss before twenty and there is a close similarity with our material when the same simple two-fold distinction is made: 38 per cent of the most and 22 per cent of the least depressed patients had lost a parent in childhood or adolescence compared with 37 per cent and 23 per cent in our series.[10]

It is unlikely that an artefact is involved: there is no reason to believe that there is much error in recording major losses (see Barraclough and Bunch, 1973) nor that the measurement of diagnosis and past loss was in some way confounded. There is no suggestion that age, previous admissions, or social class are biassing factors. Moreover, the role of constitutional or genetic factors seems unlikely to be great. While it could be argued that a constitutional disposition to develop psychotic depression could be inherited and that successful suicides among parents account for the high rate of past deaths among the psychotic group, there was only one parental death by suicide among the 114 patients. It could also be argued that in the past, serious depressive disorders in parents would have led to long periods of separation when they were in mental hospital; but this predicts an association between separation and psychotic depression – quite the opposite of that found. Another possible genetic line of explanation might develop from suggestions by a number of authors that there is a special younger group among the neurotics with sociopathic tendencies either themselves or among their first-degree relatives (Paykel, 1971; Winokur *et al.*, 1969, and Perris, 1966). These sociopathic tendencies might be held responsible both for parental divorce and for the development of depression of a neurotic character in the child later on if they are hereditable. But it is far from established that such tendencies are hereditarily rather than environmentally acquired. Thus in general we find it hard to conceive of an interpretation of the association between type of past loss and type of symptomatology that does not rest on environmental rather than genetic factors.

But if the results are not the result of artefacts and, if they are not explained by genetic factors, what is involved? So far we have dealt only with the role of loss of mother as a vulnerability factor. We need now to explain the effect of past loss in general and seek an explanation that differs from loss of mother when it acts as a vulnerability factor. We have already suggested that, in terms of symptom-formation, past loss may take the form of an enduring cognitive influence; that thinking about the loss influences the way one looks at the world – and particularly the way one reacts to later losses.[11] Loss by death may be related to psychotic-like symptoms because it tends to lead to a general attitude that one's own efforts are useless; that loss of any kind becomes like death, irreversible, with nothing to be done. Such an attitude may be particularly linked to denial of the implications of a loss and to greater 'bodily' expressions of symptoms. By contrast a person who has lost a parent and knows he or she is still alive will be likely to feel the situation less irredeemable. It is not as if an outside fate had been at work. This may give a less passive cognitive set than the death of a parent. It may also cause the separation to be seen as a rejection; if the parent is still alive and somewhere else it may seem that they have chosen to leave because the child is not lovable. Such an interpretation could prove the foundation for a life-long expectation of failure, which could become self-reinforcing. This distinction between the psychotic's sense of abandonment and the neurotic's sense of rejection would fit quite plausibly with the traditional ideas of the typical forms of psychotic and neurotic depression.

The types of enduring cognitive set predicted for the two kinds of past loss have much in common with John Bowlby's characterization of the stages of development of the child's reaction to loss of principal attachment figure: first protest, then despair, and finally detachment (1973). After a separation, it can never be ruled out as impossible that protest will finally bring about a return, however unlikely this may be. After a death it is much clearer that protest will be ineffectual. An examination of the association between individual symptoms and types of past loss does suggest that a more *protesting despair* is associated with separation and a more *retarded hopelessness* with death. Of the symptoms, retardation was one of the most important items in the discriminant function analysis. It was found in 54 per cent of the total sample but in only 30 per cent of the neurotics compared with 73 per cent of the psychotics. Retardation was particularly associated with past loss by death. Among psychotics 84 per cent with a death were retarded but only 36 per cent without such loss (p<.01). Among neurotics with a past death, 38 per cent were retarded. Among those with a past separation 27 per cent of the neurotics and 25 per cent of psychotics had retardation. It seems likely that it is retardation that largely accounts for the more general finding we have outlined. For while 82 per cent of the patients with a past death were also psychotic, as many as 75 per cent of all those with a past death exhibited retardation.

We saw in the last chapter that the association of past loss by separation with a more neurotic score on the discriminant function could not be explained by a tendency for neurotic patients to be more anxious. This hypothesis has a certain prima facie plausability given the established view that anxiety develops under conditions of uncertainty and given that separations, unlike deaths, do contain elements of uncertainty. Our data did not, however support this interpretation.

Earlier we contrasted protesting despair with retarded hopelessness. Bearing in mind Bowlby's notion of 'protest' as a response to loss, we examined various symptom items which would be considered relevant to this theme, such as suicide gestures, verbal attacks, and violent behaviour. The latter proved particularly interesting: while only 13 per cent of patients showed violent behaviour, a third with a past loss by separation did so, and only 6 per cent of those with a loss by death (p<.01). There is therefore some suggestion that symptomatology among those with a past loss by separation was often reminiscent of a gesture of protest, a desperate bid for the return of lost attention. A detailed examination of the course of the disorder before admission further confirms this. A comparison of the styles of the eleven suicide attempts among the neurotics (36 per cent of whom had had a past loss by separation) and the eight attempts among the psychotics shows that among the neurotics the attempts were less serious – often only a few pills were taken or wrists were cut with histrionic shouts but only small scratches. Most were attempts designed to be found by those close: for example, one girl who later told the psychiatrist that it had been an 'attention-seeking gesture' deliberately went to her boyfriend's flat before taking the tablets. Among the psychotics the attempts were more serious: one woman had felt suicidal for at least one month but had refrained from an attempt because she feared she would only injure herself and not succeed in dying. She finally threw herself from a fourth floor window. Often psychotics seemed to have tried to ensure that they were not discovered in time, one patient was found by chance in her gas-filled kitchen by a neighbour who did not usually call; another was only found because her daughter broke into her flat after she had not kept an appointment with a friend.

One of the items of information we detailed for every patient was the source of the idea that they should have psychiatric treatment; whether it was the husband, the woman herself, other relatives and friends, or what we called 'official' sources. The latter were probation officers, welfare officers, health visitors, the police, and doctors if the woman had not gone to them to consult about her mental state but if they had themselves noticed it and initiated the suggestion that she should seek psychiatric treatment. There were significantly more neurotics for whom the proposal had been 'officially' initiated – 22 per cent as compared with 9 per cent of the psychotics. Among the neurotic suicides as many as 73 per cent were referred by 'official' sources, while only one of the psychotic suicides was. And indeed she was very much the exception who proved the rule; she was one of the rare psychotics with a past loss by separation (there were only four) and she was not 'retarded'. Her husband, whom she suspected of infidelity, was away and she took some tablets and brandy. When they failed to have an effect she telephoned the hotel where he was staying and told him she would not be there when he arrived home. The police were informed, and came to see how she was; her cousin was summoned and then stayed one night. After her husband returned, she was taking him some tea in the morning and when he said 'thank you darling' it was too much for her: she ran straight out into the road, trying to get run over. It was only because an ambulance driver was passing that she was taken to a psychiatric department.

Referral by such 'official' sources is not only linked with what we have called the 'protest' theme among those with a suicide attempt.

Among the patients as a whole, 15 per cent had such referral; but 47 per cent of those with a past loss by separation did so and only 10 per cent of the rest. Twenty-six per cent of the officially referred neurotics were violent (as compared with 13 per cent of the rest of the neurotics). Among the psychotics with such a source of referral, however, none were violent, but the rate of retardation was lower than for the total psychotic population – 33 per cent as compared with 73 per cent. This perhaps reflects the other side of the same coin: retardation, being more akin to conventional notions of sickness, will provoke relatives and friends to suggest treatment, whereas a patient less retarded, more in the phase of protest, may be considered troublesome rather than sick by her normal contacts and only recognized as in need of psychiatric attention by someone with some expertise such as 'official' personnel.

The picture, which begins to emerge of those with past loss by separation, is in many ways consistent with the data now emerging in the neighbouring field of the study of delinquency and conduct disorders in children. Numerous studies have shown an association between a broken home in childhood and the development of anti-social problems (e.g. Bowlby 1969; Rutter 1971 and 1972). There is evidence too that broken homes are associated with attempted suicide in adult life, especially for those with personality disorder (Greer, 1964; Greer and Gunn, 1966). Frommer and O'Shea (1973a and b) found that women whose parents had separated before they were eleven had more feeding and management problems with their first babies than others, whereas loss of a parent by death at that age was not related to these aspects of infant care. Our data were insufficiently detailed to throw light on the important debate that Michael Rutter has opened up in his comprehensive review of maternal deprivation: is the experience of separation as such important or is it the discord in the home, with which such separations are highly associated, which produces the characteristic 'protest' symptomatology? Rutter and Madge's conclusion in favour of the second view (1976: 205–8) is persuasive but they are discussing the development of non-depressive antisocial disorders. In the case of depression the element of loss itself is likely to be of more crucial importance than it is for delinquency; discord alone might therefore not be expected to produce the same cognitive set of 'rejection' which we have hypothesized stems from separation. An examination of the case notes of those neurotic patients with symptoms of violence, suicide attempt, or official referral, who had not had a past loss by separation provided evidence of definite childhood experiences of rejection in five of the ten protocols; evidence of discord without such rejection appeared in only one. More work is needed to clarify this issue, but it seems plausible to suggest that it may be the very combination of the two elements, loss and tension in the home which is important in producing neurotic depressions in later life, rather than that either one or the other is crucial on its own.

It is of interest in the light of this argument about the effects of past loss that the *recent* events provoking the depressive episode under study did not relate to the type or severity of the woman's depression. It may be remembered that about three-quarters of provoking events among the patients involved a clear-cut loss. Psychotic patients were no more or less likely to have had such a recent clear-cut loss than neurotic patients. (And if age is allowed for they were only a little more likely to have suffered a loss by death in the year.) Moreover, a woman who had had a recent loss by death was no more likely to have had a past loss brought about by death. The lack of an association between the types of past and recent loss is just what would be expected if early established cognitive schemes influenced reactions to later severe events. For a woman who has earlier lost an important person by death, the emigration of her child may be seen to have death-like qualities.

One would also expect some kind of primacy effect on the way past losses influence symptom formation. If, for instance, the first loss is by death, a person will tend to see all other losses in these terms. It is possible that losses by separation would in time attenuate or even reverse the original perspective; and, of course, since we have thoughts about the past, the perspective that is important need not be formed at the time of the loss. David Copperfield lost a father before he was born:

> 'My father's eyes had closed upon the world six months when mine opened on it. There is something strange to me, even now, in the reflection that he never saw me; and something stranger yet in the shadowy remembrance that I have of my first childish associations with his white gravestone in the churchyard, and of the indefinable compassion I used to feel for it lying out alone there in the dark night.'

The measure of past loss we have used is still crude and the assumptions made about primacy will need to be tested on larger numbers. For instance, loss by death was rated for the experience of one woman whose mother died in her first year and whose father, after a struggle to cope, sent her to foster parents at the age of two; they in turn returned her at the age of seven at her father's remarriage. This experience could with equal plausibility be considered as loss by separation. It is also, of course, important to extend the work by considering a wider range of experience. What, for instance, about war-time evacuation, periods in hospital of less than one year, broken engagements, and so on?

Age and previous episodes of depression

We have already discussed a striking feature of psychotic as compared with neurotic depressed patients, namely that they are older. We have so far suggested no reason for this; it has, of course, usually been considered to be a purely physiological effect but it is by no means absurd to consider that environmental factors might also be implicated. Women in Camberwell who were fifty to sixty-five years old were much more likely to have experienced past loss than those aged twenty to thirty-five. One possible explanation is that the older women had had more time to lose husband and children; but since the majority of the past losses occurred before eighteen and the findings concerning past loss held whatever the age at loss, this can be ruled out (see *Tables* 4 and 5, chapter 14). It is more tempting to interpret this age difference as, at least in part, the result of a generational effect; improved diet, medical care, smaller families, and lack of major wars have meant that the younger generation experience far fewer deaths of close relatives in their childhood. This would be more consistent with the model:

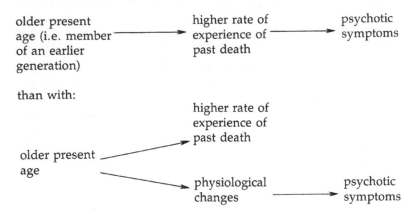

than with:

If this is true we might be experiencing a generational change in the form taken by depression – psychotic-like conditions becoming less frequent. While there is some suggestion that this may be occurring (Paykel, Klerman, and Prusoff, 1970) and that there may be secular changes taking place in the form of psychiatric disorder (Hare, 1974), there are obvious alternative explanations. Since there can at present be no direct test in the absence of evidence for a physiological link, the possibility must remain speculative. Once the present cohort of twenty to thirty-five-year-olds are fifty or over we can expect to have a clearer picture. Insofar as other kinds of major loss may be increasing, particularly from marital breakdown, there is another reason to expect a secular change in the form of depression.

We confess that we have no satisfactory interpretation for the association of a previous episode with overall severity (there is no association with the psychotic-neurotic distinction). It is of interest that it only related significantly among women without a past loss, which might be seen as suggesting some form of priority for the role of past loss. But the possibilities are too many to conclude anything other than that more research is required.

Symptom formation in the general population

At this stage we had done much better than we had dared to hope in tackling the question of symptom formation among patients treated by psychiatrists. We had entirely explained (at least in a statistical sense) the differences in overall severity between out-patients and in-patients in terms of past loss, previous episode, and severe events occurring after onset. We had further shown a remarkable association between psychotic and neurotic forms of depression in terms of type of past loss. However, when we turn to the thirty-seven women who developed depression in Camberwell we must largely report failure. We were handicapped from the start by our omission to collect information about previous episode for the whole 458 women. But leaving this aside we did not find anything to explain either differences in severity among the cases or between them and the patient series. For example, past loss did not relate to differences in overall severity among onset cases. Nor were we able to find more than a slight tendency for onset cases with 'psychotic-like' symptoms to have had a past loss through death.[12]

While in no way wishing to sidestep these negative results nor their possible implications, we do not deem them as necessarily inconsistent with the patient results. Past loss is an extremely crude measure. It is almost certain that it is not *any* past loss that is significant but loss under particular circumstances – say in terms of the kind of mourning that was possible. It might well be that in practice only a small proportion of past losses are capable of having an effect on the expression of symptoms. It follows that if a group is selected in terms of the dependent variable at issue, that is severity, by definition the subgroup of past losses will be selected that are effective in influencing severity. This is just what we have done by taking the patient group. Because they are patients, they are on average more severely depressed than cases in the general population.[13] Under these circumstances our inability to repeat our results on an unselected random sample of depressed women and therefore with an unselected group of past losses is understandable. It may well only prove possible to repeat the result on a random sample when we have identified just what aspects of past loss increase severity and influence psychotic or neurotic features.[14]

There is a second possible reason for our inability to replicate the patient results in the community series. Even if our measure of past loss had been more refined, results in the general population might have been less clear as a result of another form of selection bias. We will spell out this possibility because it has interesting implications: patients when compared with general population cases will be selected not just for overall clinical severity but for other features relevant to psychiatric referral. We saw earlier how much higher the rate of 'official' referral was among 'neurotics' than among 'psychotics' and one can speculate that this may indicate that 'neurotics' in psychiatric treatment are even less representative of community cases with depressions of more neurotic type than are psychotics in psychiatric treatment of community cases with depression of the more psychotic type. Since 'official' referral was closely associated with symptoms of protest, suicidal attempts, and past loss by separation, it is not surprising to find a much smaller proportion of the community cases than of patients characterized as 'neurotic' exhibiting these 'acting-out' symptoms. Most 'neurotics' in the general community would be identified by the absence of specifically psychotic symptoms such as retardation, or early waking or by their lesser severity. In the community, therefore, one would expect results where the neurotic depressions were related more to a *lack* of past loss by death rather than to the *presence* of a past loss by separation. A very large initial sample would thus be required to include a fair number of this particular sub-group of 'acting-out neurotics', without which the results for community cases could not be expected to replicate those for patients.

These speculations about treatment-selection factors set the results on the association of type of past loss with the psychotic-neurotic distinction in a particular perspective. We prefer to emphasize the association of past death with the diagnosis of psychotic depression, seeing it, in part, as a confirmation of Aubrey Lewis's thesis that the two-fold diagnostic distinction is really a dimension of severity. Despite the fact that our measure of overall severity was only moderately associated with this distinction, we agree with his conclusion, emphasizing the relevant concept of severity as more akin to Engel's notion of 'giving up-given up' than to the simple idea of intensity of any pattern of symptoms which underlay our measure of overall severity (see Ní Bhrolcháin, Brown, and Harris, 1977). In this respect we place particular emphasis on retardation. This symptom and several measures of severity of symptomatology are not only the factors that relate most closely to past loss by death but are also the best discriminators between the two diagnostic groups. In these terms neurotic symptoms reflect the lesser degree to which the patient has withdrawn. Thus the association between past separation and the diagnosis of neurotic depression can be seen within the same perspective. For just as a separation is less final than a death, so neurotic patients stop short of the depth of depression of psychotic patients whether they have 'acting-out' symptoms or not.

16 A model of depression

In the last chapter we outlined a theory that accounts for the results presented in chapters 6 to 14. In diagrammatic form model and theory are shown in *Figure 1*.

We will not repeat the arguments but further comments may help to clear up ambiguities – or at least set limits to them.

The model does not refer explicitly to personality dispositions. We decided that any attempt in our cross-sectional survey to distinguish personality traits from psychiatric disorder was unrealistic and we made no attempt to measure them. As academic sociologists, for understandable reasons, we gave priority to external factors such as social relationships and employment. But nonetheless cognitive set plays a critical part in our theory, and in psychological theory this would rank as an enduring personality feature. Although in the diagram separate headings have been given for 'cognitive set', 'response', and 'psychiatric disorder' it should be clear that we see cognitive set as merging into the emotional responses to events and these reactions blending with symptoms. This applies to our view of personality as a whole; while for some purposes personality traits are fittingly treated as 'background variables', it is quite in order in other circumstances to treat exaggerated traits as 'symptoms'. It is exactly this transitional position that we allot to self-esteem; as a background factor, low self-esteem can both predispose a person to a depressive reaction and, when exaggerated, become a prominent feature of the depressive disorder itself.

The model and theory are more a summary of what has emerged from our work than a claim to account completely for depressive phenomena. Nevertheless we feel the results justify considerable attention to the model, limited as it is, in the handling of depression.

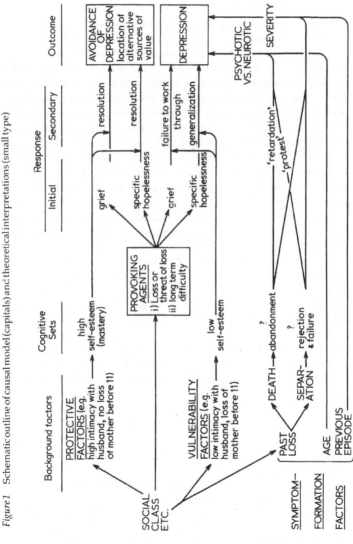

Figure 1 Schematic outline of causal model (capitals) and theoretical interpretations (small type)

For if the role of social factors is as clear as suggested by our material, attention to a person's environment may turn out to be at least as effective as physical treatment. All the same there is always likely to be a small group of depressed women for whom relevant social factors cannot be identified.

The model may be considered to beg the question of the direction of causality between self-esteem and the four vulnerability factors; causality could work either way. Women low on 'mastery', for example, might tend to choose a life-style that does not involve them in work outside the home or might fail to take action to restrict their family size; their low self-esteem may have predated the 'vulnerability factor' rather than resulted from it. Women low on self-esteem might well choose to marry men with whom it is difficult to have a confiding relationship just because they feel they will never find anyone more suitable who is willing to stay with them. Other personality features may mean that certain women find it difficult to maintain good personal relationships, even with the equable and reliable men they have married. Obviously such influences could act in both ways and be mutually reinforcing. But the question of such temporal priority should not be confused with a choice between 'social' and 'non-social'. Aspects of personality will often be the result of earlier social experience. The question is better formulated in terms of the contribution of the current environment relative to all other influences, leaving open the question of whether their source is social or non-social. In these terms the Camberwell material is enough to discredit any easy rejection of the current environment as a major influence. We have noted, for instance, the drop in 'intimacy' between wife and husband once a working-class woman has children, suggesting the importance of current influences. Equally suggestive is the finding that working-class women are only at increased risk of developing depression when they have children at home (although working-class women are more likely to have chronic conditions in all life-stages). Enough is already known about the organization of working-class family life, especially concerning the division of work and patterns of communication between husband and wife, to be confident that a good deal of the class differences in the vulnerability factors must be due to long-term cultural influences. While intensive work, ideally on a longitudinal basis, is required, it would be foolhardy meanwhile, in both scientific and practical terms, to underplay the role of the current environment – acting, we have suggested, particularly through limitations of role identities and of opportunities to find new sources of positive value. There is, in any case, the possibility that even if a woman is at risk as a result of long-standing 'personality' traits, changes in the current environment could still lessen this risk. And, of course, a strong case can be made that the higher rate of severe events and major difficulties among working-class women with children and the fact that their difficulties are of longer duration is in a large part a feature of their environment. In most instances they seemed to have been drawn into troubles not directly of their own making and about which they were relatively helpless.

Susceptibility to depression

There remain the patients who developed depression without a provoking agent – twenty-eight of the 114 – and the possibility of a fourth factor to explain such exceptions. It has been commonly argued that quite trivial stimuli can at times produce illness. While we have defined vulnerability only in terms of sensitivity to major troubles and crises, it is more usual for the term to be used to describe development of a condition with the minimum of provocation. We will use the term susceptibility to describe this tendency and thereby clearly distinguish it from vulnerability. Some of the most interesting current ideas about depression emphasize such susceptibility. Aaron Beck discusses what he calls the vulnerability of the depression-prone person as

> 'attributable to the constellation of enduring negative attitudes about himself, about the world, and about his future. Even though these attitudes (or concepts) may not be prominent or even discernable at a given time, they persist in a latent state like an explosive charge ready to be detonated by an appropriate set of conditions. Once activated, these concepts dominate the person's thinking and lead to the typical depressive symptomatology.'
> (Beck, 1967: 277)

Although somewhat akin to our notion of symptom-formation factors, they are clearly different as they are considered to increase the likelihood of depression. He goes on to suggest that the depressive-prone person has become sensitized in childhood and adolescence to certain types of life-situation – these are responsible for establishing the original negative attitudes and are the prototypes of specific stresses, which may later activate these constellations and lead to depression. He indicates that the incidents that set off the feelings and in turn depression are usually quite minor – at least in terms of the conception of threat developed in the Camberwell research. It is perhaps surprising that we have found little need to discuss such susceptibility; perhaps the nearest we have come is in terms of minor threatening events 'bringing home' the implications of a major problem. But, of course, this does not mean that the idea is irrelevant. The twenty-eight patients who did not have a provoking agent – at least as defined by us – are obvious candidates for this kind of susceptibility. And, indeed, the majority did experience something that might well have 'triggered' the depressive disorder – the woman who, for instance, had been told she had 'incurable' arthritis.

There is, in fact, evidence we have not so far mentioned that offers some support for this notion of susceptibility. Past loss, previous episode, and age of forty or over were related to overall severity at admission. We now add that the presence of all three (but not less then three) is strongly related to *absence of a provoking agent*.[1] Since the index relates to overall severity of depression, the intuitive link which many readers will have made between the notion of susceptibility and severity is supported. If necessary, room could be made in the model for a fourth factor: we would tentatively place it in the lower half of the diagram which shows the connections between these three background factors and severity of depression.

Some of the patients therefore appear to have been 'susceptible' in this sense. There are two obvious interpretations of the concept. First that some women have had their threshold lowered by a previous episode or past loss and so do not need a current loss or disappointment in order to reexperience feelings of hopelessness. Moody (1946) has reported on a patient who while in the army had been bound by a rope with his arms behind his back. He managed to escape with bound wrists and before his recapture he spent several hours with his arms tightly bound. A number of years later in the course of abreactive therapy under narcosis he developed weals with a clear pattern of rope marks around his arms. The phenomenon was observed twice and once under conditions of close scrutiny. There may in depression be some kind of 'induced sensitivity' that makes subsequent episodes more likely along the lines of this kind of 'body memory'.

A second interpretation is 'over-reaction' to particular stimuli – perhaps along the lines argued by Aaron Beck. It is of interest here that among the patients without a provoking agent those highest on this index of past loss, previous episode, and age had a smaller proportion with a 'minor' event in the three weeks before onset – 13 per cent (2/16) versus 42 per cent (5/12). The difference, however, does not reach statistical significance and its interpretation must in any case be uncertain. While the fact that those high on the index had so few minor events *could* be seen as a sign of their extreme susceptibility, it might equally be argued that they should have been more likely to succumb to minor events. The only other evidence we can produce is also unclear (though not without interest). It will be recalled that among the severe events some were considered to be more threatening than others. And yet there is no sign of any interaction between either susceptibility scores or vulnerability scores and degree of threat; that is, marked events were no more or no less likely than moderate events to have occurred to those who were more or less susceptible (or more or less vulnerable). That there is no association is somewhat surprising, although it is consistent with the general tenor of the results that the provoking agents act in a unitary manner. It is not as though moderate events less often provoked depression among the less vulnerable or less susceptible women than did marked events. But while provoking agents (either marked or moderate) were more often absent among the more susceptible women, this effect was not related to their vulnerability in the sense we have defined.

It is therefore best to end on a note of caution. While susceptibility almost certainly exists, it is at present a theoretical rag-bag – it is impossible to rule out a role for a whole range of bodily and environmental factors; and it is not unlikely that many factors will be found to be at work in such a residual group. The patients without provoking agents were too few for us to do much more than underline it as a theme that will need at some time to be incorporated into our model.

17 Summary and conclusions

Sociological studies have two broad purposes. One is to chart the impact of societies upon their members; a second is to study the societies themselves in terms of the impact of their institutions upon each other and how these relate to the impact on individuals (Boskoff, 1971). The study of psychiatric disorders can fulfill both functions. On the one hand it seeks to answer the question of whether particular political, economic, and family structures influence the rate of disorder through their impact on the individual. On the other hand knowledge about rates of psychiatric disorders can further understanding of the workings of the social systems in which they occur. In this connection depression is particularly relevant: it is not only relatively common, but it is fundamentally related to social values since it arises in a context of hopelessness consequent upon the loss of important sources of reward or positive value. A woman's own social milieu and the broader social structure are critical because they influence the way in which she *thinks* about the world and thus the extent of this hopelessness; they determine what is valued, as well as what is lost and how often, and what resources she has to face the loss.

Psychiatric disorder is common among working-class women in London but not in a rural population in Scotland. The disorders almost all involve depression or anxiety and in the urban setting, at least, are predominantly depressive. However working-class women were only at higher risk of developing depression in the year of our study when they had children at home. In explaining such findings we have viewed clinical depression largely as a social phenomenon and have developed a model which in terms of the presence and absence of three factors explains a good deal about the aetiology of *all* forms of depression. The *provoking agents* influence when the depression occurs, the *vulnerability factors* whether these agents will have an effect, and the *symptom-formation* factors the severity and form of the depressive disorder itself. The model tells us only that in some way the factors are causally linked to the disorder. It does not tell us how or why. It is important to know that a woman who has a confiding relationship, particularly with a husband, has much less chance of developing depression once a provoking agent occurs; but it is possible that the reason might have little to do with confiding as such but with, say, the way she is able to think about the marriage and value it. If this were so, confiding could only be used in the model, at least in London, because it happened to be highly correlated with aspects of marriage that were protective. We have therefore also attempted to interpret the model theoretically. What is it about confiding that is important? This distinction between creating model and theory is made for the sake of exposition. They are in practice highly interrelated activities. We have, for instance, done our best to include in the model factors that we believe are of theoretical relevance. In this sense the model is best seen as an early and relatively crude theory; it enables us to get some direct sense of what is going on and provides a framework in which we can think and test new ideas. The distinction between model and theory is, however, important in the sense that the investigator can include certain factors in the model without knowing how it is they work, so long as there is no reason to believe that their association with other factors is the result of some artefact. While it is desirable to have theoretically interpretable factors, all that is required is that they should be methodologically acceptable. In our own model we have variables that range from those about whose theoretical status we feel fairly confident (e.g. life-events) to others about which we know little (e.g. age).

In the design of the study itself we were concerned to increase as much as possible the generality of our findings. With this in mind we studied several samples of depressed women – women treated by psychiatrists for depression as out-patients and in-patients, women with depression, seen by general practitioners and women found to be suffering from affective disorders in Camberwell in 1969/71 and in 1974/75 and in the Outer Hebrides in 1975. It is helpful to bear in mind that for the task of describing the distribution of psychiatric disorder we have relied on the population surveys of Camberwell and the Outer Hebrides and for work with the model we have used the various groups of depressed women, employing each to check on the others. These independent checks of the model have given remarkably similar results with two exceptions. Not all the vulnerability factors were important for the patient groups. We have not seen this as casting doubt on the model but as reflecting the influence of an additional set of factors influencing who receives psychiatric treatment. These factors have not been incorporated into the model itself as they do not strictly concern aetiological issues. Nonetheless we give them considerable importance, not least because some of the vulnerability factors in the model also appear to influence whether treatment is received. They do so, however, in a reverse direction. That is, experiences that increase risk of depression then act, once a woman is depressed, to reduce her chances of receiving psychiatric care. A pointer to this was the finding that, in Camberwell, women with children at home were both more likely to develop depression and less likely to see a general practitioner about it. This explains why some of the vulnerability factors are not found to occur more commonly in the patient group. The second exception concerns the symptom-formation factors. These are extremely influential among the patients but much less so among the comparatively less disturbed women not receiving psychiatric care. As yet we are uncertain about the significance of this exception.

To give the results in more detail: 15 per cent of the women in Camberwell were considered to be suffering from a definite affective disorder in the three months before we saw them. About half were *onset cases* who had developed a disorder in the year before interview and practically all were depressed. In contrast *chronic cases* had been disturbed more or less continuously for more than a year. All the *cases* had experienced symptoms of a severity which, if they were to have presented themselves for psychiatric out-patient treatment in the Camberwell area, would have been sufficient, in our judgment, for them to be considered as suffering from a psychiatric disorder and to have been given treatment. An additional 18 per cent of the women were suffering from a *borderline case* condition – that is from definite psychiatric symptoms which were not considered to be severe enough to rate as cases. The ratings of *cases* and *borderline cases* were reliable, although there is clearly an arbitrary element in distinguishing the two groups. In neither were we concerned with distress, dissatisfaction, and unhappiness, although these states undoubtedly overlap a good deal with the conditions we have studied.

Our main task, the development of a causal model, could not be done without close attention to methodological issues. Only in this way could a reasonable claim be made that the factors in the model were *in some way* involved in bringing about depression. Obvious biases had to be ruled out and objections that would trivialize the model met. Measurement can be viewed in terms of meeting methodological demands (is a causal interpretation possible?) or in terms of accuracy (is the world like this?). We have been critical of a good deal of measurement in the social sciences because it manages to do badly on both counts – reliance on the narrow, though superficially attractive, technology surrounding 'standardized questionnaires' produces results about which there can be no confidence either that a causal link is present or that anything meaningful about a person's life is reflected in the data. We have devoted four chapters to questions of measurement and a summary will not be attempted here. We believe that enough has been done to rule out possible sources of bias for the claims we make about causal processes to be taken seriously. However, a general comment about our approach may be helpful. Our argument that it is change in *thought* about the world that is crucial has an awkward corollary: what is perceived by X as a change will not necessarily be seen as such by Y. In a study of children handicapped after poliomyelitis – surely a major life-event – Fred Davis notes that:

'despite the obvious and sometimes abrupt changes in the family's scheme of life occasioned by the child's handicap, it was remarkable how little conscious or explicit awareness of such changes the families demonstrated. Each time a parent was interviewed, he was asked whether anyone in the family felt or acted differently toward the handicapped, whether the child acted or felt differently about himself. Almost invariably, although sometimes after a puzzled silence, the answer came back that nothing had changed . . . Were it not for the parent's incidental remarks and unreflecting reports on specific events and situations, one might not have surmised that there had been any significant alteration in their lives.' (1963: 162)

It is clear we must accept that what is going on in a person's life, a person's perception of this, and the way change and perception of change are reported by him may all differ. The question therefore arises whose perspective do we take about life-events and the changes they entail? Is any perspective more true than another? Much will depend on what we are trying to do but it is difficult to contemplate any way of dealing with such multiple perspectives without the investigator at some stage imposing his *own* viewpoint on the world. He must use his judgment not only for methodological reasons (discussed in earlier chapters) but because the world is capable of having an impact irrespective of the meanings a person brings it. A widow of forty-five with three children faces a different world, if she wishes to remarry, than one with no children; and the meaning of her widowhood will often only slowly emerge as she faces these contingencies.

In our own research we recorded what women said they felt about incidents (including our assessment of any feelings spontaneously expressed at other points in the interview). But for methodological reasons we have placed most weight on 'contextual' ratings which were designed to record what most women would have felt given the particular circumstances – past and present – of the individual woman. But while we did this primarily for methodological reasons we also believe such judgments on the part of the investigator are essential for social science research. It is unlikely that a situation can be satisfactorily described relying only on what a person is ready and able to state about it at a particular point in time. At a minimum the investigator must take account of feelings expressed in the interview (but not necessarily recognized or freely discussed by the person) and his judgment about the situation as a whole. Our approach in no way detracts from the importance of a person's experience of his or her world – indeed it is just this that is central to our theoretical ideas about the aetiology of depression. Further, we are fully aware that we have not exhausted ways of looking at what we have studied. In future work, for example, we need to look in far more detail at the way women think about and experience their depression. It is important to know, for instance, how many women describe characteristic symptoms such as slowness and lethargy in apparently moral terms such as laziness. In our work we have attempted to provide the foundation for such studies.

We began developing the model by studying the role of life-events, building on earlier research with schizophrenic patients. There are substantial causal effects in all five main samples of depressed women – that is among in-patients, out-patients, general practitioner patients, and the first and second Camberwell samples. It was not just any life-event however unpleasant that could bring about depression. Only certain *severe* events involving long-term threat were capable of doing so. Nineteen per cent of the women in Camberwell who were not cases had at least one such event in the nine months before interview compared with 61 per cent of the out-patients and in-patients in a comparable period before onset. Since some of the latter would be expected to have had an event that was not involved in bringing about the depression, we applied a correction formula that made allowances for this. This showed that the proportion of patients with a severe event of causal importance was 49 per cent. Using the same correction for onset cases in the general community gave a figure of 53 per cent. The distinctive feature of the great majority of the provoking events is the experience of loss or disappointment, if this is defined broadly to include threat of or actual separation from a key figure, an unpleasant revelation about someone close, a life-threatening illness to a close relative, a major material loss or general disappointment or threat of them, and miscellaneous crises such as being made redundant after a long period of steady employment. In more general terms the loss or disappointment could concern a person or object, a role, or an idea.

There has been a good deal of debate about what it is about life-events that plays an aetiological role in illness. Some have argued that change itself is enough (e.g. Dohrenwend, 1973; Rahe, 1969) but probably most have emphasized the importance of the meaning of events (e.g. Lazarus, 1966; Mechanic, 1962). The Camberwell research gives an unequivocal answer – at least for depression. Change in itself is of no importance – everything turns on the meaningfulness of events. Furthermore, events involving only short-term threat although they could bring considerable emotional torment (a child nearly dying), did not contribute to the onset of depression, at least in the sense of increasing the proportion of depressed women who were involved in a causal effect. It was only events involving long-term threat, lasting at least a week but usually a great deal longer, that were significant. No other aspect of events was found to be significant once such a threat had been taken into account. Detailed measures of changes in routine and in social contacts were unrelated to risk of depression – that is the proportion of events shown to be involved in a causal effect could not be increased over and above that obtained for severe events alone when these aspects were taken into account. For change to be important it had to be associated with long-term threat which in turn usually involved loss and disappointment.

Earlier we reviewed studies that have looked at this issue; the work of Paykel and his colleagues in New Haven comes closest to meeting methodological requirements and is in general fully consistent with these results.

A good deal of previous research has assumed that the effect of life-events is additive – that two events are more likely to bring about illness than one, and three more than two. This notion seems to derive from emphasis on the importance of change rather than the meaningfulness of events. It is easy to visualize a change of residence and a change of job as summating in their effect; less easy when it is known that the job was eagerly wanted and the house-move regretted and resented. To our knowledge the question of additivity has not been systematically tested. Indeed we had a good deal of difficulty in doing so – in our case because our measure of threat of a particular event took account of other relevant events. In rating that a woman had learnt she was pregnant, we would consider not only the event itself but the fact that her husband had not long left her. In terms of this example, since the separation from husband had been taken into account in the rating of the pregnancy, 'adding' the two events at the stage of analysis was probably superfluous.

Fortunately, there were also plenty of 'unrelated' events where this kind of overlap did not occur (death of a brother and a son being sent to prison) which could be used to test for an additive effect. This showed that while there was some evidence for an effect, it involved only a handful of the patients and none of the community cases. But at this point it is important to be clear that all we had done was to demonstrate that additivity was of little significance for events having no meaningful implications for each other.

In addition to events, ongoing difficulties were common in Camberwell and certain of them were capable of playing an aetiological role. We have called them *major* difficulties; all were markedly unpleasant, had lasted at least two years, and involved problems other than health. If major difficulties are considered with severe events, using the same correction formula, the proportion of women with depression having *either* one *or* the other of causal importance increases from 49 to 61 per cent for patients and from 52 to 83 per cent for onset cases. Difficulties, although of lesser importance than events, do play a definite aetiological role in depression.

More than one major difficulty did not increase risk of depression; nor was there an increased risk when they occurred with a severe event. It is as though it is only the meaning of *particular* losses and disappointments that bring about depression. The point made earlier when discussing the additivity of events still holds: events and also difficulties often act together to produce depression but only *when they have meaningful implications for each other*. Because of the way we had measured threat we could only demonstrate this in a series of special analyses. Pregnancy and birth, for example, were associated with a greater risk of depression but it was only in the context of an ongoing difficulty, particularly bad housing or poor marriage, that risk was increased. Other examples hinged on the way women adjusted to long-term adversity. Quite minor events could at times bring about depression if they served to 'bring home' the implications of some ongoing major loss or disappointment. A woman in Camberwell, for instance, living in bad housing became depressed four weeks after her sister's engagement. Another example was the failure of long-term health difficulties, no matter how serious, to bring about depression. It was only a crisis stemming from them – a husband's stroke, for example – that did so. Indeed it almost seemed as if without such a crisis the act of caring for someone gave women a sense of purpose which might even have reduced risk of depression. In summary, a special class of event, often quite minor, could force a reassessment of the meaning and purpose of life. Adaptation and accommodation to a major loss or disappointment might go on for months, if not years, perhaps with some elements of denial and then an event, sometimes quite trivial, would 'break through' to underline the hopelessness of the position. It had been impossible to demonstrate this role of minor events in the main analysis because they, for the most part, *only* acted in the presence of a major difficulty or severe event; they could not contribute to the estimate of proportion of events and difficulties involved in a causal effect as their role was subsidiary to more obviously threatening events and difficulties.

These severe events and major difficulties are the *provoking agents* of our model. But it was insufficient to establish a causal role for such events. It was also necessary to establish just what kind of cause was involved. It was still possible to assert, for example, that our findings were of little fundamental significance as the events for the most part merely triggered a depressive disorder about to occur in any case. Fortunately a clear answer could be given for events and, by implication, for the role of major difficulties.

The 'brought forward time' index (described in chapter 7) enabled us to show that the role of severe events is formative in the sense that they bring about a condition that would not have occurred for a long period or, more likely, not at all without them. The picture for schizophrenia is different. Here a wide range of events can bring about a sudden onset of florid symptoms. The arousal of *any* strong emotion, positive or negative, appears to be enough. Events probably bring about a disorder that would have occurred before long in any case. Results for schizophrenia therefore come closer to the view that it is change itself that is important – although even here it would certainly be misguided to underplay the role of meaning. Indeed, we suspect, though cannot demonstrate, that many of the events involved in bringing about schizophrenia have a particular symbolic significance for the patient, which is often far from obvious. The basic conclusion must surely be that different aspects of events will be significant in the aetiology of different conditions. Measurement has to be flexible enough to demonstrate (not just assume) what these are. Depression and schizophrenia are unlikely to represent the only possibilities – for instance, while streptococcal infections of the throat apparently respond to much the same pattern of factors as schizophrenia there is some hint that diabetes, hypertension, and myocardial infarction as well as peptic ulcers are unduly common among those having close responsibility for the lives of other people, such as anaesthetists and air traffic controllers (e.g. Cobb and Rose, 1973). Also of relevance is the fact that severe events and major difficulties were significant in the onset of all *types* of depression, including psychotic and neurotic forms. The regrouping of patients according to the presence of a provoking agent (i.e. as 'reactive' or 'endogenous') did not reveal different clinical syndromes associated with the presence of such an agent. There was a slight hint that a sub-group of depression might exist which was without a provoking agent and which also had a high chance of having one or two of the classic somatic symptoms of endogenous depression – early waking, and appetite loss. There was also a suggestion that severely threatening events which did not involve actual loss might be associated with a marked anxiety component in the depressive episode. But at best these were small tendencies – the over-riding conclusion must be that the presence, type, and frequency of provoking agents did not relate to the form or severity of depression – essentially the same findings held for in-patients, out-patients, patients seen by general practitioners, and those seen by no one.

These findings have at a number of points been anticipated in the research literature. A more challenging claim of the model is that a provoking agent is rarely sufficient on its own to bring about depression – although it does largely determine when a disorder occurs. The need for a second kind of aetiological factor in addition to a provoking agent is illustrated by the way depression is linked to social class in Camberwell. Among those with children at home, working-class women were four times more likely to suffer from a definite psychiatric disorder (about one in five in the three months before we saw them compared with about one in twenty of comparable middle-class women). They were also a good deal more likely to experience a provoking agent. And yet surprisingly the latter explained relatively little of the class difference in depression. This can be seen in the way working-class women with children were four times more likely than similar middle-class women to develop a depressive disorder *when they had a provoking agent*. It was this greater vulnerability once an event or difficulty had occurred that had to be explained if the class differences in incidence of depression were to be understood.

It was clear that other factors, also related to social class, must be at work, and we therefore looked for the *vulnerability* factors of our model. We found that if a woman does not have an intimate tie, someone she can trust and confide in, particularly a husband or boyfriend, she is much more likely to break down in the presence of a severe event or major difficulty. Similarly she is more at risk if she has three or more children under fourteen at home and if she has lost her mother (but not father) before the age of eleven. None of these factors are capable of producing depression on their own but each greatly increases risk in the presence of a provoking agent. When they are considered together the importance of yet another factor, employment, emerges. *Table 3* in chapter 11 summarizes our findings. Women with a confiding tie with a husband or boyfriend are protected in the presence of a provoking agent whether or not any of the other three vulnerability factors are present; although risk is not negligible – one in ten with a provoking agent compared with one in 100 without. Where such a tie is lacking, risk increases when there is a provoking agent. It is greatest for those with one or more vulnerability factors in addition to lack of a confiding relationship; of particular note is the way employment halves the risk of depression among those with a provoking agent but without a confiding tie with husband or boyfriend. It was the fact that the working-class women had more of these vulnerability factors that explained most of the class differences in risk of depression. This also explains why the class differences in risk are restricted to women with children.

In summary: some of the social class difference in risk of depression is due to the fact that working-class women experience more severe life-events and major difficulties, especially when they have children; problems concerning housing, finance, husband, and child (excluding those involving health) are particularly important. Incidents of this kind are the only kind of severe event to occur more commonly among working-class women and are the most obvious candidates for the 'inner city' stresses which are the focus of much current social commentary. But most of the class difference in depression is due to the greater likelihood of a working-class woman having one or more of the four vulnerability factors and not to their greater risk of experiencing a provoking agent.

So far we have considered risk of developing depression in the year. When we consider chronic conditions the lot of working-class women is, if anything, even worse. A disconcerting number were chronic cases and this may prove to be one of the most significant findings of the Camberwell survey. In keeping with this, all forms of marked long-term difficulty were more common among working-class women and physical health problems were particularly common among those with a chronic case or borderline case condition. We have made, we believe, a reasonable prima facie case that some of the difficulties, particularly concerning housing, had served to perpetuate the psychiatric conditions, but because the onset of these conditions had preceded the year of investigation we could not definitely establish that the causal link was only in this direction; we could not rule out the possibility that the depression had also served to perpetuate the difficulty; and, of course, both processes could be at work even in the same person.

There was less depression in the rural community in the Outer Hebrides than in Camberwell. Unfortunately we did not document the rate of particular types of events and difficulties on the island and thus explore the idea that urban stresses are of a different quality. Nonetheless it is important that there were no class differences in prevalence of psychiatric disorder and no tendency for women with children to be at increased risk. These differences from Camberwell could result from the greater degree of overall protection their culture and society give these women but this has still to be documented in detail.

The comparative material raises a more general point. The Camberwell results would not necessarily be expected to occur in other urban communities or even elsewhere in London. Replication will depend on how far the conditions outlined in the model are associated with class and, even if they are, whether they have the same significance. This is the point of theory. The significance of something like going out to work is bound to depend on the broader social setting. Confirmation of the Camberwell results will therefore depend on tests of the theory as well as the model. It will be necessary to show that going out to work *does* have the same significance in different settings: and this, of course, will depend on the theoretical interpretations of the factors in the model.

In addition to the 15 per cent with a definite psychiatric disorder we have already noted that almost one in five of the women in Camberwell suffered from a borderline condition. Overall these were unrelated to class or life-stage, although chronic states were somewhat more common among working-class women. Onset of borderline conditions was strongly linked to the same provoking agents that bring about case conditions; but those who developed only a borderline condition in response to a severe event or major difficulty were more protected in terms of the four vulnerability factors. Depression in this sense is not an all or nothing matter; women are more or less successful in warding off a clear-cut depressive disorder according to the degree to which they are protected.

The frequency of borderline conditions raises the general issue of the nature of the phenomena we have recorded. The commonness of case conditions among working-class women is startling. We are fairly convinced about two things: first, that the conditions we have classified as cases are comparable in terms of severity with many of the affective disorders treated by psychiatrists at out-patient level, although we do not suggest that the distribution of severity among them exactly duplicates that of the treated conditions. They do, however, fall well within the range of conditions seen and treated by psychiatrists. Second, we are convinced that many of the borderline case conditions (as well as the cases) attend general practice surgeries and probably receive the bulk of the large quantities of psychotropic drugs prescribed there. A series of research and practical issues arise at this point about which we are much less clear. Although cases appear to be closely similar to those seen in psychiatric out-patient clinics there may well be important differences – at least for some of them. Obvious possibilities concern duration and fluctuation in the severity of the condition (although it must be remembered that half the cases had experienced much the same level of symptomatology for well over a year). A further possibility concerns differences in coping: there may well be differences both between and within the groups in reaching a decision to seek treatment either from a general practitioner or a psychiatric department. There are three obvious ways in which this might occur. First, there may be treatment barriers such as having young children. Second, the women may give different explanations of their psychiatric state. As far as we could tell (although we did not examine this systematically) the majority saw their social environment as of crucial importance – under these circumstances a woman may well be less motivated to seek psychiatric help. Third, there will almost certainly be personality factors. No one who has interviewed women at random in a general population survey can be anything but impressed by the determination of some to carry on with their lives as though little was wrong in spite of an intolerable burden of symptoms.

But even if there were some tendency for treated and untreated conditions to differ, it would still be essential to study a full spectrum of affective states for the phenomenon actually seen by psychiatrists to be understood. The issue of who is selected into psychiatric care needs to loom far larger in psychiatric research and theory (see Mechanic and Newton, 1965). That there is selection is clear: in Camberwell, for example, women receiving psychiatric care are no more likely to have children than women in the population in general and only a little more likely to be working-class. The implications of such selection may prove to be revolutionary not only where it is treatment-seeking but some other form of self-selection which has defined the target sample. For instance, it will have occurred to many readers that one of Durkheim's main findings – often replicated – runs directly counter to our own (Veevers, 1973). He found that the highest suicide rate is among childless wives and not single women and that married women with children were still lower. His interpretation is well known:

'. . . in itself, conjugal society is harmful to woman and aggravates her tendency to suicide. If most wives have, nevertheless, seemed to enjoy a coefficient of preservation, this is because childless households are the exception and consequently the presence of children in most cases corrects and reduces the evil effects of marriage.' (Durkheim, 1952: 189)

He goes on to suggest that children offer women greater protection than men because 'women profit more from children' and are 'more sensitive to their happy influence'. But it is possible that far from having a 'happy influence' the presence of children may merely determine whether suicide is or is not the outcome of an unhappiness common to all married women, whether or not they have children. A number of women in our sample told us that the only thing that prevented them from harming themselves was the need to care for their children. Similarly we found that women with three or more children at home, although as depressed as other women, were less likely to have consulted a general practitioner about their depression.

The parallel suggested between the effects of these two types of selection, treatment-seeking and suicidal behaviour, highlights the danger of drawing conclusions about suicide. Statistics concerning suicide are usually criticized for being unreliable, but as important a deficiency is their selectivity even if completely accurate: it is not clear what those who commit suicide can be said to represent. Although it is clear they are for the most part miserable people it will not do to assume that they can be used to represent all miserable people in the community and to use them to draw conclusions about the distribution of misery in the population at large. We are so impressed by this possible pitfall that we begin to doubt the usefulness of much social and clinical research with psychiatric patients – at least with the more common conditions – without parallel investigations of those *not* receiving psychiatric care (or not, for example, committing suicide). The effects of selection are likely to be so pervasive that it is not unreasonable to ask for evidence that findings are not the result of selective processes. One area where this is particularly relevant is the study of the impact of early loss of parent; the long history of inconclusive, inconsistent, and often negative findings has probably been due to the fact that early loss of a mother not only increases risk of depression but also relates to factors that make psychiatric treatment less likely.

But we still have not dealt fully with the implications of the high rate of psychiatric disorder among working-class women. Most of the women with a case or borderline case condition suffered considerable distress and there is thus undoubtedly a large overlap between our psychiatric categories and more traditional notions of happiness and dissatisfaction. Four in ten of the working-class women with a child at home expressed either considerable dissatisfaction with their marriage or notably little warmth or enthusiasm about it. Two-thirds of these women were cases or borderline cases compared with only 17 per cent of the rest of the women. Does this suggest that what we have been discussing is so common that it cannot be considered a medical phenomenon; being part of daily life it is just a particularly unpleasant form of unhappiness? To some extent this question confuses two separate issues: first, the mere frequency of a condition is not logically related to its medical or non-medical status. The frequency of hookworm infection in certain communities does not prevent it from remaining a sign of ill-health. Second, the overlap between unhappiness and depression does not mean that they are not logically distinct concepts. We did not pursue the issue of unhappiness not because it seemed less important or because a strictly clinical approach was in some way superior; we did not do so simply because it would have required measures of greater sensitivity and theoretical clarity than we possessed. To measure happiness it is necessary to be able to establish in some detail just what a woman values. We had neither the time to develop such measures nor to collect such material during the interview. As Donne suggests 'All men call *Misery, Misery,* but *Happinesse* changes the name, by the taste of man'.[1]

In future research we visualize taking the middle ground, looking both at psychiatric and more general concepts. Meanwhile the effect on the woman and her family of case, and even borderline case conditions, should not be dismissed. When psychiatrists call such states 'minor' affective disorders they refer to a comparison with major depressive illnesses, perhaps with severe retardation and delusions, not to the 'minor' amount of suffering involved or their impact on others. Personally and socially the impact can be serious, although the symptoms themselves may not rate as serious in psychiatric terms. To illustrate: as part of the life-events interview we collected details of any accident to those at home that required treatment by a casualty department or general practitioner: they included fractures, severe cuts, burns, and one death. Both social class *and* psychiatric disorder are independently related to accidents occurring to children under fifteen in the twelve months of the survey. While 9.5 per cent of the 420 children of the women with such a child at home had an accident, 19.2 per cent of the children of working-class women with a case or borderline case condition had one, 9.6 per cent of other working-class women, 5.3 per cent of middle-class women with a case or borderline condition, and only 1.5 per cent of the rest of middle-class women. The accidents were not restricted to the younger children. If anything, they were more common among the older children. That a direct causal link is involved is suggested by the fact that the rate of accidents to children among women with borderline and case conditions during periods in the year *before* the onset of their symptoms was no different from that among the children of other women.[2] The point for the present argument is that the association of accidents with psychiatric state is almost as high for borderline case as for case conditions. The full personal and social cost of such conditions is still to be documented, but we probably already know enough to see them as a major social problem.

So far we have described the two factors in our model concerned with the risk of developing a depressive condition. Some headway was also made in understanding what influences the type and severity of symptoms once a woman is depressed. This involves the third set of *symptom-formation* factors. We have in fact described two effects. One way we tried to overcome the complexity of the different characteristics of depression was to make a judgment about overall severity, taking number of symptoms, severity of individual symptoms, and degree of interference with routine and employment into account. When this was done, as might be expected, in-patients were on the whole more severely depressed than out-patients and it was this difference between the treatment groups that, in the first instance, we set out to explain. At onset in-patients and out-patients did not differ in severity; differences in severity emerged only some time after onset. A third of the patients had one or more marked worsenings of their depression which could be dated to a matter of a few days (change-points) and the entire difference in severity between the two treatment groups was associated with these changes – in-patients had more of them and when they had them they tended to deteriorate to a greater extent.

We discovered three variables that explained, at least in statistical terms, the difference in severity of the two treatment groups. First, severe events occurring *after* first onset were capable of producing a subsequent change in condition – almost as though a new 'onset' was superimposed on the existing depression. But more important were *past losses*. These were by and large losses of the immediate family in childhood and adolescence (parents and siblings) although we also included loss of children and death of a husband in adulthood if these were more than two years before onset. There is a small overlap with the vulnerability factors here as loss of mother before eleven also increases risk of depression in the presence of a provoking agent. But the overlap is not great. Loss of mother before eleven forms only about a fifth of the total experience of past loss in Camberwell and it is *any* past loss that increases severity of depressive symptoms. The results so far concern the patients but they can be extended to the general population in the sense that the amount of past loss was lower amongst women developing borderline case conditions than among cases; and the difference between case or borderline conditions seems best conceived in terms of severity. However when cases in Camberwell are considered there is *no* association between severity of disorder among them and past loss. While this may be partly due to the relatively small number of women in this group who were highly disturbed, it is more likely that future research will need to pinpoint special characteristics of a subgroup of past losses, such as unsatisfactory substitute care, which are particularly effective in influencing depression in later life.

Finally, experience of a previous episode of depression, for the patient series at least, was associated with greater severity. When considered together the three variables (that is, a severe event after onset, past loss, and a previous episode) entirely explained the difference in severity of depression between in-patients and out-patients.

But there is a second aspect of symptom formation – the classic *psychotic/neurotic division* made on the basis of the presence or absence of symptoms such as early waking and diurnal variation. The distinction has been central to much psychiatric research on depression during the last fifty years and requires separate study from overall severity in the sense that, as measured by us, the two were only moderately correlated. Much the most important factor relating to the diagnostic distinction was again past loss, but now viewed in a new way according to type of past loss. Psychotic depressive conditions were highly related to past loss by *death* and neurotic depressive conditions to past loss by *separation* – by, for example, divorce of parents or adoption of a child. Moreover when diagnosis *and* severity were considered, the latter was related to the presence of past deaths within the psychotic group and to past separation within the neurotic group. The associations of diagnosis with type of past loss are large and were not explained by factors such as age and previous episode. Furthermore the results were almost exactly repeated on a separate series of patients classified as psychotic and neurotic by another research psychiatrist.

We have now summarized the three factors of the model. In depression the role of the provoking agents is more than that of mere triggers of a condition whose aetiology lies largely elsewhere and we attribute its onset, with all its physiological components, primarily to experiences of loss and disappointment, particularly those involving the woman's view of her own identity. The range of these experiences is far broader than the bereavements held to be associated with depression. Bereavements, in fact, formed only about a tenth of the severe events (and an even smaller proportion of the provoking agents as a whole). We have therefore extended the notion of loss to include not only that of a person in ways other than death but also loss of a role and loss of an idea. This is all fairly clear from our material but from this point our theory becomes more speculative. The feelings of hopelessness, which to a greater or lesser degree follow a major loss and disappointment, will on occasion become generalized to form the central triad of the depressive experience described by Aaron Beck as the feeling that the self is worthless, the future hopeless, and the world meaningless. In arithmetical terms this occurs to one in five of the women with a provoking agent – only this proportion develop clinical depression. In our view this is because the generalization of the feelings of hopelessness has not occurred in the other four of the five. In order to explain this we have suggested that the role of the four vulnerability factors is both to lower the ongoing sense of self-esteem well before the onset of depression and thus to potentiate this generalization of hopelessness in the context of a provoking agent. Without one or more of the vulnerability factors a woman might well be able to work through the experience of loss and disappointment and find new sources of positive value, thus keeping her experience of depression within the bounds of a 'borderline case' or more often of normal grief, simple sadness, or distress.

The role of self-esteem can be seen both in a passive and in an active sense. So far, by implication at least, we have emphasized a passive interpretation – that a woman develops profound hopelessness or alternatively finds it too painful to work through her grief because of the feelings of low self-regard she brings to the loss. But the more active possibility should not be overlooked. If a woman has three or more children under fourteen living at home or has no employment outside the home, she is less able to move into new areas of activity or to make new contacts on which she can build new sources of value. The role of isolation in depression is also suggested by the ability of an intimate relationship to reduce risk of disorder. While such a relationship is likely to help provide some women with a basic sense of self-worth it also has its more active aspect. The availability of a confidant, a person to whom one can reveal one's weaknesses without risk of rebuff and thus further loss of self-esteem, may act as a buttress against the total evaporation of feelings of self-worth following a major loss or disappointment. Furthermore, the ability to talk with someone about one's feelings is a safe-guard against some sort of blanket defence mechanism of denial preventing the working through of grief. The particular importance of the intimate relationship being with a man raises questions about the value of sexuality (or at any rate some sort of physical intimacy perhaps less sexual than nurturant), but these cannot be answered without more detailed research. A sexual aspect is probably not essential for an intimate relationship to be protective; much is bound to depend on what is expected by the woman herself.

Our own interpretation of the husband as a confidant is that with the current organization of the family in urban centres, he is usually the main source of a woman's sense of achievement. It will be remembered that the risk of depression was greatest among working-class women with children at home, for whom a sense of achievement would be most closely related to their roles as mother and wife. She needs to be 'told' she is doing well to refurbish her sense of self-worth. Mary Boulton in an intensive study of women with children, in fifty London families, has described the extensive influence a husband can have on a woman's experience as a mother. A husband's appreciation is a reward in itself as well as supporting a sense of accomplishment in the way she deals with day-to-day problems of child care. His acceptance that there are difficulties and frustrations legitimizes the experiences of pervasive irritation and unhappiness felt by many women about the routine care of children and helps them to accept that this does not reflect on themselves. In general his support helps a woman to create a rewarding idea of herself. Boulton also documents that working-class husbands are more likely to fail to recognize the difficulties and frust-rations of child care. More see it as an 'easy' and 'cushy' job thereby trivializing the work and lowering their wife's sense of self-worth (Boulton, 1977).

The fourth vulnerability factor, loss of mother before eleven, we see as working in a number of ways. First, that it may have a crucial impact, in social terms, on the course of a girl's life: she may leave school earlier, make a hurried marriage, have her first child at an early age, fail to find satisfying work when she first leaves school just because she has no mother; and all this will mean that later in life she has fewer alternatives available to her when faced with loss. Second, we emphasize the impact of loss of mother before eleven on the woman's internal resources, her psychological strength, and optim-ism. On the one hand it is likely to have left her with a permanently lowered sense of her own worth. In this second sense it acts as the three other vulnerability factors in terms of ongoing low self-esteem. Third, we believe the early loss may not have been 'worked through' and a later loss is therefore more likely to revive traces of the earlier

experience which intensifies the current one along the lines of a rever-
berating circuit; of course earlier maladaptive defense mechanisms
may also be revived.

It is through this final process that we see the second and third
factors of the model as overlapping, that is, loss of mother before
eleven is included in the more general category of past loss, where it
acts not as a vulnerability factor but as a factor contributing to
symptom-formation. In order to explain the effect of past loss on
symptom formation we have postulated an intervening cognitive set
which not only influences the severity but also the type of symptoms.
Crucial aspects of this cognitive set are its fatalism and the related
degree of protest. Evidence concerning individual symptoms among
depressed patients such as violent acting out behaviour and retardation suggests that such a set may be responsible for the association of
past deaths with retarded depression where the patient has 'given up',
in Engel's sense, more completely than in the neurotic gesture of
despair. Past loss of any type can, according to this theory, influence
the cognitive set and thus act as a symptom-formation factor.

The role of severe events in producing further 'onsets' in an established depression is a special instance of the role of provoking agents
and while contributing to severity is probably best seen separately
from the other symptom-formation factors. But it does remind us of
the importance of taking into account the course of a depressive
episode and of not looking at symptoms only at first onset or at the
point of admission.

Emphasis in our theory has thus been upon the psychosocial aspects
of loss, particularly upon the appraisal of implications of event or
difficulty by the woman herself. But the model also leaves room for
other factors which we have not been able to identify with any clarity.
These may be other psycho-social factors or physiological ones. Indeed
one of the symptom-formation factors, a previous episode, is theoretically ambiguous in this sense; at this stage it is impossible to say
whether it acts upon the cognitive set, perhaps making it easier for a
woman to give up more quickly just because she has done so before, or
whether it is merely a sign that the woman has always been phy-
siologically susceptible to depression or had become so as a consequence of earlier depression. The latter possibilities would probably
work largely in a 'mechanical' way, independently of her appraisal, to
increase the severity of the disorder once it develops. Age is similarly
ambiguous. Though it plays no role as a provoking agent or vulnerability factor, it is related to the type of depression once onset has
occurred, older women being more likely to have psychotic-type
depressions. While there are undoubted physiological accom-

paniments to the aging process, a psychosocial impact cannot be entirely ignored, as the literature on the 'mid-life crisis' reminds one. Butler (1968) has speculated on the 'universal occurrence in older people of an inner experience or mental process of reviewing one's life' and believes that it can contribute to clinical depression.[3]

Leaving aside the actual processes involved, there is also room in our model for another concept, that of susceptibility. This putative fourth factor, unlike the three others of the model, implies that a woman is generally susceptible to depression (in the limiting case developing it spontaneously); but also that once depressed she will develop a more 'severe' depression. At present the notion of susceptibility has very little by way of supporting evidence although something of the kind seems highly likely. While leaving room for it in the model, we do not see it necessarily as acting only in the absence of loss; on the contrary, the analysis of the twenty-eight patients without a severe event or major difficulty suggests that *some* form of loss precedes almost all instances of depression. One important area to explore in future is just such patients without severe events or major difficulties before onset. Research might also profit from a special selection of patients with hallucinations and delusions. Under a tenth of our patients had hallucinations and the figure was only a little higher for delusions of any kind. In view of the rarity of these and of pathological guilt among the general population cases, there is much to be said for seeking out such symptoms in future work. Meanwhile it is reasonable to rest some faith in these results that have emerged from a sample of patients unselected for anything except onset within the last year. They suggest that social factors play a formative role in the majority of onsets of depression at all treatment levels and with diverse symptom pictures and that they also enhance both vulnerability to loss events and severity of the condition once it occurs; that the processes by which they have this impact work through the person's appraisal of their meaning for her and her life plans; and that the somatic symptoms of depression are the sequelae of the basic cognitive appraisal. The results as a whole focus attention on the importance of attachment theory for the understanding of depressive phenomena. But this does not mean, of course, that they just have implications in terms of individual psychology. The social class differences have much wider implications. The possibility that there exists a special group of 'inner-city stresses' with attendant inner-city disorders sets the results firmly in the context of the discussion of 'urban crisis'.

One point raised by these broader factors is the significance of the accelerating and unbalanced outflow of population from the centre of London – particularly of the more skilled and mobile. How far has it tended to leave a relatively more disadvantaged group of people in our inner cities? It is perhaps worth recalling that our two-fold social class division is arbitrary and that three more or less equal social categories give a progressive gradation of psychiatric disorder. Our discussion of working and middle class is no more than a way of speaking; the effect appears to be a straight forward function of 'standing in society' and, as we have seen, appears to be entirely explained by differences in the distribution of the provoking agents and vulnerability factors of our model. The question of population movement can be viewed in economic and material terms or in terms of some notion of personal inferiority. The latter theme, of course, has always been present when discussing the poor and disadvantaged. Given some of its unpalatable political implications, it seems pointless to spend time on the matter until the necessary research has been done. Quite straightforward comparative research would take us a long way. Would our findings hold in 'newer', less disadvantaged populations when individual women had been matched for the experience of comparable 'factors' in the model? *Table 3* in chapter 11 is again central; we suspect that, although the distribution of women among the various risk groups would differ, reflecting the overall greater advantages of a 'newer' population, the rates of psychiatric disorder *within* the various risk groups would be the same as for the women in Camberwell. This, after all, can already be seen when comparing class groups within Camberwell itself. While we are content to leave the matter for empirical enquiry it is difficult to deny that the implication of the model as a whole is that major improvements could be obtained by changes in the environment – sadly, however, well-intentioned intervention in terms of traditional 'social work' might not prove very helpful (Geismer *et al.*, 1972; Goldberg, 1973).

These general comments overlay an uncomfortable awareness of how much there is still to be done before the model can be said to have been satisfactorily linked to broader social processes. Sociology has always had its own brands of psychology although often disguised. We have, in effect, developed a social psychological theory of depression and at the same time made a reasonable case for the relevance of wider social processes, leaving more obscure than we like the details of this influence. Just how much, for instance, of the difficulty of women with young children stems from the circumstances of their task and how much from a sense of doing work that is undervalued in a society geared to reward through employment? How many of the marital difficulties associated with working-class life stem from the physical problems associated with rearing young children and how many from wider values linked to sex-roles? It is not particularly helpful to point out that to some degree all are probably involved. While we know enough about family life in London to give some answers – for instance, about class differences in the amount of cooperation between husband and wife in child-rearing and household tasks – it would nonetheless at present be speculative to link them with our model (see Oakley, 1974; Ginsberg, 1976; and Boulton, 1977).

It is perhaps unnecessary to emphasize in any case just how many of the theoretical interpretations that we have used still wait to be firmly established. Further research can go in a number of directions. It can expand the time dimension by documenting earlier experiences more carefully, for example tracing long-term class differences in experience more systematically, particularly in ways of coping with crises in early life. Alternatively, work can document the present more sensitively – the things a woman has and would like to have that make her life meaningful and how these interact with the 'factors' in our model. This will involve establishing how far some women are more protected, not because they avoid fundamental crises, but because of the greater variety of their lives and a greater input of 'positive' experiences, which enable them to hope for better things more easily. The middle-class woman can more often travel, visit friends at some distance, or buy a new dress; she has perhaps greater confidence and skills in seeking out pleasurable experiences; and also a stronger belief that she will eventually achieve certain goals of importance. Adjustment in adversity may prove to be largely a matter of how to sustain hope for better things.

As well as provoking guidelines for further research, these results as they stand can provide the kernel of a radical critique of the broader cultural, political, and economic system and, more narrowly, of the role of the medical and other helping professions. They have implications that concern not only the optimum organization of the family but also the role of women in the wider economy and the values given these functions by the media and society at large. They also suggest that no single avenue of intervention is likely to provide the best answer for a condition with such complex aetiology. Once it can be accepted that in many cases a combination of chemotherapy and psychotherapy needs supplementing with social changes, such as work or regular meaningful activity outside the home, the role of medical and social agencies in the treatment of depression should emerge in a new perspective. Instead of competing for priority in explanation and treatment, each would contribute information and recommendations to the other, thus giving what would be truly psychosomatic attention to a troubled person instead of just treatment to a 'sick' woman or solace to a stricken mind. Under such circumstances the issue as to whether depression was or was not an 'illness' would become a pointless linguistic wrangle as unimportant as the discussion as to whether water at 85°F is hot or not hot but merely warm. In the end in such debates the contestants usually abandon the dichotomous label in favour of a dimensional type of description, in this example the Fahrenheit scale. At the moment it is impossible to dismiss it as such, as a sterile controversy, without appearing to be cowardly evading important moral decisions which seem to flow from asserting or denying it to be 'illness' – the decision, for instance, about when a person requires attention or privacy or compulsory treatment of some kind. And yet it is important to come out into the open and say that in some sense it is a non-issue, because by focussing on that alone, discussion can often afford to miss the details of exactly those important moral and practical issues that underlay the original furor. These are issues that concern both the genesis of the condition, and so in some sense involve the problem of free will and responsibility, and its management and outcome, thus involving stigmatization and the distribution of social resources to relieve the genuine distress of those involved. When these issues are confronted directly, the vaguer issue of illness/non-illness loses its importance. Meanwhile although our results leave no doubt of the relevance of the notion of illness for at least some with a depressive disorder, the term should be used sparingly, for it is an easy trap in which clear thinking can be snared by dualistic fallacies.[4] For it is difficult to maintain that our borderline cases should not attend general practice surgeries just because their symptoms, not having passed the threshold of caseness, do not qualify them to be considered as ill.

The results of this study suggest that the understanding of untreated depressions can be of great help in the understanding of those that have reached the treatment setting, and thus that even severely disturbed in-patients might benefit if physical treatments were supplemented by what might be called social therapy designed to raise their sense of self-esteem and increase the alternative sources of value available to them in the long term. The number of depressed women not seen by psychiatrists is large and of those not seen, or, in effect, not given serious attention by their general practitioner, is not inconsiderable. This is one, but, of course, not the only reason why the issue of treatment must be considered side by side with the issue of prevention. The implication of these results for the latter can only be the need for wider social and political changes which would mean that fewer people experienced provoking agents and fewer people were vulnerable in the first place. These findings provide backing for many reforms in our current social organization, increases in the number of nursery school places and the number of part-time employment opportunities for women being some obvious candidates. They point, too, to the large areas of loneliness and isolation which exist amid our so-called affluence, and to the important role they play in determining family health. To combat these, and to build a sense of mastery and self-esteem, which will render every member of the community more resilient to the buffets of experience, requires more than comforting talk in a surgery, although even this is all too often not available.

While these results show that things are not well there are no grounds whatsoever to suggest matters are getting *worse*. We just do not possess the necessary evidence about the past. If we were to speculate we suspect things have improved; certainly what little evidence we have from the two Camberwell surveys five years apart could be seen as some hint of this. But for an understanding of what is going on and what might be done we have no doubt that more must be known about the effect of particular social contexts on particular psychiatric disorders (and for that matter physical disorders). After all, 'integration' into the small-scale community in the Outer Hebrides is not, apparently, without cost in terms of psychiatric disorder other than depression. We must not, in any case, lose sight of the fact that the particular form of psychiatric problems is likely to change – both in time and space. Only theoretical understanding of what is going on can help in these circumstances.

We do not suggest withdrawal from these wider concerns. Research on psychiatric or medical disorders should not be divorced from moral and political awareness. Whether we like it or not, the finding that so many working-class women in Camberwell were psychiatrically disturbed is not a sterilized neutral fact. But, at the same time, if the problems are too broadly stated there will be a danger that little will be forthcoming in the way of worthwhile knowledge about both origins of depression and treatment and preventive strategies.

Future research will need to focus on the role of the immediate social context, on individuals and their households, and on how they get caught up in a crisis or difficulty, try to cope with it, and the resources they have for this. But at the same time the possibility of spelling out broader links must be pursued. There is a somewhat uneasy division of labour here. Both individual-orientated and society-orientated studies are required; both are part of sociology and both are essential. The need is for each to remember the other. It is too easy for the broader approach to ignore the complexities of the individual's immediate social milieu and for the more detailed approach to get lost in the intricacies of the individual personality.

Part VI
Appendices

Appendix 1
Examples of caseness
and borderline caseness

1 Chronic case of depression

Mrs A. was a 54-year-old married woman who lived in a high-rise council block in Camberwell. She worked as a part-time office cleaner in the early mornings. Mrs A's husband suffered from chronic relapsing schizophrenia and, although in regular employment when well, he was very withdrawn, odd in his habits, and unable to sustain a close relationship. They had one son who was married and living in Surrey but they had little contact with him or any other relative – Mrs A had no close friends.

She has been unhappy and dissatisfied with her life for many years and did not think she had been really well since her twenties. She had a previous history of two 'nervous breakdowns', both treated at home by her family doctor, one during the last war which suddenly followed a report that her husband was missing, and the second 14 years ago. Her descriptions of both episodes suggested depressive episodes.

For the past four years Mrs A had been chronically depressed. Her mood fluctuated but she had been feeling particularly low during the few weeks before interview. She said 'I feel as if I want to go to bed and never wake up' – the future looked bleak and unchanging and she had contemplated suicide from time to time. This was on the whole a fleeting thought: she felt she must keep trying to look on the bright side. She felt mentally and physically exhausted and neglected her housework and knitting. 'I can't be bothered with anyone. I'm in a dream, everything vague.' She felt she could not concentrate on any work or leisure activity since she was constantly worrying over trivial matters which made her feel keyed up and tense. She got off to sleep quite easily with the aid of 'Sonalgin' (Barbiturate and Phenacetin), but woke frequently through the night and finally woke in the early hours, unable to get off to sleep again. She felt at her lowest at this time of day. Her appetite had been poor for a year and she never enjoyed her food, but in the last month she had lost 4 or 5 lbs. Mrs A attributed her depression to her unhappy marriage and her mild, grumbling osteoarthritis.

2 Onset mixed case of depression and anxiety

Mrs B was 18 years old, worked full-time as a telephonist, and was married to a 19-year-old labourer. They had a 2-year-old baby who was born prematurely after a difficult labour and had been obviously spastic since birth. Mrs B said she had always been a nervous, jittery person and indeed during the interview she moved restlessly round the room, fidgetted, and was anxiously overtalkative. She felt that she had become much worse since her baby was born and now found it impossible to relax. She felt anxious about being left alone in the house with the baby and often had a dry mouth and butterflies in the stomach. On one occasion recently she felt so frightened she picked up the baby and rushed out of the house to the fresh air in a panic. Even with her husband in the house she hated being in a different room from him and slept with the hall lights on so that she would not feel afraid to get up in the night alone.

During the last two years she had had bouts of depression lasting only two or three days, but three months before interview she began to feel more seriously depressed and tearful. Her anxiety symptoms worsened and she began to panic in shops, crowds, and in buses. Her regular tension headaches worsened and she described them as 'unbearable – like clamps round my head'. She was unable to concentrate on work or housework and stopped away from work for three weeks. She felt extremely tired and slept very heavily, waking late and feeling unrefreshed. She had lost interest in food and had lost 1½ stones in 2 months – she had been overweight after the baby's birth and wanted to lose weight but had never been successful before. She found herself 'flying off the handle at everyone' and withdrew from even her husband's company. 'I felt I was in a maze, closed in, tucked up inside myself.' The future looked black but she did not actively contemplate suicide. She took a handful of prescribed 'Motival' tablets on an impulse one day. Her GP referred her to the Emergency Clinic but she did not keep her appointment. Five or six weeks after the onset of severe symptoms, her depression began to lift and at interview she was mildly depressed but chronically anxious.

3 Chronic case depression

Mrs C was well until her husband's death in an accident 2 years ago. Shortly after this she became very depressed, became completely anergic, and took to her bed. She lost her appetite and 18 pounds in weight and complained of early morning wakings. She said she completely lost interest in her surroundings and neglected the children. Her GP suggested she go into hospital but she made a great effort to look after the children properly. Her symptoms continued until about six months before interview when she began to regain a few pounds in weight. However, she continued to feel tired most of the time and felt her housework took too long to do – sometimes she rested one to two hours in between her domestic chores. She felt moderately depressed most of the time, though this was less severe than 6 months ago. 'I just keep going, thinking there must be someone worse off than myself.' She was no longer able to enjoy herself and felt she did not care what happened to her. Whereas she used to be a very sociable person, she had lost interest in visiting relatives and now only saw her father. Her concentration had improved in the past few months and she was now able to read books for fairly long periods of time. She still had difficulty getting off to sleep and woke between 6 and 7 a.m. She felt mentally tense and nervous every few days and this could be very intense and distressing.

4 Onset case depression

Mrs W was 57 years old, previously widowed and separated from her second husband. She lived on her own as a tenant of her in-laws, and worked full time in a clerical job. Three months before interview, she began to have pain in her stomach. She went to her GP 'glad that this time it was physical not mental', since she had two previous admissions to mental hospital. However, after a Barium meal, she was told that the pains were probably due to 'nerves'. Six weeks later the pains went away but she began to feel depressed – this was about six weeks before the interview. She had feelings of hopelessness and suicidal thoughts, although did not make a suicide attempt (she had a history of three previous overdoses). At the same time she became tearful and became preoccupied with paranoid ideas about her relatives; for example she would not go through their part of the house to use the toilet, but went to the public lavatory down the road since she felt her relatives were against her in an unexplained way. Her thinking was muddled but she had not interpreted this as being due to outside influence. She felt exhausted and lacking in energy and could not get through her housework. She lost interest in going to her Ladies' Darts Club and in meeting people but continued to take a pride in her appearance. She had increased her consumption of alcohol during this past three months and had experienced periods of amnesia. She was being treated with Largactil by her GP.

5 Chronic borderline case depression

Mrs E was 56 years old and had been married for 30 years to an unskilled labourer. She had an unmarried daughter living at home who was chronically handicapped with schizophrenia, and a married son who lived out of London and whom she saw infrequently. There was constant bickering and friction between Mrs E and her husband caused by resentment because he took no interest in their sick daughter and she felt she had had to carry all the burden of coping with the daughter's erratic behaviour and frequent relapses. She said she had felt 'fed-up' and miserable for the past couple of years and no longer looked forward to going out socially or to holidays like she used to – she said she could not be bothered to meet people any more. She was often preoccupied with the responsibility of her daughter. 'I've got this for life.' She did not enjoy her food and had a poor appetite but had not lost weight recently. Most nights she had difficulty getting off to sleep but then slept through until morning. She had no diurnal variation of mood and had not lost interest in her home or her appearance; her concentration remained unimpaired. She was still hopeful that things might improve in the future and had never contemplated suicide. She had always suffered with asthma which had become worse over the past 2 years – she felt that the tiredness and breathlessness of her chronic chest complaint was also getting her down.

6 Chronic borderline case depression

The subject was a 60-year-old widow who had been well until her husband's terminal illness with severe chronic asthma. For the two years before his death 8 years ago she nursed him at home and at that time felt moderately depressed. When he died she became severely depressed for many months and was prescribed psychotropic medication by her general practitioner. Since then she had had recurrent episodes of depression lasting up to 2 months, when she became very miserable, lethargic and withdrawn, and anorectic. She had marked sleep disturbance and diurnal variation of mood. In the year before interview she had not had an episode as severe as this but had felt moderately depressed much of the time. She felt unhappy and low and was often tearful, although she could pull herself out of it temporarily with an effort. When feeling down she wanted to stay away from neighbours but still appreciated her family being with her. She worried a good deal about her family in case anything should happen to them too but knew that this was unreasonable. She continued to feel at her worst in the mornings and habitually woke early at 4 or 5 a.m., however she usually got off to sleep again. She was taking Valium and Sodium Amytal from her GP and felt she would 'collapse without them'.

7 Onset borderline case depression

Miss D was a 20-year-old unmarried girl living with her mother in the bottom half of a house. The upper half of the house was occupied by her father, who was legally separated from her mother. There was no contact between the two parents. Miss D's brother also lived in the house and was in contact with both 'sides'. Miss D worked as a semi-skilled photographer's printer and had recently been going out regularly with a boyfriend; she also had a fair number of girlfriends, but all other relatives lived abroad.

Six months before interview, her mother aged 60, was admitted to hospital with a severe stroke. She returned home an invalid, about a month before interview, and since then Miss D had felt she must stay in more than she would really like. Neither her father nor brother gave her any help with her mother or the housework. A social worker had recently suggested the council might be able to provide a home help. Miss D was a girl who had always lacked self-confidence and was a 'worrier'. She had often felt 'tensed up' in her muscles and went through periods of sleeping badly. However, two months ago, she began to worry a great deal about her mother, found she disliked being alone in the house. She felt very miserable and cried more than usual and lost her appetite – she lost 7 lbs in weight. This episode was short lived and by the time her mother came home she was feeling better. She had no additional symptoms during her 'depression'.

8 Onset borderline case depression

Since hearing of her sister's suicide attempt several weeks before interview, the subject had been feeling miserable and crying easily. She was a rather nervous and tense person in general with a fear of heights and lifts but she had been feeling more tense and anxious since the news. She was preoccupied with the thought of her sister's suicide attempt, but could turn her attention elsewhere with an effort and was able to concentrate on most things, although her reading was a little impaired. She felt tired and drained of energy but continued to cope efficiently with the housework and her children and didn't lose interest in meeting her friends. Her appetite and sleep were unaffected.

Appendix 2
Clinical ratings

All of these items were rated for mental state at 'admission', for the point a year prior to admission and for all change-points occurring including onset. Most of the symptom items are quite straightforward, but some examples of scale-points in section 2 (severity ratings) are given for clarification.

1 Symptom data

Depressed mood

1 crying
2 feeling miserable/looking miserable, unable to smile or laugh
3 feelings of hopelessness about the future
4 suicidal thoughts
5 suicidal attempt
6 diurnal variation – worse in the morning
7 diurnal variation – worse in the evening
8 increased morbid interest – not associated with worry

Elated mood

9 unusual cheerfulness/excitement
10 uncharacteristic attempt or actual taking on of new responsibilities

Over activity

11 restlessness – e.g. pacing up and down, fidgeting, wringing hands

12 thoughts racing through mind
13 talkativeness
14 increased output in purposeful activities

Fears/anxiety/worry

15 psychosomatic accompaniments
16 tenseness/anxiety
17 specific worry
18 panic attacks
19 phobias

Thinking I

20 feelings of self-depreciation/nihilistic delusions
21 delusions or ideas of reference
22 delusions of persecution/jealousy
23 delusions of grandeur
24 delusions of control/influence
25 other delusions, e.g. hypochondriacal worry
26 auditory hallucinations
27 visual hallucinations

Thinking II

28 pre-occupational thinking
29 obsessive thinking
30 pre-occupational behaviour
31 obsessive behaviour

Under activity

32 slowness of thinking/speech
33 slowness of action, i.e. retardation
34 feeling tired/complains no energy/getting up late/falling asleep on chair
35 stupor

Drive

36 increased appetite
37 loss of appetite
38 increased libido
39 loss of libido

Sleep

40 initial insomnia of more than one hour (10 nights or more in a month)
41 waking early (2+ hours earlier, 10 nights or more in a month)
42 middle insomnia
43 increase in weight
44 loss of weight

Socially unacceptable behaviour

45 irritability
46 verbal attacks
47 violence/destructive behaviour
48 odd/bizarre behaviour

Effect on day-to-day routine

49 being less talkative/not answering back
50 avoids seeing friends and relatives/draws the curtains
51 loses interest in things (work, hobbies, family)/sitting around doing nothing
52 loss of interest in personal appearance
53 inability to make decisions

Employment or housework/child care

54 impaired performance
55 stopping work

2 Severity Ratings

56 overall severity (1 severe – 5 mild)
57 severity of depressive mood (0 nil – 3 marked)
58 ,,   ,, elated mood   ,,
59 ,,   ,, anxiety   ,,
60 ,,   ,, hallucinations/delusions/ideas of reference
                                     (0 nil – 3 marked)
61 ,,   ,, preoccupational thinking   ,,
62 ,,   ,, overactivity   ,,
63 ,,   ,, retardation   ,,
64 ,,   ,, appetite disturbance (0 marked decrease – 3 nil – 6 marked increase)

65   ,,   ,,   sleep disturbance (0 nil – 3, 4 marked)
66   ,,   ,,   socially unacceptable behaviour (0 nil – 3, 4 marked)
67   ,,   ,,   effect on day-to-day routine
68   ,,   ,,   impact on employment/household tasks   ,,
69   number of new symptoms since last change point
70   total number of symptoms

Examples of overall severity ratings – 6 (least) to 1 (most)

In some 'high' and 'low' examples of the individual scale points are given.

point 6 — nil
She normally had some difficulty with sleep (041).

point 5 — low
She was restless, fidgety, had constipation and always thought people were looking at and talking about her (047).

She had been unhappy for a long time and often had periods of depression quietness, lack of energy, and irritability (044).

point 4 — low
She was miserable, felt lost, and did not know what to do. She could not swallow or eat, had weight loss, slept badly, and had the shakes (039 at first change point, C1).

point 4 — high
She was moody, irritable, unreasonable, and would not talk, stormed out of the room – incidents that were infrequent and over quickly. She shut herself in her room occasionally, drew the curtains for the rest of the day. She would be all right when she got up. She got on badly with her parents. She coped less with her job – her boss ticked her off. She cried and found herself banging into cars at traffic lights (042 at C1).

point 3
She looked miserable and depressed. She lacked energy – and would drop off to sleep. She was slower at doing things and did less around

the house. She was quieter and sometimes did not answer. She lost interest in bingo and betting. She worried about her job – she had been getting very forgetful at work and had complaints about this. She would wake up at night and had difficulty getting off to sleep again. She was irritable and lost interest in her appearance. Her appetite decreased. She would worry about the psychiatric treatment of daughter. At the levelling-off point (the week before A) she became very much quieter and more depressed (040).

point 2 — low
She cried in public. She was very miserable and worried about how depressed she was becoming. She was tense and panicked during the night when she could not sleep. She was restless, fidgety and could not concentrate. She had a specific worry over her friend's marriage, also over marriage in general, and her boyfriend. She panicked when she had to face people. She could not get off to sleep and would wake at 5 a.m. She avoided college friends. She lost interest in her college work, and tended to put off decisions about things she had to do. She gave up college a week before admission (038).

She was terribly depressed and upset. She cried on and off nearly every day. She said life was not worth living, several times. She was very tensed up and her usual lack of energy became worse. She also became very slow. Her appetite substantially decreased. She lost interest in her clothing and her children and lost affection for them (044 at C1).

point 2 — high
She had bad 'turns' and feared a stroke and fainting. She was scared to go out because of this. She had feelings of hopelessness and that life was not worth living, and thought of taking something. She had almost no energy and became slower and more tired, and could hardly manage any housework. She sat around 'going to pieces'. She lost interest in her home and hobbies. She became withdrawn and did not want to see people because she felt they were against her, and were talking about her. Occasionally she heard voices. She slept badly and her 'turns' woke her up. She was restless and fidgety. She suffered from indigestion and went off her food. Frightening thoughts raced through her mind and she could not stop them. She felt something awful was going to happen and became all worked up. She lost interest in her appearance (036 at C2)

point 1 — low

She was very depressed and cried a lot. She had feelings of hopelessness and thoughts of harming herself. She became very harsh with her children and shouted at them and hit them (most unusual for her). She became listless and paid no attention to what was said to her. Certain thoughts occupied her and she could not stop a 'horrid voice' at the back of her mind. She worried about her husband's misconduct. She had cold sweats and her hands had become very clammy. She did not want to go out because she felt that people were watching her. She had difficulty with sleep until 2 a.m. She became tired and everything was too much of an effort. She sat and stared, and did not want to be bothered with anything. She had paralyzing feelings in her arms, and was indecisive. Her appetite decreased a bit. She suffered from retardation and was slow in doing things: she went into her bedroom and just wanted to sit there or lie on the bed. She had a general loss of interest, e.g. in shopping and her appearance. She managed only bare necessities of household and child care activities. She lost affection for her children (041).

point 1 — high

This involved an attempted suicide or gross retardation, e.g. staying in bed all day. Subject had been depressed and anxious for a few weeks, staying in bed more than two hours longer than usual, losing interest in her appearance, her housework and her knitting, with substantial loss of sleep and appetite. Just before admission she said life was not worth living and wanted to stab herself. A few days later she wounded herself quite seriously on the neck with a knife. She tried to hide the wound from her daughter and husband, becoming agitated and saying she did not want them to be blamed for it, or sent to prison. She was found the next day with the gas on, reading a book on methods of suicide (018).

Appendix 3
Examples of events
by type and severity

Brief examples of events in ten general categories are given, each divided into *severe* and *non-severe* (in terms of long-term threat). For explanation of ratings of severity see chapter 6. For each example the actual scale ratings are given for both long- and short-term threat: short-term threat is given first. (Scale points are: 1 = marked, 2s = moderate subject-focussed, 2o – moderate other-focussed, 3 = some, 4 = none or little.)

In order to avoid bias the examples have been chosen randomly from the first Camberwell series (500s are cases). Some of the events could have been included in more than one of the ten categories and there is inevitably an arbitrary aspect to some of the allocations.

Deaths

Severe

564 – Subject's father died age 81. She was married and he had lived with her for 7 years (1–1).
324 – Neighbour/confidant of subject died aged 84: subject and neighbour lived in the same block of flats and saw each other several times a week. Subject was not directly involved in death (1–2s).

Non-severe

507 – Subject's grandmother who looked after her when she was 10 (after she lost her mother) died in Ireland (1–2o).
302 – Subject's neighbour (not a confidant) collapsed and died: subject was directly involved in the death (1–4).

394 – Subject had to tell her husband that his sister had died (2s–4).

Illness to subject and accidents

Severe

348 – Subject had a stroke and was taken to hospital – still could not move her hand properly at interview. Age 63 (1–1).
328 – Subject had a haemorrhage in her nose, and was rushed to hospital. It took a week to bring it under control. She was in hospital three weeks (1–2s).
641 – Subject had car crash – her car was 'written off'. Subject was badly hurt, lost seven teeth, had a broken arm and ribs. She said it was her fault: she had been drunk (1–2s).

Non-severe

341 – Subject, in late twenties and with no children, had a miscarriage a week after learning she was pregnant – the pregnancy was unplanned (2s–4).
394 – Subject experienced cramp pains at night and fainted in kitchen. General practitioner took her off 'pill' and said everything would be all right (2s–4).
370 – Subject was in a car accident. In a rainstorm a woman 'walked into the car'; her husband was driving. The woman left hospital the same evening as the accident. There were no police charges (2s–4).

Interaction changes

Severe

553 – Subject's husband was sent to prison for two years; subject was pregnant (1–1).
515 – Subject's friend and only confidant left to live in Ireland; she had seen her three times or more a week (2s–2s).

Non-severe

377 – Subject's parents had a quarrel and her mother came to stay with her: she only remained a few weeks but had planned to stay much longer (2o–2o).
325 – Subject's husband went to Portsmouth to work for about three months: he did not come back at weekends (3–3).

392 – Subject's friend moved to North London; she still sees her occasionally but has only a fraction of their previous rate of contact (3–3).

Important news, decisions, and disappointments

Severe

508 – Subject was threatened with eviction for not paying rent: husband said he had been paying an 'agent' and it was not clear whether husband or 'agent' was to blame. In general the family were poor and had £150 in debts (1–1).
501 – Subject heard that her teenage nephew had cancer of the spine; five months before another nephew had cancer. Both were close companions of her teenage son. Subject was drawn into the crisis (1–2s).

Non-severe

301 – One of subject's two daughters who lived locally said she was going to move to a new town with her husband and children: the decision however was not finalized (3–3).
372 – After discussions with her husband subject decided that she would give up her career as photographic model and perhaps go to university (4–4).

Miscellaneous crises involving lost pets, burglaries, etc.

Severe

564 – Subject found out her husband had made a 'sexual advance' to someone at work. The young woman was married and her family was involved in the resulting crisis (1–1).
501 – Subject's son, aged 15, was charged with housebreaking and put on probation. It was his first offence. A policeman came to see her and her son went to court a week later. He had left his name and address with the dealer who had taken the goods he had stolen. The whole incident was totally unexpected (1–2s).

Non-severe

301 – Subject's son-in-law was arrested for assaulting a policeman while he was drunk (later he was sent to prison for six months) (2o–2o).
308 – Subject's 16-year-old son announced that he planned to leave

home to live alone. Her husband 'took a week to talk him out of the idea' (2s–4).

325 – Subject's dog whom she had had 4½years had to be given away as dogs were not allowed in their new home (3–3).

318 – Subject's son said he wanted to get engaged. Subject's husband thought he was too young and discussed it with him for 2 to 3 days (3–4).

Illness to others and accidents

Severe

323 – Subject's father was admitted to hospital with 'transient strokes' and she was told that he would 'probably die this time' (1–1).

Non-severe

305 – Subject's brother living in Derbyshire had 'nervous breakdown' and admitted to hospital. Her mother is 'a schizophrenic' (1–2o).

334 – Subject's friend attempted suicide. Subject saw her several times a month. Subject was told of her admission by the hospital and had to tell her friend's husband (1–3).

308 – Subject's daughter had acute appendicitis and was taken to hospital. She made a good recovery (1–4).

632 – Subject's 8-year-old son knocked 'in air' by a car. He was not injured but was extremely difficult in his behaviour for three months afterwards (1–2o).

312 – Subject's son fell from window and was in hospital for three days (2o–3).

Role change to subject

Severe

384 – Subject left her husband and she and her mother (they had all been living together in mother's house) went to stay with friends. She intended the separation to be permanent (1–1).

371 – Subject found out she was pregnant by fiance and said she had 'never dreamt it would happen'; her whole life plans were 'shattered' – she could not go on a secretarial course and the marriage date had to be brought forward (1–2s).

Non-severe

377 – The birth of subject's first baby. No problems (1–3).

391 – Planned birth of subject's second child and stopping work (3–4).

Job changes

Severe

508 – Subject's husband was sacked after only three weeks in his new job. Subject thinks that he was sent a bad reference from his previous job. He had recently been sacked from another job. The family were in debt (1–1).

416 – Subject left her job because her son was starting school and she had to be at home for him in his holidays. Her husband gave her very little money and the giving up of her job led to great tension as the financial difficulties were made much worse (1–1).

406 – Subject was sacked soon after restarting her job as an invoice typist after being away two years: she was told she had not enough experience. Because her husband was in poor health they relied more than average on her money and were saving for a home (2s–2s).

Non-severe

415 – Subject's husband was made redundant. There had been no warning. He had had two previous jobs in the year. He felt he could always get a job as an electrician, but he helped out in his mother's shop for a bit (over Christmas). There were some money worries but they were not severe (4–3).

350 – Subject's husband changed to nightwork (4–3).

322 – Subject's son started his first job after leaving school (4–4).

635 – Subject had been a home help for years. She left the job because a change in policy meant she could not look after people she knew personally (2s–3).

418 – Subject gave up her part-time job she had had for four years (4–4).

Residence changes

Severe

565 – Subject and her family moved in order to get away from very difficult neighbours: they could not really afford the cost of the new flat (2s–2s).

Non-severe

567 – Subject and husband moved to a new flat: the rent was very high but they thought they could use their savings and not stay long. They planned to move eventually to a New Town (2s–3).

Role changes to others

Non-severe

375 – Subject heard that her daughter's husband had left her: he had regularly 'beaten her up' (1–2o).
379 – Subject's husband threw up his university course just before he was about to go into teaching practice (2o–2o).
424 – Subject's daughter broke off her engagement (3–4).

Appendix 4
The brought forward
time index: T_{BF}

This appendix is the work of Julian Peto.

N.B. The term 'event' is used in the statistical sense in the Appendix, and is thus applied both to life-events and to the occurrence of onsets.

We begin with a few definitions:

1 Event rate

By event rate we mean the rate $r(t)$ at which random events occur at a particular point in time (t). (We write r as $r(t)$ to emphasize that it may vary with time.) This rate is equal to the limit of the expression

$$r(t) = \frac{\text{probability of an event occurring in the interval from } t \text{ to } t + dt}{dt}$$

when dt approaches zero. If the rate is constant, it is the average number of events occurring in a given period. The probability of an event occurring in the interval dt is thus simply $r(t).dt$.

2 Poisson process

If an event rate is constant, the expected time to the next event is the same from any point in time. If you receive telephone calls at a constant rate of two per hour, for example, the average time from one call to the next will evidently be half an hour. However, if you start measuring from any point in time (you might for example wait until you have not had a call for half an hour before starting your clock) the average time to the next call will still be half an hour. This is similar to the coin-tossing problem, where the probability of getting heads on the eleventh throw is still 50% even if the last ten throws were tails.

A process with a constant event rate r (we use r rather than r(t), since the rate does not vary) is called a Poisson process. The average time T_{AV} to the next event is the reciprocal of the rate, i.e.

$$T_{AV} = \frac{1}{r} \tag{i}$$

We can also calculate the probability Pr(n) that exactly n events will occur during a fixed period of length L. This is

$$Pr(n) = \frac{(r.L)^n.e^{-r.L}}{n.^1} \tag{ii}$$

the probability that no events will occur is therefore

$$Pr(O) = e^{-r.L}$$

and the probability that one or more will occur is

$$1 - Pr(O) = 1 - e^{-r.L} \tag{iii}$$

3 Community life-event rate

If we observe the proportions of a group of people with 0,1,2, etc., life-events during a fixed time, these will not obey the Poisson formula (equation (ii)) unless different individuals suffer events at roughly the same rate. The Table gives the numbers in the first community sample in the depressive study reporting 0,1,2,3,4, and 5 severe events during the year preceding interview and expected numbers for a Poisson process with the same mean.

Table 1   *Proportion of severe life-events in community sample in the 12 months before interview and expected number based on Poisson distribution with same average*

observed no.	no. of events	expected no.	average event rate in 12 months
144	0	125.2	
45	1	70.6	
20	2	19.9	
7	3	3.7	
2	4	0.5	$\frac{124}{220} = 0.56$
2	5	0.1	

The data are based on 220 subjects

We are able to use the year as a whole and there is no falling off in either marked events or moderate subject-focussed events. In the 6 months furthest from the interview there were 32 marked and 32 moderate subject-focussed events and in the 6 months nearest interview 29 and 30 respectively. We have therefore adopted the average rate of severe events as 0.56.

The Poisson does not fit well perhaps because different individuals suffer different life-event rates and some events may generate further events. If we assume a Poisson distribution and base our rates on p, the proportion with one or more events, using the equation derived from equation (iii) when L = 1, that is,

$$r = \log_e \frac{1}{(1 - p)} \tag{iv}$$

we should underestimate r by 25 per cent.

We therefore assume that each individual suffers life-events at a constant rate, but recognize that different individuals have different rates.

4 A model of the onset process

Consider a particular patient, whom we shall denote by i. We suppose that he suffers an underlying 'spontaneous' illness process, giving him an onset *rate* $s_i(t)$ at age t which varies through his life. If he suffers a life-event at age t, there is a certain *probability*, $O_i(t)$, that it will provoke an onset that would not otherwise have occurred. We could base our study on any arbitrary functions $O_i(t)$ and $s_i(t)$, but to make the model more sensible we assume that vulnerability to events varies with degree of 'latent illness', i.e.

$$O_i(t) = c_i.s_i(t), \text{ where } c_i \text{ is some unknown} \tag{v}$$
$$\text{constant characteristic}$$
$$\text{of the } i^{th} \text{ patient.}$$

We also assume that he suffers life-events at an unknown constant rate r_i.

5 The brought forward time

The assumption in equation (v) imposes an upper limit on $s_i(t)$; since $O_i(t)$ is a probability it cannot exceed one, so

$$s_i(t) \leqslant \frac{1}{c_i}$$

at any time. If we assume that $s_i(t)$ equals l/c_i, i.e. that the spontaneous onset rate always takes this maximum value, we shall minimize our estimate of the expected time from any point to the next spontaneous onset. In fact in equation (i) if the rate is l/c_i, this will be simply c_i. If the particular patient's onset were provoked by an event, we should thus say (if we know c_i) that the smallest possible estimate of the expected time from that onset to the next spontaneous onset he would otherwise have suffered is c_i. This is precisely the minimal estimate of the brought forward time which we seek, i.e. if the ith patient suffered a provoked onset, the expected time T^i_{BF} by which the provoking event advanced his onset obeys the inequality

$$T^i_{BF} \geqslant c_i. \tag{vi}$$

We therefore call c_i the ith patient's 'brought forward constant'.

6 Probability of provoking onset

We shall in what follows assume for simplicity that when an event provokes onset the onset occurs immediately. This is not a critical assumption. We estimate x, the proportion of onsets that were provoked, from the proportion h with one or more events during the 'causal period' before onset, whose length equals the longest delay between provoking event and consequent onset. Since h will be the same, for a given causal period, whether the accumulation of events is distributed throughout the period or concentrated just before onset, our estimate of x will not be affected. The equation for x (page 130) in terms of h and p is

$$x = \frac{h - p}{1 - p} \tag{vii}$$

Consider again the ith patient. The probability that he will suffer a spontaneous onset during the short interval of length dt starting at age t is $s_i(t).dt$, while the probability that a life-event will occur and provoke onset during this interval is $r_i dt$, the probability that he will experience such an event at all, multiplied by $O_i(t)$, the probability that such an event at age t will provoke onset. Thus the total probability that he will suffer an onset for either reason during this interval is

$$s_i(t).dt + r_i.dt.O_i(t)$$

which combined with (v) gives:

$$\text{Probability of onset in this short interval} = s_i(t).dt + r_i.dt.c_i.s_i(t)$$
$$= s_i(t).dt.(1 + r_i.c_i). \tag{viii}$$

Since the probability that a provoked onset will occur during this interval is $r_i.dt.O_i(t)$, which equals $s_i(t).dt.r_i.c_i$ by (v), the probability that an onset occurring in the interval was provoked is

$$\frac{s_i(t).dt.r_i.c_i}{s_i(t).dt.(1 + r_i.c_i)}$$

which equals

$$\frac{r_i.c_i}{1 + r_i.c_i}.$$

Since this expression is independent of time it is constant and equals the probability that any onset he suffers was provoked. Denoting this constant probability by x_i,

$$x_i = \frac{r_i.c_i}{1 + r_i.c_i} \tag{ix}$$

7 Estimate of minimum brought forward time

If we have observed n patients who have suffered onset, the proportion of onsets which were provoked, x, will in expectation be the average probability for the observed group, i.e.

$$\text{Expected value of } x = \frac{1}{n} \sum_{i=1}^{n} x_i = \frac{1}{n} \sum_{i=1}^{n} \frac{r_i.c_i}{(1 + r_i.c_i)} \tag{x}$$

We shall ignore sampling fluctuation, and assume that

$$x = \frac{1}{n} \sum_{i=1}^{n} \frac{r_i.c_i}{(1 + r_i.c_i)} \tag{xi}$$

We can estimate the average event rate r of the community from our comparison sample. We assume that the individuals' life-event rates are different, and estimate r as in the *Table 1*, from the number m in the community sample, and the number of events k they suffer in a fixed period T, since

$$r = \frac{k}{T.m} \text{ in expectation.} \tag{xii}$$

It is this estimate of r that is used in the present work.
(If the distribution of events (see *Table 1*) in our community sample were nearly Poisson we might prefer to estimate r from equation (iv) by

$$r = \log_e \frac{1}{(1-p)} \qquad \text{(xiii)}$$

to avoid introducing extra parameters).

It is a fundamental assumption of our method that the life-event rates of patients are similar to those of matched controls from the community (see discussion on p. 119). We therefore assume that

$$\text{Expected value of } \frac{1}{n} \sum_{i=1}^{n} r_i = r.$$

Ignoring sampling fluctuation, we shall put

$$\frac{1}{n} \sum_{i=1}^{n} r_i = r \qquad \text{(xiv)}$$

r is of course the average life-event rate in a group matched for age, sex, family size, etc., rather than in the whole population.

We wish to find a conservative estimate of T_{BF}, which is the average time by which the onsets of those patients whose onsets were provoked were brought forward by life-events. Since x_i (equation (ix)) is the probability that the ith individual's onset was provoked, and T^i_{BF} is the average time by which it was brought forward if it was provoked,

$$T_{BF} = \frac{\sum_{i=1}^{n} x_i . T^i_{BF}}{\sum_{i=1}^{n} x_i} = \frac{1}{n.x} \sum_{i=1}^{n} x_i . T^i_{BF}.$$

Therefore (equation (vi))

$$T_{BF} \frac{1}{n.x} \sum_{i=1}^{n} x_i . c_i. \qquad \text{(xv)}$$

We seek the minimum value that T_{BF} can take for any values of the different onset rates r_i and 'brought forward constants' c_i of our patients. We must therefore find the values r_i and c_i ($1 \leq i \leq n$) which minimize the right hand side of equation (xv) and satisfy equations (xi) and (xiv). Since for each equation the expressions being summed are the same function of r_i and c_i, it follows by symmetry that our estimate of T_{BF} will be minimized if we assume that r_i and c_i do not vary between patients.[1] Thus $c_i = c$, some constant, for all i, and $r_i = r$ (equation (xiv)) for all i.

Thus (equation (xi))

$$x = \frac{r.c}{1 + r.c}$$

and hence

$$c = \frac{1}{r} \cdot \frac{x}{1 - x} \cdot$$

Equation (xv) reduces to

$$T_{BF} \geq c,$$

so we conclude that

$$T_{BF} \geq \frac{1}{r} \cdot \frac{x}{1 - x} \cdot \qquad \text{(xvi)}$$

Substituting for x in terms of h and p (equation (vii)),

$$T_{BF} \geq \frac{1}{r} \cdot \frac{(h - p)}{(1 - h)} \cdot \qquad \text{(xvii)}$$

r can be estimated from equations (xii) or (xiii). If events tend to generate further events we shall observe clusters rather than isolated events, but the analysis may be applied in the same way, regarding clusters as single 'events'. The estimate of r from equation (xii) will then be too high, and our estimate of T_{BF} will be still more conservative. If we use the length of the causal period as our time unit, as we do in chapter 7, and measure r accordingly, the result will be in these units, and must be multiplied by the length of the causal period. However, the result will in expectation be unaffected if we use a longer causal period, since r will change proportionally, and x will have the same expected value. If we observe over too short a period we shall exclude some provoking events, reducing h, and hence x. The result will then be still more conservative.

It might seem possible, since T_{BF} is an average over the provoked group of patients, that a few of the proportion x had their onsets advanced enormously, while the remainder were triggered. This is not

---

1 It is straightforward to establish this formally by introducing Lanrange multipliers (see e.g. Courant and Hilbert (1953: 165)), and to check that this extremum is the minimum.

so. If we assumed that 5% of these patients were perfectly well when the events provoked their onsets, so their onsets were brought forward by a life time, we could subtract 5% from x and recalculate T_{BF} for the remainder. If x were 34 % and r were .015 per three weeks (our 'marked event' results) T_{BF} would only be reduced from 2 years to 20 months.

Appendix 5
Interview schedule
for events and difficulties

Note: (i) At the first stage of the depression project questions about events were asked separately from those about difficulties.
(ii) The 'questions' are often in the form of a reminder to the interviewer of what to cover in questioning.

* * *

A Once an event has been established, question in detail about incidents leading to it, or stemming from it e.g. decisions preceding a job change or a marriage.

B Make sure to relate each event to (i) change-points; (ii) other events or difficulties.

C Make sure the respondent knows the range of people included in the terms 'close relative' and 'close friend'. Remind them from time to time during the interview both about these terms and about the 12 month period.

Now I'd like to ask about the last 12 months:

Section I – Health

Has anyone in the family been ill?
What about you? Your husband or children or parents? etc.
How serious was it? An emergency?
Anyone off work because of it? For how long?

Has anyone been admitted to, or left, hospital during the last 12 months?
For what illness?
Was it a routine admission, or an emergency?
How long for? What changes were involved for you?
What is the medical outlook?
If someone outside household – How involved were you?

Have any relatives or close friends died?
Were you involved at all? Did you expect it? Were you present?

Any surgical operations in the last 12 months?
e.g. to self, child, or parent.

Have you had any bad news about an illness that's been going on for sometime?

Are there any chronic health problems?
For yourself or close relatives?
e.g. Does anyone suffer from:–
any chest troubles
high blood pressure
heart trouble or stroke
varicose veins or piles
asthma
tuberculosis
chronic bronchitis
gall bladder or liver trouble
stomach ulcer
any other chronic stomach trouble
kidney trouble or trouble passing water
arthritis or rheumatism
nervous trouble of any kind
diabetes
thyroid trouble
blackouts, fainting attacks, or dizzy spells
repeated trouble with back or spine
chronic skin trouble
hernia or rupture
epilepsy (or fits)
migraine
trouble with periods or other gynaecological trouble

Have you any relatives who are a worry to you for other reasons?
e.g. because of old age or incapacity, or a drinking or gambling
problem, a mental handicap, or anything else at all?

S's own past health (a special section)

I'd just like to ask you about your health in the past:

In your life have you had any operations?

When? What?
   hysterectomy?
   sterilization?
   D & C?
   abortions?
   removal of cyst?
   breast removal?

Have you ever had any serious illness?

When? What?

Or did you have any other childhood problems?
   e.g. problems at school or in your family?

If over 38 what about the change of life (menopause)? Have you had any problems associated with that?

In the last 12 months:

Has there been any nervous trouble (apart from yourself) in the family?
   Has anyone been treated at a psychiatric O.P. clinic or hospital?
   Has this ever happened in your family outside the 12 months?
   Has there been any attempted suicide?

Have there been any accidents?
   On the road, or in the home? etc.
   What about the children?
   Have you been involved in or witnessed any road accidents?
   Or anything like that?
   Probe: How serious?
      How far were you involved?
      Have you ever been in a serious accident?
      When? What?

Has there been any pregnancy in the family? Any miscarriages?
   If (i) married 16–45, or (ii) married women under 35 with a regular boyfriend in the last 12 months (otherwise use judgment), ask:
   What about you, have you been pregnant? Or worried that you might be?

Any babies born? Anyone lost a baby? Any grandchildren arrived?

Section II – Role changes

Has anyone in the family got married in the last 12 months?
   What about your brothers, sisters, parents, children, friends?

Anyone engaged?
   What about your brothers, sisters, parents, children?
   When was this? When was it decided upon?
   When was it first made official?
   Was it expected?

Has anyone close retired for good?
   e.g. husband, parents?
   Was this expected? What changes did it bring? e.g. financial,
   routine changes, etc.?

Or has anyone separated from or divorced their husband or wife?
   Were you involved at all?
   Did you expect it to happen?
   What about your brothers or sisters?

Anyone started school or college?
   e.g. begun school for the first time?
   Gone away to University?
   How did you feel about this?

Anyone taken any important examinations or qualifications?
   What were the results?

What about friends? Have you made any new friends?
   (of either sex, at all?) **Probe for new opposite sex relationships.**

Or lost someone you were close to?
   Why was this?

*Have there been any big changes in the amount you see of your friends or
relatives?*

   Ask if appropriate:–
Do you have a boyfriend at all?

Have you thought of getting engaged or married?
   i.e. in the last year or to someone in past years

What happened?

Would you like to get married, do you think?

   For older, single or widowed subjects:– (use tact!)
Have you ever considered marriage?

Or been engaged?

How long ago was this? Do you have any regrets about it now?

Section III – Leisure and interaction

Have there been just the————————of you at home during this 12 months?

Has anyone come to stay? For how long?

Has anyone left the household at all? Permanently?

Is there anyone you see much less of?
Why is this? Do you miss them?

What do you do with your leisure time?
Get brief list of hobbies, T.V. watching time, etc.
Collect list of joint activities with other household members.

Do you feel you have enough leisure time?

Are there things you'd like to do but can't?
Why is this, i.e. short of money, transport, etc.
Can you get a babysitter if you need one?

Do you invite friends home at all?

Have you had any difficulties with friends? Or been worried about them at all?

Have you had a holiday in the past 12 months?
How did it work out? Did you have a good time?
Anything unexpected or important happen when you were away
or on your return?

Section IV – Employment

A. For subject

Do you enjoy your job?

Has anything happened at work?

Have you been off work at all or put onto a new job, or changed jobs?

Has anyone you worked with closely left in the last 12 months?
If so, check:
1 Seen regularly and frequently at work?
2 (a) Extra-work involvement – seen out of work hours?
   (b) Close relationship required by job?

(c) Effect on subject's job?
3 Extent of separation.

How do you get on with your workmates?

Have you had any trouble or difficulties with them?

Were there any other difficulties at work?
Probe for events or long term difficulties
e.g. long hours, low pay, travel etc.
What do you like about your job?
Is there anything you don't like about it?
Probe:
Promotion
Responsibility
Wage increases

Is there other work that you would have liked better?
If yes: Why?

Have you felt that the demands made on you at work were too great?
Probe:
Deadlines to meet
Not enough training/information?
Bad physical conditions

Are you a member of a trade union? Do you get proper sick pay when ill? Are there any times in your work when you don't know what is expected of you?
Pause. . . . For instance when one person wants you to do one thing and someone else wants you to do something different?
Probe:
Supervisors
Colleagues
Juniors (if applicable)
If there are any difficulties, have you ever thought of asking to be transferred to another section/department?

Have you been expecting any changes in your job?

How do you feel about the future, do you think you'll stay in this job?
Might you leave for any reason? **If relevant, probe for threat of HAVING to give up work for any reason.**
If relevant, probe uncertainty of e.g. chances of promotion, or graduation + time duration of promotion or of student or trainee ·
role

Have you done different types of work in the past?

Have you ever in your life had to give up a job, or been dismissed from a job?

B. *For head of household i.e. subject's husband or father*

Has your husband/father been working all this last 12 months?
Work history for last 12 months. Why left, when arranged, etc.

Any time off through sickness? redundancy? strikes?

Has he had any promotion in his job? **(Applies only to chief wage earners)**
Collect periods of unemployment in the last 12 months lasting 4 weeks. For 'important' members of household.

Does he have any problems in his job at all?

Is he a trade union member?

If you (or your husband) lost your job, how easy would you find it to get another?

Has he any qualifications or special skills?

Section V – Housing

How long have you lived in your present home?
Changes in subject's residence over last year.

Do you own it yourself?

Do you like living in your present house/flat?

Can you tell me if any of the following have been a problem in your house/flat?

Interviewer use judgment

Not enough room? **Obtain number of rooms, excluding bathroom (kitchen = 1 if big enough to have a meal in).**

Sharing facilities? Self-contained? Have you a fridge, a freezer, washing machine, central heating, etc.?

Do you feel it's private enough?
Trouble with repairing the house – anything wrong with roof, dry rot, damp walls, rats, etc. **Check** problems about getting it done, payments, etc.

Have you approached the landlord/council about this?

Have there been any problems with the landlord – any restrictions – that sort of thing?
Where relevant: did this affect you?

Have there been any problems, that you know of, about paying for the house – keeping up with the rent/mortgage?

Do you qualify for a rebate? Do you get it?

What about the neighbourhood? How do you get on with the neighbours? Have there been any difficulties with them? Have you fallen out with any neighbours who used to be friends or acquaintances?

Have you ever felt cut off in your present home – too far from friends or work?

Have you considered living anywhere else? What have you done about it? **If relevant, probe uncertainty of e.g. moving, or likelihood of leaving home.**

Section VI – Money

May I ask a little about financial circumstances?

Have you had any money worries? Especially in last 12 months? **If yes:** Have you tried to borrow from anybody? Have you thought of trying to earn more?

Have you gone without things you really need?

Does everyone here contribute to household expenses (inc. children over school age)?

Where relevant, e.g. students: Do you think your parents should help you out a bit more?

Do you get free school dinners? **If no:** could you get them if you wanted to?

Have you been getting any social security benefits?

Section VII – Crises

Has there been any crisis/emergency? **Pause** Any crisis involving your husband/wife/son(s)/daughter(s) etc.?

Has there been anything in the home? Such as a burglary or fire? Or being attacked in the street? Has this ever happened to you at any time in your life? How old were you?

Have you had to break any bad news to anyone?

Have there been any legal troubles, or having to go to court?

What about notice of eviction or any HP difficulties?

Have you or anyone in the family had any contact with the police at all?
Or any contact with any social agency such as welfare officer, marriage
   guidance counsel?

What about your mother, sisters, parents, children, friends?
If children over 5, have your children ever been in any trouble like that at any
time?

Have any of your relatives had any crises or troubles with which you've had to
help – e.g. has anyone gone to stay with an ill relative?

Or any in which you've been involved?

What about friends? Have there been any troubles or difficulties concerning them in the past year? **Pause:** Have any died; or some other
   crisis?

Have you lost any pets?
   Any more general disappointments in the last 12 months? e.g. child
   failing an exam.

Section VIII – Forecasts

Have you or any member of the family had any unexpected news in the last 12
months about anything that has happened or is going to happen?
   Pause:
   For example, sometimes a family will get a letter saying they are
   going to be rehoused, or they might perhaps get notification of
   redundancy.
   Anything like that.
   Give time to think.
   Refer to possibly relevant events already established.
Sometimes people learn unexpected things about others close to them, such as
discovering their child has been stealing at school, or their husband/wife has
been having an affair, or their boyfriend/girlfriend has been seeing someone
else. Have you had anything happen like this? . . . *news that shook you at all?*
   Anything like that at all?

Section IX – Marital

(Cover before and after psychiatric onset)

Have you and your husband both been living at home during this time?

   If negative response:
Have you been separated for any length of time during the last 12 months?

Have either of you ever considered a permanent separation or divorce? *

How well would you say you and your husband get on in general?

Would you say there are any problems about your relationship?

How often do you and he have quarrels or tiffs?

What are they usually about? e.g. disagreement about children, about money etc.)

Do you feel you can talk to him quite easily?

Do you talk to him about things that worry you?

Do you wish you could confide in him?

When he has problems or worries does he talk them over with you?

Are you an affectionate person, do you think?

What about your husband, is he demonstrative?

What about the sexual side of things – have there been any difficulties or problems about this?

Do you like doing the same things when you are together?

How do your parents get on with him? (**Probe** for any tension here)

And what about his parents – *do you get on with them?*

Section X – Interaction with parents

(Especially for single girls, but use briefly for all whose parents are alive. Question before and after onset)

How do you get on with your parents?
    Who do you feel closer to – your mother or your father?

How would you say you got on with your mother?
    Is she easy to get on with?

Is she an affectionate person?

Does she show interest in you – in the things you do?
Probe: Quarrels and sources of tension

---

* Coping probes should be used at these points – Have you tried to talk things over with – ? Have you sought help or advice from anyone else? Confided in anyone about it?

Would you say there's any tension or difficulty between the two of you?
Do you ever avoid her – or try to keep out of her way?

Do you feel you can confide in her?

If yes: Do you find it helpful to talk things over with her?
If no: Would you like to be able to confide more in her?

Do you feel you have to tell your mother about things you do? For example, do you feel you must tell her where you're going – or if something happens to you like a rise in pay?

Repeat questions above for father, and other household members where appropriate

Does either parent treat you as younger than you are?
Does you mother/father tell you if (s)he disagrees with things you do?
How much do you feel you can get on with things without interference from your parents?
Do your parents say anything about the sorts of clothes you should wear? – or the way you have your hair, anything like that?
Are there any (other) things like this your parents keep reminding you about? Or anything they keep telling you to do – or complain to you about?

For everyone: *How would you say your parents got on together?*
Are there any difficulties between them?
Did/do they quarrel at all? – or have periods of not speaking to each other?

Section XI – General

Has anything particularly disappointing happened over the last 12 months that you haven't mentioned already?

Have you had to make any important decisions over this time?

You will have gathered by now that we're interested in anything upsetting, important or exciting that has happened to you. **Pause:** *Exciting in a pleasant or unpleasant way*

Has anything given you special pleasure?
e.g. a visit from a relative, a holiday, child winning a prize, a present, new car, etc.

Anything turned out better than expected?
     e.g. financial windfall? Relationships improving in some way?

In your life so far:-
Are there things you wish had turned out differently?
Or any regrets you have?
     e.g. over education, training, marriage?
What if anything gives you special fulfilment or satisfaction in your life?

Section XII – Resources section

Finally, I'd just like to ask one or two questions now about what would happen to you if one of these emergencies did occur:
Do you know anyone who could look after the children for you if you were called away in a hurry? Have you ever helped anyone else out in this way?

Do you know a lawyer you could contact? Have you ever contacted him?

How easy would it be for you to get, say, £100 quickly? By selling something or drawing on savings?

Have you got a bank account? How easily could you get an overdraft?

Have you or your husband taken out a life insurance?

What plans do you have for your retirement? What sort of pension will your husband get, and will he take it up?

   Probe for the stability of these resources, both objective and subjective.

Some suggested probes to cover each event/difficulty

Events

Basic description

   1 *PLACE* in and outside household

   2 *PROPINQUITY* – rate of contact

   3 *SOURCE/INDEPENDENCE*
          How long had it been planned?

4 *ACCEPTANCE*
> How did you feel about it?
> Were you pleased?
> Would you have preferred it not to happen?

5 *RELEVANCE FOR LIFE GOALS*
> At the time, how important did it seem to you?
> Has it prevented you from doing anything you'd planned to do?
> Has it strengthened any of your plans for the future?

6 *ROLE CHANGE*
> Did it make you feel any differently about yourself?

Preparation

1 *EXPECTEDNESS OF OCCURRENCE/TIMING SPECIFIC WARNING/TIMING REFERRED TO IN SPECIFIC WARNING*
> You said you expected it, but did you expect it to happen at that particular time?

2 *WARNINGS – GENERAL AND SPECIFIC*

3 *AVOIDABILITY*

4 *AVOIDANCE BEHAVIOUR*

5 *MANOEUVRABILITY* (After event)
> Could anything have been done to alter the course of events?

6 *PREVIOUS EXPERIENCE OF ANY SIMILAR SITUATION*
> – nature and time.
> How did you cope before?
> Was it successful/unpleasant/difficult in any way?

7 *SYMBOLIC SIGNIFICANCE*
> Can you think of any reason why you may have found this upsetting?
> Have any close relatives experienced anything similar to this?
> What happened?

8 *EMOTIONAL/PRACTICAL PREPARATION*
> After you knew it was going to happen, but before it happened did you worry? What about? When started?
> Did you wonder at all what would be involved? What would happen afterwards?
> Did you talk it over with anyone?

Did this help/make you less worried/give you any ideas how to deal with it?
Before it happened did you do anything to make it easier?

Immediate reactions

How did you feel about it at the time it happened?
Can you say more?

1 *PHYSICAL DANGER*
Were you frightened you might get hurt?

2 *ANGER/DEPRESSION* etc.
Did you feel angry/depressed?

3 *THREAT TO SELF ESTEEM*
Did you feel let down at all?
Were you at all ashamed?
Did you think less well of yourself?

4 *TIME DURATION CRISIS ASPECTS* (if any)
How long did you think it would be before you'd know how things were going to turn out?
How long did you think it would be before X would be out of danger/difficulty?

5 *EMOTIONAL COPING*
Going back to the time it occurred, did you feel: you could cope/overwhelmed/fairly calm about it/that you could handle the situation?

6 *ABILITY TO COPE DURING WEEK OF EVENT*
Was there anyone available to help?
Were there any difficulties about . . . e.g. your wife coming home?
Did your routine change that week?
Did you manage to carry on as usual?

7 *PRACTICAL COPING*
What have you done since it happened?

Implications

1 *EXPECTED TIME DURATION*

2 *INTERACTION CHANGE*
Did this mean you saw more or less of any close relative/friend?
How often did you see them before/after?

3 *IMPLICATIONS OF INCREASED INTERACTION*
Was there anything about the new relationship that worried you?

4 *ROUTINE CHANGE*
How has your day-to-day life changed?
Did you change any other routines?

5 *HABIT CHANGE* – no. changed hours, length time previous habit, no. times made change before.

6 *PAST/FUTURE REWARD*
How well did you get on with . . . ?
                          like your job?
What did you feel about the future – Did you expect to enjoy . . . ?

7 *NEW SKILLS*
Did you have to learn anything new?

8 *MATERIAL PROBLEM* Financial/Space

9 *SUBSTITUTES*

10 *DECISIONS*
Did you have to make any decisions on the spot?
Have you had to make any decisions since the event – as a result of it?
Did you find it difficult?

11 *CONFLICT IN NORMS*
Did you see this as interfering with any other things you should be doing?
Did you feel unsure about what was the right thing to do?
Did you feel uneasy about deciding to do X? Why?

12 *TENSION BETWEEN S AND X, OR X AND Y*
How well have you got on with . . . since – ?
Did it cause a lot of tension?
Was there any tension between X and Y after this?
If Yes   Did it upset you a lot?
             Did you have difficulty managing it?
             Did it interfere with anything?
How long were you expecting it to last?

13 *CONTROL OF INFORMATION*
Did you feel you had to hold anything back after this happened?
Did you feel you could talk freely about it?

Help

1 *AVOIDABILITY*
How did you feel you should help – become involved?
How strongly?
Did anyone at home make you feel you ought to help?
Did anyone at home have any views about . . . ?

2 *JOINT EXPERIENCE*

3 *SUPPORT* positive/negative/ambivalent: practical/emotional
Reactions of others: panic/in control
Did the people at home know about it?
How did they feel about it?
What did they say – do about it?
Did they help/encourage you/hinder at all?
Was there anyone who you feel could have helped and didn't?
Or taken an interest and didn't?
Did anyone talk it over with you? Give any practical help?
What about the people involved with you?
How did they react at the time?

Difficulties

1 *Timing of difficulty/uncertainty etc. and length of exposure to difficulty up till C3*
Check (i) Whether B to C1 : C1 – C3 : or both
(ii) How long difficulty/uncertainty been going on.

2 *Reported Severity*
How much did you worry about this?
How much did this bother you?

3 *Amount of time with the problem (if clear external focus)*
check no. hours/day.

4 *Amount of time problem on S's mind*
For problems without clear external focus
How often would this be on your mind?
For problems with clear external focus
When you weren't (e.g. with X), how often would this be on your mind?

5 *Uncertainty/Likely time duration of uncertainty*
(see Qs in main schedule)

6 *Optimism/Pessimism concerning outcome*
How did you think things would turn out?
Were you expecting this to improve?

7 *Expected time duration of difficulty at C1*
How long did you think it would be before (e.g. X would be overcome)?

8 *Help/Support*
Read with related chronic difficulties together.
Has anyone tried to help you with_____?
Collect details e.g. Who? How often? Type help (practical/emotional)? When did it stop?
Did you feel anyone took an interest in how you were managing?
Who? (**if not mentioned**): What about spouse/parent?
Did you talk about any aspect of it with anyone?
Who? (**if not mentioned, ask about spouse/parent**) How often?
if necessary, ask:
How did your husband/wife/mother/father/boyfriend feel about it?
Was he/she sympathetic?
Was there anyone who made things worse?
Was there anyone you expected to be sympathetic who wasn't?

Appendix 6
Examples of difficulties by type and severity

As with events the difficulties have been selected randomly and are presented under three heading; *health, household,* and *other.* In brackets we give the rating on the 6-point scale of severity – 1 (high) and 6 (low). The first rating is the contexual rating used for most of the analysis: the second is the general rating that took into account the degree of unpleasantness and distress 'reported' by the subject which at times differs from the first rating.

Health

319 – Subject is married, aged 34, with one child. She had to leave school early because of rheumatic heart disease and has been an invalid since then. She said she had been told on several occasions by her doctors that 'she would not last the year' (most recently 4 months before interview). She has to live a very restricted life: she does not get up until noon and often does nothing because she feels so weak. She says her doctors are considering a major operation (1.1).

614 – Subject is 60 and lives with her husband. Her husband had had a coronary thrombosis 2 years earlier. He was in hospital for six months and then resting at home for three months. He had been back to work for a little but then told to have another extended period at home. As he was told to take things very easily he had recently changed his job and had much less pay. She said he had complained of feeling useless and bored at the new job, but had recently felt somewhat better about it. He is on a strict diet and takes 'blood tablets'. She worries a good deal about his health and their future (2.2).

432 – Subject has diabetes and since she has to cook her own meals, she has to live within easy access or her work. Her husband wants to have a child – she has been told that she would have to go to hospital 10 weeks before it was due. Her husband is very unwell (rated 1.1 on his health) and this would mean leaving him at home alone (3–3).

Household

505 – Subject is 25 and lives with her husband and three children (aged 1, 2, and 3) in one room with one bed. The room is very damp and they share a kitchen. They have extremely poor relations with their landlady who has accused them of stealing food, etc. The landlady's children often make a great noise when her children are trying to sleep; but nonetheless the landlady makes a great fuss about the noise subject's children make (1.1).

386 – Subject is 52 and has been married 34 years and has two children at home. She has a very poor relationship with husband. She never goes out with him: 'He's a moody type of man, he's very jealous.' They have long periods of not speaking at all and confide absolutely nothing. There has been great trouble over one of her sons: her husband says that she is much too soft with him (he's recently had trouble with the police). He shows her no affection – for example, the last time she was in bed unwell he offered no help at all. 'He's a dark horse: he keeps stores of money for his own things.' 'I'm not wicked . . . but if God did take him before he was too old, deep down I wouldn't miss him a great deal' (2.2).

569 – Husband's drinking worries her. He goes out drinking every night and comes home 'the worse for drink'. He then fidgets all night long and 'will rant and rave and curse on'. She says she tries to ignore him and they often have periods of not talking for three days. He is however no longer violent. Their disagreements are mainly about the children – she feels he is too hard on them. She is no longer interested in sex 'I just no longer want to be touched' (2–2).

376 – Subject is 46 and lives with husband and a daughter of 20. Her son left home 2 years ago before he married and they never see him at all. He left after a row with his father about the girl he was going to marry (3–3).

Other difficulties

506 – Subject is 32 and lives alone with five children aged 5, 6, 7, 8, and 13. She has not seen the man she used to live with for several years. She does not work and lives on 'National Assistance'. She is behind with rent and hire purchase payments and has been 'chivvied' by creditors. She says she does not worry very much: she has a 'welfare lady' behind her but she does find it difficult to feed and clothe the children (2–3).

416 – Subject is 40 and lives with her husband and son of 6. 'We never get out of debt however much we scrimp and save.' Her husband has been ill a good deal and had been off work for 1½ years. At the time of the interview he had been back at work for 7 months but they still have debts of £46. She does not see any way they can be cleared (2–2).

312 – Subject cannot read or write and never went to school and 'cannot get the plum jobs'. She feels inferior because of this, but does not worry about it. She can do a knitting pattern (3–4).

514 – Subject is 57 and lives with her husband. He has trouble with his leg and is often off work (he has been off 6 months in the last year). He does not get any sickness benefit from work and this makes things 'quite tight' and for some time they have been living off her wage (3–3).

Notes

Chapter 1

1 Most research workers in the socio-medical field will have their own choices here. We might mention research by Cobb and his colleagues on rheumatoid arthritis in women, Lee Robins on sociopathic personality, and that by Rutter and his colleagues on the relation of psychiatric disorder in children to psychiatric disorder in their parents.
2 For an excellent account of issues surrounding psychiatric diagnosis see Zigler and Phillips (1961).
3 We also refer later in this book to work with schizophrenic patients. For a similar discussion of the nature of schizophrenia see Wing and Brown (1970).

Chapter 2

1 Bornstein et al, 1973; Clayton et al, 1968, 1972, 1974.
2 The inter-rater reliability was .79 (product moment correlation).
3 We are grateful to Professor John Copeland for his help with this.
4 Dr Ray Prudo played a large part in making these ratings.

Chapter 3

1 Robert Merton uses the term empirical generalization in much the same way as we use causal model: 'An isolated proposition summarizing observed uniformities of relationships between two or more variables' (Merton, 1957: 95).
2 Studies, not reviewed later in detail, that have looked at life-events and depression are Parker et al., 1959; Sethi, 1964; Forrest, Fraser and Priest, 1965; Hudgens, Morrison and Barchaa, 1967; Leff, Roach and Bunney, 1970; Beck and Worthen, 1972; Cadoret et al., 1972.
3 However, these effects are likely to be small. This is confirmed by a comparison of the occupation of any male 'head of household' of women in the

first survey with that provided by the 1961 census for men in Camberwell – 67 per cent were manual workers and 12 per cent unskilled which is very close to the census figures of 69 per cent and 13 per cent respectively.
4 Numbers of patients making contact with out-patient and emergency clinics in Camberwell in the years 1965–70 and number of contacts made.

	1965	1966	1967	1968	1969	1970
patients*	1,729	1,743	1,964	1,970	2,089	2,080
individual contacts	8,197	7,773	8,643	9,338	10,008	10,047

*Unduplicated total of patients within each separate year (see J. K. Wing and A. M. Hailey, 1972: 153).

5 We are indebted to Dr John Macleod the general practitioner on North Uist without whose generous help the Island survey would not have been possible.
6 The shortened versions of the PSE differed marginally between the two surveys, the first being based on the eighth edition and the second on the ninth edition.
7 We are grateful to Dr Elaine Murphy for carrying out this analysis.

Chapter 4

1 In the later study of depression the only change was the inclusion of loss of 'confidants'.
2 Because events can be complex they are not always mutually exclusive; to deal with this we developed simple rules for classifying them in one rather than another category. This, however, occurred only rarely (e.g. the death of a mother-in-law normally excluded because it did not involve a 'close' relative or someone in the household but in this instance included because her death created the problem of caring for her ailing husband). If an event could be included in terms of the 'rules' for one and not the other it was always included.
3 In the later depression study we included deaths of 'confidants'.
4 For confidants the rate of contact had to be at least once a week.
5 For details see Brown and Birley (1968); and Birley and Brown (1970). The instrument has now also been used to study physical disorder (e.g. Connolly, 1976).
6 Occasionally we classified as 'independent' events brought about by the subject. Most of these had been planned at least 3 months ahead and arranged to occur on a definite date (such as a wedding), or were the result of the subject placing himself in the hands of some agency at least 3 months beforehand and being unable to predict the date of the event (such as hospital admission for a routine operation). In such cases the actual date of the event is most unlikely to have been influenced by the insidious onset of illness. In all a definite commitment had been made more than 3 months before; and neither the commitment nor its fulfilment seemed in any sense unusual or the result of a developing mental disorder. In a few instances we

included hospital admission in which the person had sought help in an emergency – one patient, for example, because of quickly developing blindness due to an eye infection.

7 There was a third category of 'illness related' events that occurred after onset. When we came to look at the relationship between life-events and change-points after onset of depression (see chapter 13) these were excluded, since we had every reason to believe they were the direct consequence of the depression, for example, losing a job through 'slowness' or a suicide attempt.

8 It may be objected, continuing with this example, that this will prove wasteful by including in the basic unit too many events demanding no change of skill (and by implication no anxiety). If this is likely to be so it is possible to define the *unit* in a way that it has only a *probabilistic* relationship with qualities of interest – in the present instance, the need to develop new skills. Thus, if we believed that the development of new skills was important, we might decide in the definition of our unit to exclude changes involving the same type of work (for instance, a car mechanic going to another garage). In general the aim of drawing up a definition should be to ensure that the unit correlates reasonably well with qualities that we think might be of importance in the research problem we are tackling. To return to our example: the definition would probably still give us sufficient instances of changes of job with *and* without the demand for new skills to enable us to test whether such a demand has the significance we have visualized. The approach is flexible because it allows us to do this and also to explore other qualities. The correlation between unit and quality should be moderate. If the correlation is too low we risk collecting a good deal of data of little intrinsic interest; if it is too high we will run into the kind of circularity that we set out to avoid.

9 As would be expected there was a considerable amount of variability in the score allocated to the descriptions by the different raters; but this variability is conveniently by-passed henceforth through using only the average of the distribution of each set of scores. The high correlations usually obtained when comparing the results from different calibration studies are irrelevant for this point – and are indeed explained by it (e.g. Masuda and Holmes 1967; Kamaroff, Masuda and Holmes, 1968; Mendels and Weinstein, 1972). The correlations are high because the *average* scores are used, again ignoring the considerable variation obtained for most items *within* each study.

10 We have not attempted a comprehensive review of other instruments; as far as we are aware other methods developed for use in the general population are open to the same broad objections. Most have been heavily influenced by the Holmes and Rahe instrument though some appear to have been amended sufficiently to avoid some of the criticism of the SRE (e.g. Paykel, Prusoff and Uhlenhuth, 1971).

11 We use the word possible here as it is unnecessary for bias to be actually present – only that it may well be present and cannot be ruled out by any procedures employed or by convincing argument.

12 The arrow from R to X in *Figure 1* (and later in *Figure 2*) represents a causal link: in *Figure 1*, for instance, that the investigator's or the subject's knowledge of Y brings about X. This convention can be confusing if it is not realized that the arrow is a way of representing the fact of contamination. Of course R cannot really influence X as such (which has already happened

in this instance); but it can bring about X *as rated or reported* and this is the critical point since we know of factors such as life-events *only insofar as they are measured*. Contamination can therefore be seen as linking two causal systems: that of the 'real' world and that produced by the measurement process itself.

Chapter 5

1 The amount of agreement between the accounts of patient and relative when describing the *same* event ranged from .74 for the rating of all self-reports of threat (long-term), .89 for the expectancy of the event occurring when it did, to almost total agreement for scales dealing with more obvious aspects such as amount of change involved in daily routine or in face-to-face contacts with others.

The overall agreement between *separate* interviews on the contextual long-term threat of particular events was only 0.66. Since we found that the inter-rater reliability for this rating was only 0.75 the overall agreement would be influenced by this. Reliability can be improved by using the agreed ratings based on the meetings of all investigators. When this was done reliability improved and, as expected, the agreement between ratings based on the separate patient and relative accounts rose from 0.66 to 0.85 – a quite acceptable level of agreement.

Therefore as with the schizophrenic study we concluded that the reliability and validity (in the sense of cross-respondent agreement) of the measures concerning events was usually good and always acceptable.

Chapter 6

1 As noted already in chapter 3, it makes no sense to include in such comparisons women in Camberwell with a definite psychiatric disorder. If there is a causal link between the psychiatric disorder and events, they will have a higher rate of events and their inclusion would only serve to reduce, unnecessarily and misleadingly, an association between events and onset of depression.

2 The focus rating was discussed in the last chapter (see page 94). A car accident, for example, would be rated as subject-focussed if the respondent was either alone in the car or with another person; it would not be rated as subject-focussed if, say, the respondent's husband was involved but she was not. We strongly suspect that dividing moderate events in this way simply introduces a new point on the severity of threat scale. If 'severe' events are seen as the top two points on a 5-point scale of threat the reader will, we believe, have caught the essence of the distinction. In reading the descriptions of events we had no doubt that moderate events that focussed on the subject (either alone or jointly with someone else) were on the whole more threatening than those focussed only on another person. By incorporating the focus rating into the 4-point threat scale we have, in effect, tended to ensure that events involving persons outside the subject's household will be included in the 'severe' category only if they are particularly threatening (i.e. rated 'marked'). The classification of 'severe' events has therefore a certain conceptual untidiness. To try to change it at a

late stage would have risked introducing bias. There is, however, no reason why in future a 5-point scale of threat incorporating this distinction should not be developed. (It should not prove difficult.) Finally it is important to note that four separate surveys (patient, first Camberwell, second Camberwell, and general practice) independently confirm the validity of the distinction between the two kinds of moderate long-term threat. In all four it is only 'moderate subject-focussed' events that are associated with onset of depression.

3 Results for onset cases were 100 and 168 severe events and non-severe events respectively per 100 women (35 for marked and 65 for moderate, subject-focussed events). Rates for women attending a general practitioner were similar.

4 It will be remembered that we asked about events in the 12 months before 'admission' and too few patients had onset near enough to their admission for weeks 49–52 before their onset to be included.

5 Onset among patients occurred on average 14 weeks before 'admission': we have added to this a further 3 weeks to take account of the delay between 'admission' and interview, meaning that length of recall was on average 17 weeks longer than for normal women. This means that an average of 14 weeks before onset fell into the period of under-reporting and only 5 weeks of that for normal women. A correction requires adding 22 non-severe events which give a rate for the patients of 194 (221/114).

6 Those with at least one severe event in the two categories are:

	independent events		possibly independent events		possibly independent events for women without independent event	
	n	%	n	%	n	%
patients	57	50	26	23	13	11
onset cases	21	57	7	19	4	11
normal women	60	16	18	5	15	4

7 In order to compare the two sets of results we used a 'percentage ratio' which expresses the differences between proportions in a way that takes account of differences in the absolute size of the pairs of percentages that are compared (see Galtung, 1967: 198–204). The ratio is:

$$\frac{\% \; 'a' \; - \; \% \; 'b'}{\% \; 'a' \; + \; \% \; 'b'}$$

For instance, it takes account of the fact that for most purposes we will not want to consider a difference between 10 and 20 per cent of the same order as one between 60 and 70 per cent, although both involve a difference of 10 per cent. The percentage ratio is 45 per cent for patients and normal women with three or more severe events of any kind and 52 per cent for patients and normal women with two or more 'unrelated' events, suggesting the latter is, if anything, the stronger effect

8 Several analyses were carried out all based on the principle of allocating arbitrary weights to events based on the contextual threat ratings. Some of

the analyses excluded 'related' events (e.g. learning a husband has cancer and his death) and others included them. No matter what method or weights were used we were unable to increase our ability to 'predict' onset.

9 We would not rule out tackling the issued of such 'symbolic' appraisal in future research. In the example discussed it is possible that the interpretation of the first event, her father's death, had no direct aetiological role – it may indeed have been a *result* of her depression (in spite of her insistence that she had had the thoughts before it). But this is in principle the same type of problem tackled by the contextual ratings and it might be possible to overcome such possible reporting 'bias' by again ignoring in our judgments what a woman said she felt and her psychiatric state.

10 These conclusions are confirmed by the relatives' accounts. Not only was there a high agreement with the patient's account, but the comparison showed no tendency for the patient to exaggerate in her reports the intensity of her feelings at the time.

Chapter 7

1 We would not always make this assumption. For example it might not be justified in the case of drinking and car accidents: in this instance heavy drinking is equivalent to our 'events' and car drivers who have accidents might well be heavier drinkers (i.e. have a higher rate or 'events') than the general population.

2 The inclusion of psychiatric 'cases' in this instance should not be confused with their exclusion in the last chapter in the initial test for the presence of a causal link between life-events and onset. As we have already noted, it would obviously be misleading to include them in the comparison between patients and normals.

3 We are indebted to Julian Peto for the mathematical development of the solution to these problems.

4 The length of the causal period is used as the unit of time for convenience but in expectation approximately the same result would be obtained if any *longer* period were used, and h, p, and r were defined accordingly. It is therefore not important to determine the exact point before onset at which the conditional rate returns to the true patient rate to calculate the brought forward time, although if too short a period is taken, the resulting estimate will be even more conservative.

5 It may be useful to go through this particular calculation. The average time period covered for patients was 38 weeks and this was therefore also used for the community sample. Therefore:

time period = 38 weeks = causal period

h = proportion of patients with at least one severe event before onset = $70/114$ = .614

p = proportion of total general population with at least one severe event in the 38 weeks before interview = $114/458$ = .249

r = rate of severe events per 38 weeks for total general population sample (taking 38 weeks before interview) = $162/458$ = .354

Using $T_{BF} = \dfrac{h - p}{r(1 - h)} \cdot 1$ time period $= \dfrac{.614 - .249}{.354\,(1 - .614)} \cdot 38$

$= 101.5$ weeks $= 1.95$ years

It will be recalled that severe events are marked events and moderate subject-focussed events. When these are considered separately their T_{BF}'s are 105 and 71 weeks respectively.

6 Schizophrenic patients were of both sexes but the population comparison group drawn from the depression study consists only of women. We used this comparison group rather than the original employed in the schizophrenic study to avoid the formidable undertaking of re-rating events in terms of long-term threat, which was not used in the earlier study. The rate of events among the 'normal women', however, is very close to that found in the comparison group of men and women used in the original schizophrenic study.

7 In the general population on average 8.4 per cent had a severe event in any one 9-week period.

8 So far we have suggested that the effect of severe events most often occurs within 9 weeks of their occurrence although at times they can probably bring about clinical depression after a good deal longer. There is evidence that events some distance from onset were also capable of speeding up the development of depression in the sense of reducing the average *time* elapsing between severe event and onset when patients had more than one severe event. Two-thirds (19/28) of patients with more than one severe event had one within three weeks of onset compared with only a third (15/42) of those with one event (p<.01). The presence of an earlier severe event appears to bring about onset more quickly when the next severe event immediately before onset is considered. For the week before onset the proportions were 54 per cent for the 28 patients with multiple events and 24 per cent for the 42 with just one event (p<.01). There is the possibility that the result is due to an artefact: that the earlier event had already 'caused' onset and at the same time led to a subsequent severe event which in fact was of no direct causal importance. The reduced time would then only be apparent. For instance, the woman's depression may have already been determined by the fact that her husband said he was to leave home and was not influenced by his actually leaving three weeks later. However, since the result was exactly the same for those with multiple events who had an 'unrelated' event outside the three weeks (14/20 – 70 per cent) as for those with only a 'related' event (5/8 – 63 per cent), a case can be made for a 'speeding up' effect.

9 The calculation for T_{BF} for cases for a 9-week period is as follows:

$h = .568$, $p = .084$, $r = .085$, time period $= 9$ weeks

$T_{BF} = \dfrac{.568 - .084}{.085\,(1 - .568)} \cdot 9$

$= 117.7$ weeks $= 2.26$ years.

10 The study has been reported in a series of papers: Paykel *et al.*, 1969, 1970, 1971, 1974 and Uhlenhuth and Paykel, 1973; Paykel, 1973. A good introduction by Eugene Paykel (1974) can be found in *Life Stress and Illness*, edited by E. K. Eric Gunderson and R. H. Rahe.

11 Data on rates of events are not given in these two studies and the value of r

was therefore based on the Poisson approximation using those with at least one event in the 6 months (see Appendix 4).

12 Eugene Paykel has discussed the magnitude of the effect of life-events in terms of the epidemiological concept of *relative risk* (MacMahon and Pugh, 1970). A direct measure is possible in the Camberwell study. Since 24.7 per cent (24/97) of the women with a severe event and 4.0 per cent (13/322) of the women without a severe event developed depression the relative risk is 6.2 (i.e. 24.7/4.0). This, as Paykel points out, is an easily interpretable measure of the magnitude of a *causative* association; an estimate can also be easily calculated when only the proportion with an event are known for a patient and comparison group (Paykel, 1977). Using the patient data and Camberwell material for normal women this estimate of the relative risk of depression based on severe events in the 38-week period is 6.3:

provoking agent	patients	normal women
present	a	b
absent	c	d

$$\text{relative risk} = \frac{a.d}{c.b} = \frac{61.80}{39.20} = 6.3$$

However, the estimate of relative risk for schizophrenia based on any kind of event in 3 weeks before onset and a similar period in the original comparison group is 6.4 (i.e. 60.81/40.19) which is almost exactly comparable to that for depression. Since the index of relative risk does not discriminate between the two conditions it clearly does not deal with the same question as T_{BF}, that is the distinction between triggering and formative effects.

Chapter 8

1 The inter-rater reliability of two raters on the six point scale of contextual severity is .84.

2 We refer to difficulties rated on the top 3 points of the six-point severity scales. There was close agreement between the contextual and general threat scales:

		normal women general threat						patients general threat					
		1	2	3	4	5	6	1	2	3	4	5	6
	1	17	4	1	1	0	0	27	0	0	0	0	0
	2	3	66	7	8	1	0	2	50	0	1	0	0
contextual	3	0	15	108	14	3	0	0	19	57	3	0	0
threat	4	0	8	31	214	26	3	0	2	19	69	4	0
	5	0	0	15	54	284	14	0	0	8	32	74	1
	6	0	0	2	11	25	186	0	0	1	3	31	30

	1–3	4–6
1–3	<u>221</u>	27
4–6	56	817

	1–3	4–6
	<u>136</u>	4
	30	244

3 Rates per 100 women of minor difficulties (i.e. rated 4 to 6) are:

	A. *type of minor difficulty*		B. *non-health minor difficulties by whether there is also a major difficulty*	
	health	non-health	major difficulty	no major difficulty
patients	126 ⎫	125 ⎫	130 ⎫	118 ⎫
	⎬ 133	⎬ 117	⎬ 126	⎬ 106
onset cases	159 ⎭	95 ⎭	124 ⎭	70 ⎭
normal women	141	90	92	89
difference depressed and normal women	−8	+27	+34	+17

4 The rate per 100 women of all non-health difficulties rated 1 to 3 lasting less than 2 years is:

	less than 1 year	1 to 2 years
patients	30.7	20.2
onset cases	18.9	35.1
normals	13.6	11.0

However if difficulties either leading to or caused by a severe event are excluded the differences are much reduced – 15.8, 10.8, and 11.3 respectively for difficulties of less than 1 year and 15.8, 27.0, and 9.9 respectively for those lasting between 1 and 2 years. Further, since in most instances women with such difficulties *also* have a major difficulty, their inclusion makes no difference to conclusions about the size of an aetiological effect ('x') for patients and only slightly increases it for onset cases. Larger numbers are required to settle the matter: but since we can see no theoretical reason why difficulties lasting less than 2 years should not play an aetiological role, we believe we have probably been too conservative in excluding them.

Chapter 9

1 The argument for the respective contributions of events and difficulties runs as follows: the percentage of patients having *either* a severe event or major difficulty is 75.4 per cent (86/114), compared with the total general

population figure of 36.2 per cent (166/458). The corrected proportion, x, for patients with an event or a difficulty is 61.5 per cent, an increase of 12.9 per cent over the x when just events are considered. The x for difficulties whether or not there is a severe event is 30.6 per cent. These figures allow the calculation of the separate contributions of events and difficulties: events independently contribute 61.5 per cent minus 30.6 per cent, i.e. 30.9 per cent; difficulties independently contribute 12.9 per cent and therefore the contribution of the joint effect of events and difficulties is 17.7 per cent (i.e. 61.5 per cent − 30.6 per cent + 12.9 per cent). The independent contribution of severe events is thus somewhat more than twice the size of the independent contribution of difficulties. The joint effect of events and difficulties is quite sizeable – larger than that of difficulties alone and just over half the independent contribution of events. For onset cases the independent effects of events and difficulties are 48.6 per cent and 26.1 per cent respectively and the joint effect 10.4 per cent.

2 The period before onset was on average 38 weeks for patients and for onset cases; and a comparison of 38 weeks before interview was therefore taken for 'normal' women. The period was 41 weeks for general practice patients. Chronic cases are excluded: 21 of the 39 are positive on 1, 2 or 3.

3 It is of interest that 'unrelated' difficulties and 'unrelated' events show only a small and statistically non-significant association, suggesting our judgments about 'relatedness' are valid. A positive association would not, however, have disconfirmed the validity of the ratings: women with an event may have been more likely for other reasons to have a difficulty and vice versa. The association of 'unrelated' events and difficulties among women in Camberwell is:

		number of 'unrelated' difficulties		
		0	1	2+
number of	0	288	51	3
'unrelated'	1	65	25	6
events	2+	14	6	0

4 The data are, as follows, based on women with at least one severe event or major difficulty, using those occurring before onset for patients and onset cases and those occurring in the 38 weeks before interview for normal women:

	number of events and difficulties		
	1	2	3+
A *a severe event and/or major difficulty of any kind*	%	%	%
patients (86)	36 (31)	26 (22)	38 (33)
onset cases (33)	52 (17)	24 (8)	24 (8)
patients and cases (119)	40 (48)	25 (30)	34 (41)
normals (114)	66 (75)	20 (23)	14 (16)

| | number of events and difficulties | | |
	1	2	3+
B 'unrelated' events and/or difficulties only	%	%	%
patients (86)	56 (48)	23 (24)	16 (14)
onset cases (33)	61 (20)	24 (8)	15 (5)
patients and cases (119)	57 (68)	27 (32)	16 (19)
normals (114)	75 (86)	21 (24)	4 (4)

This table should be compared with *Table 2* in chapter 6.

5 In relation to *Table 2* note, (i) only one event (that with the greatest threat) has been taken for each woman; (ii) since the events for normal women occurred in the course of one year their proportions have been adjusted accordingly; (iii) among onset cases in the community there were four women involved in a pregnancy/birth before the depression. Two had an associated severe event. One of these was due to a husband being sent to Borstal for two years a short while after she learnt she was pregnant. Results for these onset cases in the four rows of *Table 2* are 5.4 per cent (2/37) for non-severe threat, and 2.7 per cent (1/37) and 5.4 (2/37) for the two types of threat associated with pregnancy or birth.

6 The rates of health difficulties per 100 women are:

focus and severity	chronic cases	normal women	onset cases	patients
marked subject	33.3	6.3	8.1	8.7
marked other	23.1	11.5	5.4	12.3
minor subject	100.0	56.8	75.7	48.2
minor other	143.6	84.3	78.4	76.3

Chapter 10

1 See Dohrenwend and Dohrenwend, 1969. More recent statements by these authors were published in 1974b and 1975.

2 Women in Camberwell by life-stage and marital status are:

	younger	−6	6—14	15+	older	total
single	22	–	–	–	14	36
married	34	105	91	64	88	382
widowed/ separated/ divorced	3	4	2	8	23	40

A third of the *older* group had children living away from home.
Age is not importantly related to prevalence of psychiatric disorder and the differences that occur seemed best explained by factors related to life-stage and class. Prevalence figures for caseness in the year are:

18—25	26—35	36—45	46—55	56—65
%	%	%	%	%
7	22	17	14	20
(5/72)	(22/101)	(16/95)	(14/102)	(18/88)

The lower rate among the youngest group is related to the fact they have no chronic cases.

3 Here we give rates of psychiatric disorder for the three months before interview as we believe they are a more accurate estimate of the prevalence of disorder than those for one year. But in dealing with onset of disorder we use the whole year as this gives a greater number of onset cases on which to base our research for aetiological factors. The basic data for the cases shown in *Figure 1* are:

	younger	−6	6—14	15+	*older*	
working class	2/17	18/58	12/55	9/41	14/69	55/240
middle class	3/42	2/51	2/38	2/31	5/56	14/218

While this simple social class dichotomy is usually used, for all important tabulations we have also looked at a three-fold division and this shows in each instance the same order of difference. For example, for the present result 24 per cent of the 'low' status, 12 per cent of the 'intermediate', and 7 per cent of the 'high' are cases.

4 The proportion of cases among women with children at home are:

three or more children under 14 at home	all women child under 6			working-class women child under 6		
	yes %	no %	%	yes %	no %	%
yes	40 (10/25)	23 (5/22)	32 (15/47)	56 (9/16)	31 (5/16)	44 (14/32)
no	12 (10/84)	11 (20/143)	13 (30/227)	21 (9/42)	20 (16/80)	20 (25/122)
total	18 (20/109)	15 (25/165)		31 (18/58)	22 (21/96)	

5 The basic data for these results for the three months are:

	younger	*child at home*	*older*
		onset cases	
working	1	21	3
middle	2	3	4

	younger	*child at home*	*older*
		chronic cases	
	(excluding cases who had recovered in the last three months)		
working	1	18	11
middle	1	3	1
		total women	
working	17	154	69
middle	42	120	56

6 The basic data for borderline cases in the 3 months for class and life-stage are:

	younger	*−6*	*6—14*	*15+*	*older*	
working class	3/17	10/58	9/55	8/41	15/69	45/240
middle class	10/42	6/51	11/38	2/31	9/56	38/218

Five per cent (12/240) of working class and 6 per cent (14/218) of the middle class are onset borderline cases and 14 per cent (33/240) and 11 per cent (24/218) chronic.

7 This is a ratio produced by dividing the suicide rate of the unmarried by the rate for the married for each sex separately. Ratios of more than 1.0 indicate a relatively lower rate for the married. The separate ratios for men and women can then be compared. In this way he showed, for example, that in nineteenth-century France, while married men with children when compared with unmarried men without children had a coefficient of preservation of 2.9, for married women the same comparison provided a coefficient of only 1.89. The index was 1.50 for married men without children, and for women without children it was 0.67 i.e. married women without children actually had a higher suicide rate than single women of the same age (see Durkheim, 1952: 197–98).

8 For three-quarters of the 40 who were widowed, separated, and divorced the woman's current or last occupation level was the same as her husband's 'usual' occupation when she had lived with him. This rule did not therefore make a great deal of difference.

9 Brown, Ní Bhrolcháin, and Harris (1975: 241) gives an account of this social status index.

10 For example see Hollingshead and Redlich (1958). For recent compilations of social class differences see Reid (1977) and Westergaard and Resler (1976).

11 The agreement between the *Bedford* and *Goldthorpe-Hope* measures of class based on women with children at home is:

		Goldthorpe-Hope	
		high status	*low status*
Bedford	*high status*	105	41
	low status	15	113

The results for the *RGO, Bedford,* and *Goldthorpe-Hope* measures were similar for two-fold and three-fold divisions. The two-fold results in terms of prevalence of caseness in Camberwell per 100 women with children at home are:

	'high status'	'low status'	
RGO	3.4 (3/88)	22.6 (42/186)	low = skilled manual and below
Bedford	6.8 (10/146)	27.3 (35/128)	low = semi and unskilled manual (RGO) without 16+ years education of husband or wife or possession of a car *and* a telephone
Goldthorpe-Hope	5.0 (6/120)	25.3 (39/154)	low = 23 to 35; high = 1 to 22

Lazarsfeld and Barton (1951) have coined the term 'interchangeability of indicators' to describe the way in which different measures of the same concept, although modestly correlated, can give essentially the same results.

12 Ritter and Hargens (1975) showed that a woman's own occupational level (if she was working) was as important as her husband's occupation in predicting how far she saw herself as 'middle class'. But they were dealing with a woman's views about class and the point cannot be necessarily generalized to other 'dependent' variables. (And, of course, there are difficulties about what to do when a woman does not go to work.)

13 For example, for women with children at home in Camberwell the prevalence of psychiatric disorder was:

		woman's 'peak' occupation high %	low %	
	high	4 (4/77)	5 (2/38)	5 (6/115)
husband's occupation	low	17 (8/42)	28 (31/112)	25 (39/154)
		10 (12/119)	24 (36/150)	

The study by Ritter and Hargens, mentioned in note 12, also checked to see whether an occupational scale developed for men (Duncan's socio-economic index) could be used to grade woman's occupations. They showed that taking account of the woman's occupation (by a discriminant function analysis giving optimal predictive weights to each occupational group) gave practically the same result as using the original measure. This suggests that it is reasonable to use classifications, such as that of Goldthorpe and Hope developed primarily for 'male' occupations, to rank 'female' occupations.

14 We obtained the usual occupation of the father of the women in Camberwell and it was therefore possible to compare the prevalence of psychiatric disorder by past status with that by the current position based on husband's or own occupation. (Ten women whose social class had been based on father's current occupation were excluded.) Father's usual occupation was unknown for 5 per cent of the women and this included six of the cases. Results for the remainder show that current status is much more highly related to psychiatric disorder than past status. Where the current status is non-manual, father's occupation is unrelated to prevalence of disorder – 8 per cent (6/75) for manual and 10 per cent (8/82) for non-manual father. Where current status is manual the rate of disorder is somewhat lower when father was non-manual than when he was manual – 14 per cent (6/43) and 22 per cent (50/223) respectively (p<.01). Not too much can be made of this result except a general confirmation that a woman's current environment is of major importance in influencing risk of depression – although the hint that the past can play some role should not be ignored and we return to this in later chapters.

15 The chart in Appendix 3 follows this ten-fold scheme and gives examples of events of all degrees of threat.

16 For *younger* women 31 per cent (13/42) of middle-class women and 47 per cent (8/17) of working-class women have a severe event, and 36 per cent (20/56) and 30 per cent (21/69) respectively of the *older* women.

17 The 47 per cent is reduced to 32 per cent when only marked non-health difficulties are considered.

18 The basic data in terms of rate of difficulties per 100 women are:–

	A. *severity 1 to 3 non-health*	B. *severity 1 to 3 health*	*A+B*	*severity 4*	*severity 5 and 6*	*total*
younger	54	22	76	86	186	348
child	53	30	83	84	157	324
older	27	40	69	86	160	315

19 The figures are 9/30, 12/48, 30/55, 18/32, 28/51 respectively for the five life-stages.

20 A. The data in terms of women having at least one severe event/marked difficulty are:

	middle class	*working class*	*ratio*
	%	%	
severe event	43 (93/218)	55 (132/240)	1 to 1.28
marked difficulty of less 2 years (excluding any resulting from a severe event)	14 (30/218)	13 (31/240)	1 to 0.93
marked difficulty 2 years +	24 (53/218)	42 (101/240)	1 to 1.75

B. Marked difficulties lasting 2 years or more by type are:

	Goldthorpe-Hope	high status	low status
Household	10 (22/218)	25 (61/240)	1 to 2.52
Health	13 (28/218)	22 (53/240)	1 to 1.73
Other	2 (5/218)	5 (13/240)	1 to 2.37

C. Severe events by type are given in *Table 3*.

Chapter 11

1 Of those who experienced a major difficulty or a severe event, the proportion becoming a case was 15 per cent (7/53) for those reporting 'marked' support, 20 per cent (13/64) 'some', and 28 per cent (13/46) 'none' (n.s.). Where the support differed between particular severe events or major difficulties we took the least favourable report.

2 The standard questions were: (i) If you had a problem of some sort who would be the first person that you would want to discuss it with? (ii) What about your . . . husband (*pause*). Mother, (*pause* etc.), sister, father, brother? What about any friends? Are any of them close enough for you to be able to confide in? And would you feel you could tell them anything? Or most of any troubles that you might have? (iii) Is your husband easy to talk to in general about things? Does he ever get bored or stop listening? Or say that women are always worrying about things that aren't really important?

3 The measurement of communication between husband and wife is particularly difficult and there must be doubt how far it can be accomplished by interviewing (see Rutter and Brown, 1966: 259). We do not claim our rating is a measure simply of communication; it certainly contains an attitudinal component and also probably tends to pick up general qualities of the relationship.

4 For women with an event or difficulty and without children, 10 per cent (3/31) in 'a', 16 per cent (3/19) in 'b', and 27 per cent (3/11) in 'c' or 'd' developed depression compared with 11 per cent (6/57), 32 per cent (9/28), and 50 per cent (9/18) for women with children.

5 There is a slight and non-significant association between loss of father before eleven and psychiatric disorder. This is explained by the fact that a number of women with loss of a mother before eleven also lost a father at about the same time.

6 The percentage of the 458 women who developed psychiatric disorder in the year by number of children living at home and employment is:

severe event or major difficulty		no severe event or major difficulty	
3 children less 14	less 3 children	3 children less 14	less 3 children
9/21	24/143	0/20	4/235
43	17	0	2
p < .05		n.s.	

severe event or major difficulty		no severe event or major difficulty	
not employed	employed	not employed	employed
18/74	15/90	3/97	1/158
24	17	3	1
	n.s.		n.s.

Total number of children, regardless of their ages or whether they live at home, does not increase vulnerability once three or more children under 14 living at home has been taken into account.

7 The distribution of the three vulnerability groups by social class, excluding chronic cases, is:

	'A'	'B'	'C'	
working class	123	68	18	209
middle class	158	47	5	210
	281	115	23	419
			$p < .01$	

8 The proportion who developed depression by vulnerability categories A, B and C, social class, and presence of provoking agents is:

	'A' 'a' intimacy	'B' 'non-a'	'C' 'non-a' + 3 or more children under 14 or early loss of mother
	%	%	%
(i) *with provoking agent*			
working class	12 (5/41)	20 (9/44)	83 (10/12)
middle class	9 (4/47)	22 (4/18)	50 (1/2)
(ii) *without provoking agent*			
working class	0 (0/82)	8 (2/24)	0 (0/6)
middle class	2 (2/111)	0 (0/29)	0 (0/3)
(chronic cases excluded)			

9 Percentage of women with a loss of parent before 17 among those who were cases at any time in the year (76) and the remaining women (382) is:

age at loss	loss of mother		loss of father		loss either	
	cases	normals	cases	normals	cases	normals
	%	%	%	%	%	%
0 to 10	22.4	6.0*	17.1	11.5	34.2	13.6*
11 to 16	0.0	2.1	2.6	5.0	2.6	6.0

* p < .01: other differences not significant

10 Age and class differences in the proportion of women in Camberwell with a past loss are:

	middle class	working class
	%	%
18–40	23 (25/110)	32 (34/107) n.s.
41–65	38 (41/108)	51 (58/133) p < .05
	p < .05	p < .01

Further details giving the type of loss are given in Brown, Harris and Copeland (1977: Figure 1). All comparisons (e.g. note 9) have been standardized for these age and social class differences.

11 The percentage of women in Camberwell who suffered an onset of psychiatric disorder in the year of study by whether they had a severe event or major difficulty and the presence of past loss (chronic cases excluded) is:

	A: any past loss		B: other past loss (excluding 30 women with loss of mother before 11)	
	yes	no	yes	no
severe event or major difficulty	%	%	%	%
	22 (15/67)	19 (18/97)	15 (8/53)	19 (18/97)
none	3 (2/76)	1 (2/179)	3 (2/60)	1 (2/179)

Fifteen per cent of the patient and the general Camberwell population with a past loss had more than one. Since such multiple losses do not contribute to the processes discussed in this chapter and later they have been ignored.

12 The data are:

Provoking agent	A. working-class vulnerability factors			B. middle-class vulnerability factors		
	0	1	2 +	0	1	2 +
yes	16	46	35	19	37	11
no	48	47	17	54	67	22
	gamma .51, p < .05			gamma .14, n.s.		

Results for intimacy alone are comparable.

13 Our reasons for believing that the higher rate of past loss among patients does not indicate that it raises the risk of depression are as follows. The basic one is that statistical manipulation shows that such loss does not behave as though it were a vulnerability factor. If it had acted in this way, patients with a past loss should be particularly likely to have had a severe event or major difficulty since it is only by their presence that a vulnerability factor leads to depression. However, although loss of mother before 11 conforms to this expectation (A below), other past losses do not (B below):

	A		B*	
	loss of mother before 11	no loss of mother before 11	other past loss	no other past loss
	%	%	%	%
per cent with a provoking agent	92	75	70	74
(n = 114)	(12)	(102)	(48)	(54)

*Excluding 12 patients who had lost a mother before 11.

If past loss does not act as a vulnerability factor, how are we then to explain the greater proportion of patients with a past loss? Two possibilities occur to us, both involving the issue of selection into psychiatric care:

(i) Let us assume that those patients with previous contact with a psychiatrist have a somewhat increased chance of contacting a psychiatrist about any further depressive episode. (This might be due to an increased risk of a new episode of depression or simply to a greater chance of seeing a psychiatrist about a subsequent episode.) Some of the previous episodes would be expected to have been brought about by loss of a child or husband that we have counted among 'past losses'. It follows that patients with a previous episode would be expected to have a raised rate of past loss. The argument is supported by the fact that a fifth of the 52 patients with a previous episode had lost a child or husband in adulthood (when it might well have been the provoking agent for the previous episode) compared with only 8 per cent of patients without a previous episode (p<.02).

(ii) We will show in a later chapter that past loss plays an important role in determining severity once a person has developed depression; since patients tend as a group to be more severely disturbed than cases in the general population, they would be again expected to have a somewhat greater frequency of past losses.

14 The percentage of patients, onset cases, and normal women with various vulnerability factors is:

	loss mother	'non-a' intimacy	not employed	3 + children under 14
	%	%	%	%
patients (114)	11	65	46	8
onset cases (37)	22	70	57	24
normal women (382)	6	34	39	8

	loss mother	'non-a' intimacy	not employed	3+ children under 14
general practice (34)	13	65	47	9
Row 1 vs 3	n.s.	p < .01	n.s.	n.s.
Row 1 vs 2	n.s.	n.s.	n.s.	p < .01
Row 2 vs 3	p < .05	p < .01	n.s.	p < .01

Results for women with children when considered alone are broadly comparable.

15 Both correlations are significant:

| | intimacy | | | 3 children under 14 | |
early loss mother	'a'	'b'	'c'/'d'	yes	no
yes	10	5	11	7	19
no	174	58	19	35	215
		gamma = .56			gamma = .40

Other associations are 3+ children and lack of employment, .10; low intimacy and lack of employment, −.03; 3+ children and low intimacy, −.06; early loss and lack of employment, −.08. Results for women with children are the same except for a small correlation between low intimacy and lack of employment, .20.

16 The figures for chronic cases are: 73 per cent (16/22) attended a general practitioner for their psychiatric condition for those with less than three children under 14 at home and not working, 60 per cent (6/10) for those working with less than three children under 14, and 86 per cent (6/7) for those with three or more children under 14.

Of the 37 onset cases, 49 per cent (18/37) had not received any help from their general practitioner: five had consulted him but not told him about their psychiatric symptoms (they had reported 'migraine', dizziness, rashes, amenorrhea, and a heart condition). Seeking advice was highly related to the woman reporting a previous episode – 94 per cent (15/16) and 19 per cent (4/21) respectively (p<.001). There was no association with social class, life-stage, or 'intimacy context'. Forty-six per cent (17/37) had been given a psychotropic drug such as 'librium', 'valium', or an antidepressant. Very much the same results emerged concerning treatment given for the chronic cases.

17 Using the three Goldthorpe-Hope categories the percentage class distributions are:

	high (1 to 17)	intermediate (18 to 31 excl. 26)	low (32 to 35 + 26)	
normal women (382)	32	36	32	(100%)
all cases (76)	15	27	58	(100%)
patients (114)	24	46	30	(100%)

Since our patients were specially selected for onset in the year we cannot be absolutely sure that they would resemble a *random* sample of depressed patients in Camberwell, and so too much weight should not be placed on this result. However, preliminary results from a study of all women receiving psychiatric care, based on the Camberwell Register, suggests that the result is broadly correct. An alternative explanation is, of course, that many cases in the general population are 'not really' psychiatrically disturbed, only 'unhappy' and these unhappy women are mostly working class. Since we do not believe there are any clinical grounds for such a conclusion we have not considered this possibility in the text.

Chapter 12

1 Dating of onset is more difficult for borderline cases than cases and this discussion should be seen as approximate. We have done our best to deal only with events that we considered definitely occurred before onset.

2 Those 'high' on vulnerability were (i) 'non-a' on intimacy and not employed or (ii) 'non-a' on intimacy and with early loss of mother before 11 or three children under 14, irrespective of whether or not they were employed. Those 'low' on vulnerability were (i) 'a' on intimacy or (ii) 'non-a' on intimacy who were employed and had no other vulnerability factor. The index is in line with the discussion of the relative importance of high intimacy and the other three vulnerability factors in chapter 11.

3 Exclusion of the period after onset of case or borderline case conditions makes no difference to these results.

4 The basic data are 11/39, 7/56, 1/68, and 18/295 respectively.

5 Brown, Ní Bhrolcháin, and Harris (1977b) contains a discussion on social class, deprivation, equality, and depression (*Sociology* 11: 527–31).

6 When severe events directly resulting from a major difficulty are excluded, the proportion with a severe event among chronic conditions is 24 per cent (23/95) and 19 per cent (55/295) among normal women.

Chapter 13

1 Forty-five per cent (33/73) of in-patients and 24 per cent (10/41) of out-patients had a second change-point and 10 per cent (7/73) and 2 per cent (1/41) respectively a third. Severity of disorder was rated '1' (high), to '5' (low). Only patients rated at onset as '3', '4', or '5' on overall severity changed to a more severe rating by the time of admission. Of the 40 in-patients with a rating of '3', '4', or '5' at onset one moved 4 points, six 3 points, fifteen 2 points, eleven 1 point, and seven remained unchanged – compared with three out-patients moving 2 points, seven 1 point, and fifteen unchanged. The average movement for in-patients was 1.58 points (63/40) compared with 0.52 (13/25) for out-patients (p<.05). The data for overall severity is:

	(high) 1	2	3	4	(low) 5	total	average score
admission							
out-patients	3	15	21	2	0	41	2.54
in-patients	16	50	7	0	0	73	1.86
			p < .001				
onset							
out-patients	3	13	16	6	3	41	2.83
in-patients	8	25	22	15	3	73	2.73
			n.s.				

2 This recording of 'change-points' in depression is to our knowledge the first systematic attempt to examine the course of the disorder and it is possible that we have exaggerated the 'quantum' nature of the changes. There was certainly a good deal of gradual deterioration *between* change-points. However, our impression has been that the development of depressive disorders treated by psychiatrists often involves marked and discrete periods of deterioration (and sometimes improvement). In any case we have only concluded that *differences* in severity of depression between in-patients and out-patients can be explained by what occurs at these points of the change; it is not claimed that a certain amount of further deterioration does not also take place.

3 Patients with a severe event after onset and before a change-point were only a little more likely to have had one before onset: 65 per cent (15/23) of those with a severe event before a change-point had one before onset compared with 42 per cent (11/26) of those without – n.s. Three patients were excluded from this calculation since time between onset and later change-point was so short.

4 The difference is statistically significant – p<.001. For the comparison we used 49 'periods' before a change-point and 75 between onset and a change-point. Only periods of at least 4 weeks in length were used: they ranged from 4 to 44 weeks and averaged 14 weeks. We used four periods: onset – second change-point (C2), C2 – third change-point (C3), onset – 'admission', or C2 – 'admission'. Periods of less than four weeks were excluded and this meant omitting one 'onset – C2', one 'C2 – admission', and 15 'onset – admission' periods.

5 If the presence of *any* event is taken as long as it has some degree of threat, 69 per cent (34/49) of periods before a change-point and 28 per cent (21/75) of other periods after onset have at least one event. When allowance is made for the fact that the comparison group has somewhat shorter periods, the proportion with an event of causal significance, x, increases from 37 per cent for severe events to 44 per cent for all threatening events (i.e. severity 1 to 3, any focus, short or long term threat), suggesting that minor events do little or nothing to bring about change-points.

6 The data for this score are based on previous episode, past loss and presence of a severe event after onset are:

	score		
severity at admission	2 or 3	1	0
high (1/2)	36	39	9
low (3/4)	4	13	13

p < .001

When we turn to overall severity at *onset* the association of past loss is much the same (gamma = .39 at onset and .47 at admission), but the presence of a previous episode is much less highly related to severity at onset than at 'admission' (gamma =.28 compared with .58). The third factor, the presence of a severe event after onset is, of course, only capable of influencing severity at admission.

7 The data are:

	score			
	0	1	2	3
% with severity rating '1' or '2' at admission	18%	52%	82%	100%
	(3/17)	(14/27)	(14/17)	(4/4)

The association of the score with treatment status is:

	0	1	2	3
in-patients	5	15	⌞16 20 4⌟	
out-patients	11	12	⌞2 2 0⌟	

gamma = .72, p < .001

When severity at 'admission' is controlled this association disappears (gamma =.02), indicating that the difference in severity between the two treatment groups is entirely due to these three factors (or factors related to them).

8 Per cent of patients with ratings of '1' or '2' on severity at admission are:

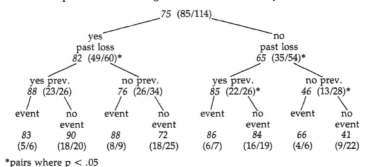

*pairs where p < .05

9 The argument is as follows: if the presence of a previous episode acted as a vulnerability factor, more patients with an episode would be expected to have a severe event or major difficulty. This would be because a vulnerability factor acts only through provoking agents. However, patients with a previous episode do not have a greater proportion with a severe event or major difficulty.

	previous episode	no previous episode
	%	%
per cent with a severe event or major difficulty	71 (37/52)	79 (49/62)

Chapter 14

1 The data on severity and diagnosis are:

severity rating at 'admission'	psychotic	neurotic	total
	% (n)	% (n)	% (n)
1 (high)	19 (12)	12 (6)	16 (18)
2	65 (41)	47 (23)	57 (64)
3/4 (low)	16 (10)	41 (20)	27 (30)
	100 (63)	100 (49)	100 (112)

Severity x pychotic/neurotic: p < .01, gamma .41

2 Although we take this point up in the next chapter, a fuller discussion of this issue and full details of the statistical analyses have been given in Ní Bhrolcháin, Brown, and Harris (1977). Inter-rater reliability for the various clinical scales used in this report was satisfactory, generally reaching a product-moment correlation of at least .80.

3 One of us independently rated the patients once the analysis had been done. The overall agreement with the original rating by the psychiatrist was 78 per cent. Agreement about the least psychotic patients was only 58 per cent compared with 85 per cent for the rest; this is consistent with our general impression that the 'overlap' between the two conditions is greatest among the 'least psychotic' half of the psychotic group. The ratings by the psychiatrist have been used in all analyses, unless we refer to the scores on the discriminant function.

The 17 items and their weights are set out below:

	weights	psychotic	neurotic	p
retardation	2.166	73%	31%	.001
waking early	1.623	56%	22%	.05
severity of obsessions/preoccupations*	1.047	82%	63%	.05

	weights	psychotic	neurotic	p
severity of impact on employment/ household tasks*	0.644	84%	65%	.05
middle insomnia	0.557	52%	37%	.2
diurnal variation, worse in the morning	0.532	45%	31%	.2
initial insomnia	0.487	69%	55%	.1
loss of weight	0.412	48%	31%	.1
loss of appetite	0.147	81%	63%	.05
severity of effect on day-to-day* routine	−0.069	71%	55%	.1
slowness of thinking/speech	−0.147	44%	20%	.05
severity of appetite disturbance**	−0.253	35%	47%	.1
overall severity***	−0.538	16%	41%	.01
impact on decision-making	−0.545	60%	47%	.2
verbal attacks	−0.681	29%	43%	.2
specific worry	−0.762	53%	65%	.2
total number of symptoms	−1.106	58% N=62	39% N=49	.05

* These items, originally 4–5 point scales, have been dichotomized at the best
  discriminating point. All other items are binary ratings.

** Dichotomized at marked and moderate loss vs. little or no loss or some gain in
  weight; weight gain was very rare.

*** Severity is rated from 1 (severe) to 5 (mild) and dichotomized at the best discrimin
  ating point. On the dichotomization, 0 represents therefore high and 1 low overall
  severity. The other severity scales are rated in the intuitively obvious way – a high
  score representing high severity, etc.

4 Fifty-eight per cent (36/62) of the psychotic (P) and 65 per cent (32/49) of the
  neurotic (N) group had a severe event before onset. Even those with a
  markedly threatening event did not differ: P:39 per cent (24/62) and N:41
  per cent (20/49). A slight difference appears in the proportion with a major
  difficulty – P:40 per cent (25/62) and N:55 per cent (27/49) although this is
  not statistically significant. The proportions having either a severe life event
  prior to onset or a major difficulty are P:71 per cent (44/62) and N:80 per cent
  (39/49). (The total for the discriminant function was 111 since one protocol
  was lost and two patients with definite manic symptoms were excluded.)
5 See Brown, Ní Bholcháin, and Harris (1977) for details. In fact, in terms of
  the aggregate data, only one patient with an event was added to the
  neurotic and subtracted from the psychotic group.
6 It might be objected that the traditional dichotomy has generally considered discrete events to be 'precipitants' and that ongoing difficulties of
  the kind included as provoking agents are not eligible for this role in the
  debate despite the evidence for their aetiological role in depression. In fact
  we carried out similar analyses defining 'endogenous' and 'reactive' in

terms of severe events alone. There were five items on which the groups differed significantly at admission, and two items at onset. Once again the items associated with the 'endogenous' group were of the type predicted by those who support the traditional two-fold division.

7 When the various possible types of loss were considered in detail these differences held for each, with the exception of loss of father by death where there was only a small difference between the two diagnostic groups. Since the numbers involved are small for the particular comparisons, little importance need be given at this point to this one exception. Of patients having a past loss by death, 82 per cent (37/45) are psychotic; of those having suffered loss by separation 73 per cent (11/15) are neurotic. Of those having neither, 41 per cent (21/51) are psychotic and 59 per cent (30/51) neurotic. Numbers in a previous account of this research were slightly different as we have now changed the discriminant function from a 23- to a 17-item analysis to conform with certain technical statistical requirements.

8 In our patient series we found complete agreement between the past losses obtained by interviewing patients and relatives and those recorded in the Maudsley in-patients records. In order to conform to the criteria of our own series we excluded five patients of Kendell's who were foreign or had marked manic symptoms or an important physical element such as epilepsy. Kendell's patients were a little younger – 57 per cent were under 40 at admission compared with half of our series.

9 The data are:

severity at 'admission'	any past loss		'effective' past loss	
	yes	no	yes	no
severity 1/2 (high)	49	35	43	41
severity 3/5 (low)	10	20	5	25
	gamma = .47		gamma = .68	

10 Another analysis took account of the degree of psychotic and neurotic features according to the 17-item discriminant function scores. It shows that 'effective' loss is particularly related to overall severity among the extreme psychotic and extreme neurotic halves of the two diagnostic groups, that is in the diagnostically most typical groups. The percentage with past loss, counting only deaths for psychotic patients and only separations for neurotic patients is:

	severity of symptoms at admission		
	1 (high)	2	3/4 (low)
	%	%	%
A. extreme psychotic/ neurotic quartiles*	90 (9/10)	55 (17/31)	14 (2/14)
B. less extreme psychotic/ neurotic quartiles	50 (4/8)	41 (13/32)	19 (3/16)

* These groups have been defined by taking the extreme and less extreme psychotic

and neurotic halves of the two diagnostic groups using the rankings of the 17 item discriminant function scores i.e. group A are the most psychotic and most neurotic patients. Top row $p < .05$; bottom row, combining columns 1 and 2 $p < .01$.

11 An excellent and straightforward account of the logic of such analyses is given by Rosenberg (1968). *Figure 3a* is an instance of testing for an 'intervening' factor and *3b* for an 'extraneous' factor. The data are:

	previous episode		*no previous episode*	
	psychotic	*neurotic*	*psychotic*	*neurotic*
−39	8	10	9	29
40+	26	5	19	5
	gamma = −.73		gamma = .85	

	Age −39		*Age 40+*	
	psychotic	*neurotic*	*psychotic*	*neurotic*
previous episode	8	10	26	5
none	9	29	19	5
	gamma = .44		gamma = .16	

Zero order gammas
Age x P/N: .87; previous episode x P/N .47; age and previous episode .46
Partial gammas
Age and P/N controlling previous episodes .81
P/N and previous episodes controlling age .32
Age and previous episodes controlling P/N .33

12 Within the psychotic group 81 per cent of those aged between 18 and 39 are in the top two severity categories and 85 per cent of those over 40. There is, on the other hand, some association within the neurotic group: of those under 30, 73 per cent are in the top two categories and 37 per cent of those aged over 30 ($p<.05$). However these figures are interpreted, they cannot explain the association between age and diagnosis by postulating severity as an intervening factor. The proportions at the top two points of the 5-point scale of severity are 73 per cent of those aged 18 to 29, 67 per cent 30 to 39, 77 per cent 40 to 49, and 73 per cent of those 50 and over.

13 Age at first onset was almost always defined by the first contact with medical services – an unsatisfactory measure but the only possible one with our present data. Five patients had a past loss *after* their first episode of psychiatric disturbance and it is possibly misleading to include them. However, results are hardly affected if these losses are excluded: 68 per cent of the most psychotic, 42 per cent of the least psychotic, and 14 per cent of the neurotic patients had a past loss through death ($p<.01$); and none, 10 per cent and 22 per cent respectively, had a past loss by separation ($p<.01$).

14 Although the measure of family history which we did have was almost certainly inadequate, it is perhaps worth recording that when we examined

its relationship with age at first onset it did emerge in the predicted direction: more of the early onset group had a positive family history of mental illness than of the late onset group (p<.05). This history involved not just alcoholism and sociopathy, but also depression. For, of those with depression in either first or second degree relatives, 76 per cent were in the early onset group.

15 We divided the 112 patients into three categories on the basis of criteria derived from the clinical interview. In the first (n=62) the symptomatology was considered to be wholly depressive with little or no anxiety component; in the second (n = 29) there was anxiety accompanying the depression but the intensity was not such that had these anxiety symptoms been present on their own without depressive symptoms, the women would have been considered any more than an example of borderline caseness; in the third group (n = 21) the anxiety symptoms were of such proportions that even in the absence of her depressive symptoms the patient would have been likely to be accepted for psychiatric treatment, for her disabling phobias or her frequent panic attacks.

This categorization might well be criticized for amalgamating under one heading of 'anxiety' diagnoses such as anxiety neurosis (ICD 300.0) and phobic neurosis (ICD 300.2) which are traditionally kept separate. One of the reasons for doing this was the small numbers remaining if this further distinction was made; and there appears to be some justification for this amalgamation in that none of the results presented was substantially changed when further subdivision was attempted contrasting depressions with a phobic anxiety component and those with a free-floating one. Another failing in the categorization was its omission of a specific dating of the anxiety component. For patients and onset cases the depressive component was, by definition, of less than twelve months duration, and we did little analysis with the chronic cases precisely because of this uncertainty about the dating of onset. Among the patients and cases the anxiety component had often been present at a borderline case level of severity or lower at the beginning of the year, but was greatly exacerbated with the onset of the depression. Anecdotally, however, we can report that these anxiety symptoms were often very longstanding, dating from adolescence. At this level a range of problems may arise, for example over the boundary between a trait and a symptom, and the relationship of the former to provoking agents, which our data is not sufficiently detailed to answer.

16 Only 14 per cent of the case anxiety/case depression group were in the more extreme half of the psychotic group on the 17-item discriminant function score, compared with 24 per cent of the case depression/borderline anxiety, and 34 per cent of the case depression alone groups. Conversely 62 per cent of the case anxiety/case depression, 45 per cent of the case depression/borderline anxiety, and 37 per cent of the case depression alone groups were in the two neurotic quartiles. Similarly for the measure of overall severity, 9 per cent of the case anxiety/case depression, 10 per cent of the case depression/borderline anxiety, and 31 per cent of the case depression alone were rated 1; while those with a rating of 3 or under were 42 per cent of the case anxiety/case depression, 31 per cent of the case depression/borderline anxiety, and 19 per cent of the case depression alone.

17 Thirty-eight per cent of the case anxiety/case depression group were in the

young life-stage without children, as compared with 14 per cent of the case depression/borderline anxiety and 17 per cent of the case depression group.

18 The basic tables for these results are:

	focus of health difficulties		
	subject (S)	both S and O	other (O)
patients*			
with anxiety	3	0	7
without anxiety	6	1	4
chronic cases			
with anxiety	3	6	5
without anxiety	4	2	2
chronic borderline cases			
with anxiety	6	1	11
without anxiety	8	0	4

* Patients were all onset, not chronic conditions, by definition. These results apply only to marked difficulties. For cases and borderline cases moderate health difficulties are also included in these tables.

19 Twenty-two of the 39 chronic cases had some sort of moderate or marked health difficulty of more than two years duration. Of these, 20 involved some loss of activity, and of these 14 were subject-focussed and six other-focussed health problems. Among the 32 chronic borderlines with such health difficulties there were 20 with loss of activity involved; again 14 were subject-focussed and 6 other-focussed. Figures were even clearer for onset cases. A similar tendency (for a loss element to be associated with chronicity and focus on the subject) was found for loss of role, although the overall number of health difficulties entailing such a loss was much smaller for each group.

Chapter 15

1 Others have also believed that loss *in itself* is not crucial in the aetiology of depression – for example Gaylin (1968: 16–22).
2 It is perhaps unnecessary to add that our emphasis on the importance of a husband is simply taking cognisance of life in Camberwell as we saw it. At the time of our work serious consideration of alternatives to traditional patterns of marriage were rare. One woman of 28 did live with her husband *and* her lover in the same house and apparently did well; another had had a series of lovers over the previous five years with her husband's approval – but with far less happy consequences. We are convinced for most women in Camberwell these were, at most, very distant fantasies.
3 It has been suggested on various occasions that loss of a parent is not itself as important in the aetiology of depression as the discontinuity and social upheaval that may result. We therefore considered the experience of women in the general population who had lost a mother before 11, dividing

them into 23 who had lost continuous contact with their father at some time soon after the loss of their mothers and sixteen who had maintained a continuous contact with their fathers (or in rare cases another person such as a grandmother who had already been living with them). (For one woman the information was not available.) Discontinuity *per se* did not relate to the development of depression; 30 per cent of those with discontinuous contact were cases compared with 56 per cent of those in continuous contact. Examination of the data from our own *patient* series confirmed this result (and also patients of R.E. Kendell's – see Chapter 14). Though our measure of continuity is crude, it is possible that too much weight has been given in the literature to discontinuity of contact as the crucial aetiological factor as against the loss itself. However, the emphasis on discontinuity is understandable, as it is very highly related to loss of mother before 11. In the general population most experiences of discontinuous contact among those who lost *either* parent before 17 resulted from a loss of a mother before 11 (88 per cent). But it is important to note that nearly half of the losses of mother before 11 were followed by continuous contact, usually with a father. Future research must bear this asymmetry in mind.

4 Personal communication from John Birtchnell, 1977.

5 See Parkes 1972, Chapter 8. There is an increase in mortality among widowers in the first year of bereavement (Young, Benjamin and Wallis, 1963; Rees and Lutkin, 1967) and health may well be affected for as long as two years. The increased mortality (at least in British widowers over 55) seems particularly due to mortality from coronary thrombosis and arteriosclerotic heart disease (Parkes, Benjamin and Fitzgerald, 1969). Two studies have shown deterioration in self-reported health in a considerable proportion of recently widowed women (Marris, 1958; Parkes, 1970); and in England, at least, there is a rise in the number of consultations.

6 The rate of such deaths for the total Camberwell sample is 6.1 per cent, and the proportions involved in a causal effect ('x') are 4.7 per cent for patients and 7.9 per cent for onset cases, compared with 49 and 53 per cent respectively for all severe events.

7 When the wide definition of events is used, including any incident a woman reported as welcome, the number of 'positive' events reported in the first Camberwell series by middle-class women is 1.89 and by working-class women is 1.64 (standardizing for differences in life-stage); the average for onset cases when standardized for life-stage is 2.01 compared with an average of 2.10 for the rest of the sample. The frequency of such events does, however, relate to life-stage, declining over the five life-stage groups: the averages are 3.42, 2.22, 1.96, 1.46 and 1.19. To give some idea of the types of events involved, we have divided them into three broad groups: 'material' (purchases, winning at bingo, etc.), 'achievements' (son passing examinations, learning to crochet, etc.) and 'social' (making a new friend, the birth of a grandchild, taking a holiday, etc.). Thirty-six per cent of 'positive' events involved material possessions, 26 per cent were achievements and 38 per cent were 'social'; there were no class differences in the frequency of the first two categories. However middle-class women mentioned social events more than twice as often – an average of 0.37 per person compared with 0.16 (p<.05).

8 The most comparable study is one carried out by a team at the Institute of Psychiatry who interviewed families of ten-year-old children on the Isle of

Wight and in an inner London borough: 12 per cent of mothers on the Isle of Wight had shown psychiatric disturbance in the 3 months before interview and 28 per cent of those in London – figures quite close to our own for women in that life-stage (Rutter *et al.*, 1975; Rutter and Quinton, 1977).

9 A fuller account of North Uist and these results is given in Brown *et al.* (1977b). See pages 368–72 for a discussion of the differences in anxiety – other conditions.

10 The four other studies do not separate data for men and women. Three give similar results to those just quoted (Beck, Sethi, and Tuthill, 1963; Sethi, 1964; Munro, 1966) and one does not show a difference, although a measure of unsatisfactory family relationships in childhood does relate (Abrahams and Whitlock, 1969). Like us when we used the *total* community series as a comparison group, none of the five studies obtained an association between early loss of a mother or a father and the occurrence of depression as such. As we have explained in chapter 13, we think this may well reflect the number of women currently, let alone formerly, depressed who had also lost a mother who had not been excluded from the comparison group. The study by Sethi (1964) includes loss of a sibling: however the inclusion of non-depressed patients in his 'no or low depression' group confuses the issue of the role of loss in symptom-formation in depression. Two other studies are relevant. Wilson, Alltop, and Buffaloe (1967) found that depressed patients who had lost either parent by death before the age of 16 had an elevated score on the psychotic but not the neurotic scales of the MMPI. A study by Forrest, Fraser and Priest (1965) did not find any difference in childhood bereavement before the age of 15 between a neurotic and psychotic depressed group. The fact that they were a highly selected group of patients taking part in a drug trial may have some bearing.

11 Lichtenberg (1957) has discussed loss and depression in somewhat similar terms and Becker (1974) some cognitive approaches to depression.

12 The severity distribution of the highest point during their episode for the 37 onset cases is 3 = '5' (low), 16 = '4', 15 = '3', 1 = '2' and 2 = '1' (high). We made no attempt to rate cases in the general population as psychotic or neurotic. However, to see whether there was any indication of a similar tendency, we distinguished cases who showed either: (i) early morning waking or (ii) slowness or retardation, symptoms associated with a rating of psychotic on the discriminant function analysis. Fifty-two per cent with one of these symptoms had had a loss by death, compared with 39 per cent of the women with neither symptom. The difference, although in the predicted direction, is not statistically significant.

13 Of the patients 73 per cent (81/111) were on severity points 1 and 2 and of the onset and chronic cases 8 per cent (6/76). This is almost certainly an exaggerated estimate of the difference between the two groups; while cases were interviewed at a random point in time of their disorder, patients were interviewed at the point of their 'admission' which is likely to be the time of greatest severity and disturbance. This is bound to some degree to exaggerate differences in severity.

14 It is the danger of selecting a sample in terms of a dependent variable that is usually discussed (e.g. Blalock, 1961). However, it is perhaps too little recognized that, as a welcome by-product of such a procedure, a crude measure such as 'past loss' can be recognized and isolated. This can be

done just because the selection makes the crude measure valid and sensitive for the particular non-random sub-sample in a way that would not have emerged in a random sample. The shortcoming is that one must live with uncertainty as to whether the results are replicable on a random sample until the indicator has been refined in further research and appropriate theory developed. It is possible to derive a more general principle about the sensitivity of indicators from this. The fact that a measure produces the same results for both a non-random and a random sample offers strong evidence that one is working not only with a valid measure but with a sensitive and accurate one – this holds, for example, for our measures of loss of mother before 11 and for the two provoking agents.

Chapter 16

1 Forty-three per cent (9/21) with all the three and 20 per cent (19/93) of the rest were without such a provoking agent (p<.05).

Chapter 17

1 *John Donne, Complete Poetry and Selected Prose*, 'Devotions Upon Emergent Occasions', XIII (ed. John Hayward), London: The Nonesuch Press, 1932.
2 The basic data are 24/125, 12/125, 2/38, and 2/132 respectively – p<.001. For full details see G. W. Brown and S. Davidson 'Social Class, Psychiatric Disorder of Mother and Accidents to Children' (1978).
3 Experiences in the past are reappraised and the process is triggered by the awareness of approaching and inevitable death. He suggests that endogenous as opposed to the reactive depressions 'may owe their existence to the inner process of life review'. Although no one has so far adequately documented such processes it is important to keep in mind their possible existence (Butler, 1968: 486).
4 For a brilliant and entertaining exposition of the pitfalls of dualistic thought cf. Robert Pirsig's *Zen and the Art of Motorcycle Maintenance* (1976), especially p. 320.

References

Abraham, K. (1911) Notes on the Psychoanalytic Investigation and Treatment of Manic-Depressive Insanity and Allied Conditions. In *Selected Papers on Psycho-Analysis*. London: Hogarth, 1927.

Abrahams, J. J. and Whitlock, F. A. (1969) Childhood Experience and Depression. *British Journal of Psychiatry* 115: 883–88.

Acker, J. (1973) Women and Social Stratification: A Case of Intellectual Sexism. *American Journal of Sociology* 78: 936–45.

Ainsworth, M. D. S. (1967) *Infancy in Uganda; Infant Care and the Growth of Attachment*. Baltimore, Md.: The Johns Hopkins Press.

Ainsworth, M. D. S. and Wittig, B. A. (1969) Attachment and Exploratory Behaviour of One-Year-Olds in a Strange Situation. In B. M. Foss (ed.), *Determinants of Infant Behaviour*, Vol. 4. London: Methuen.

American Psychiatric Association (1965) *Diagnostic and Statistical Manual for Mental Disorders*. Washington: A.P.A.

Andersen, R. and Delliger Kasper, J. (1973) The Structural Influence of Family Size on Children's Use of Physician Services. *Journal of Comparative Family Studies* 4: 116–29.

Aries. P. (1962) *Centuries of Childhood*. London: Cape Publishers.

Arnold, M. B. (1961) *Emotion and Personality, Vol. 1: Psychological Aspects*. London: Cassell.

Ausubel, D. (1961) Personality Disorder Is a Disease. *American Psychologist* 16: 69–74.

Baker, M., Dorzab, J., Winokur, G., and Cadoret, R. (1971) Depressive Disease: Classification and Clinical Characteristics. *Comprehensive Psychiatry* 12: 354–65.

Barraclough, B. M. and Bunch, J. (1973) Accuracy of Dating Parent Deaths: Recollected Dates Compared with Death Certificate Dates. *British Journal of Psychiatry* 123: 573–4.

Bart, P. E. (1974) The Sociology of Depression. In Paul M. Roman and Harrison M. Trice (eds.), *Explorations in Psychiatric Sociology*. Philadelphia: F. A. Davis.

Bartlett, Sir Frederick (1932) *Remembering: A Study of Experimental and Social Psychology.* Cambridge: Cambridge University Press.

Beck, A. T. (1967) *Depression: Clinical, Experimental and Theoretical Aspects.* London: Staples Press.

—— (1971) Cognition, Affect and Psychopathology. *Archives of General Psychiatry 1:* 495–500.

Beck, A. T., Sethi, B. B., and Tuthill, R. W. (1963) Childhood Bereavement and Adult Depression. *Archives of General Psychiatry 9:* 295–302.

Beck, J. C. and Worthen, K. (1972) Precipitating Stress, Crisis Theory, and Hospitalization in Schizophrenia and Depression. *Archives of General Psychiatry 26:* 123–9.

Becker, E. (1964) *The Revolution in Psychiatry.* New York: The Free Press.

Becker, J. (1974) *Depression: Theory and Research.* Washington: V. H. Winston.

Benedek, T. (1938) Adaptation to Reality in Early Infancy. *Psychoananlytic Quarterly 7:* 200–15.

Berg, I. A. (ed.) (1967) *Response Set in Personality Assessment.* Chicago: Aldine Press.

Bernard, J. (1968) The Eudaemonists. In S. Z. Klausner (ed.), *Why Man Takes Chances.* New York: Doubleday.

Berthoud, R. (1976) *The Disadvantages of Inequality.* London: MacDonald and James.

Bettelheim, B. (1967) *The Empty Fortress: Infantile Autism and the Birth of the Self.* New York: The Free Press.

Bibring, E. (1953) Mechanisms of Depression. In P. Greenacre (ed.), *Affective Disorders: Psychoanalytic Contributions to their Study.* New York: International Universities Press.

Birley, J. L. T. and Brown, G. W. (1970) Crises and Life Changes Preceding the Onset or Relapse of Acute Schizophrenia: Clinical Aspects. *British Journal of Psychiatry 116:* 327–22.

Birtchnell, J. (1970a) Early Parent Death and Mental Illness. *British Journal of Psychiatry 116:* 281–8.

—— (1970b) Recent Parent Death and Mental Illness. *British Journal of Psychiatry 116:* 289–97.

—— (1970c) Depression in Relation to Early and Recent Parent Death. *British Journal of Psychiatry 116:* 299–306.

—— (1972) Early Parental Death and Psychiatric Diagnosis. *Social Psychiatry 7:* 202–10.

—— (1975) The Personality Characteristics of Early Bereaved Psychiatric Patients. *Social Psychiatry 10:* 97–103.

Blalock, H. M. (1961) *Causal Inferences in Nonexperimental Research.* Chapel Hill: The University of North Carolina Press.

Bloor, M. (1976) Bishop of Berkeley and the Adenotonsillectomy Enigma. *Sociology 10:* 43–61.

Blumenthal, M. D. (1971) Heterogeneity and Research on Depressive Disorders. *Archives of General Psychiatry 111:* 659–74.

Bornstein, P. E., Clayton, P. J., Halikas, J. A., Maurice, W. L., and Robins, E. (1973) The depression of Widowhood after Thirteen Months. *British Journal of Psychiatry 122:* 561–6.

Boskoff, A. (1971) Process Orientation in Sociological Theory and Research. *Social Forces 50:* 1–11.

Boulton, M. (1977) The Rewards and Frustrations of Motherhood. (Unpublished manuscript)

Bowlby, J. (1951) *Maternal Care and Mental Health. W.H.O. Monograph No. 2.* London: H.M.S.O.

—— (1960) Separation Anxiety. *International Journal of Psycho-Analysis* 41: 1–25.

—— (1961) Processes of Mourning. *International Journal of Psycho-Analysis* 44: 317–40.

—— (1971) *Attachment and Loss 1: Attachment.* Harmondsworth: Pelican Books.

—— (1973) *Attachment and Loss 2: Separation: Anxiety and Anger.* Harmondsworth: Pelican Books.

Brenner, M. H. (1971) Economic Changes of Heart Disease Mortality. *American Journal of Public Health* 61: 606–19.

—— (1975) Trends in Alcohol Consumption and Associated Illnesses, Some Effects of Economic Changes. *American Journal of Public Health* 65: 1279–92.

Breuer, J. and Freud, S. (1895) *Studien über Hysterie.* 1. Auflage. (s. 5–6). Leipzig und Wien: Deuticke.

Briscoe, C. W. and Smith, M. D. (1973) Depression and Marital Turmoil. *Archives of General Psychiatry* 29: 812–17.

Brown, G. W. (1959) Experiences of Discharged Chronic Schizophrenic Mental Hospital Patients in Various Types of Living Group. *Milbank Memorial Fund Quarterly* 37: 101–31.

—— (1974) Meaning, Measurement and Stress of Life Events. In B. S. Dohrenwend and B. P. Dohrenwend (eds.), *Stressful Life Events: Their Nature and Effects.* New York: John Wiley.

Brown, G. W. and Birley, J. L. T. (1968) Crises and Life Changes and the Onset of Schizophrenia. *Journal of Health and Social Behaviour* 9: 203–14.

Brown, G. W. and Davidson, S. (1978) Social Class, Psychiatric Disorder of Mothers and Accidents to Children. *Lancet* (in press).

Brown, G. W. and Rutter, M. (1966) The Measurement of Family Activities and Relationships: A Methodological Study. *Human Relations* 19: 241–63.

Brown, G. W., Birley, J. L. T., and Wing, J. K. (1972) Influence of Family Life on the Course of Schizophrenic Disorders: A Replication. *British Journal of Psychiatry* 121: 241–58.

Brown, G. W., Harris, T. O., and Copeland, J. R. (1977) Depression and Loss. *British Journal of Psychiatry* 130: 1–18.

Brown, G. W., Harris, T. O. and Peto, J. (1973) Life Events and Psychiatric Disorders. Part 2: Nature of Causal Link. *Psychological Medicine* 3: 159–76.

Brown, G. W., Ní Bhrolcháin, M., and Harris, T. O. (1975) Social Class and Psychiatric Disturbance Among Women in an Urban Population. *Sociology* 9: 225–54.

—— (1977) Psychotic and Neurotic Depression. III. Aetiological and Background Factors (unpublished).

Brown, G. W., Bone, M., Dalison, B., and Wing, J. K. (1966) *Schizophrenia and Social Care. Institute of Psychiatry, Maudsley Monograph 17.* London: Oxford University Press.

Brown, G. W., Monck, E. M., Carstairs, G. M., and Wing, J. K. (1962) Influence of Family Life on the Course of Schizophrenic Illness. *British Journal of Preventive and Social Medicine* 16: 55–68.

Brown, G. W., Sklair, F., Harris, T. O., and Birley, J. L. T. (1973) Life Events and Psychiatric Disorders. Part 1: Some Methodological Issues. *Psychological Medicine* 33: 74–87.

Brown, G. W., Davidson, S., Harris, T., Maclean, U., Pollock, S., and Prudo,
    R. (1977) Psychiatric Disorder in London and North Uist. *Social Science and
    Medicine*.
Butler, R. (1968) The Life Review: An Interpretation of Reminiscence in the
    Aged. In B. Neugarten (ed.), *Middle Age and Ageing: A Reader in Social
    Psychology*. Chicago: University of Chicago Press.

Cadoret, R. S., Winokur, G., Dorzab, J., and Baker, M. (1972) Depressive
    Disease: Life Events and Onset of Illness. *Archives of General Psychiatry 26*:
    133–6.
Campbell, D. T. and Stanley, J. C. (1966) *Experimental and Quasi-Experimental
    Designs For Research*. Chicago: Rand McNally & Co. *Reprinted from Handbook
    of Research Teaching* (1963). American Educational Research Association.
Cannel, C. F., Fisher, G., and Bakker, T. (1961) Reporting of Hospitalization in
    the Health Interview Survey. *Health Statistics*, Series D, No. 4. (Reprinted
    in *Vital and Health Statistics*, 1965, Series 2, No. 6.) US Department of
    Health, Education and Welfare. Public Health Service.
Carney, M. W., Roth, M., and Garside, R. F. (1965) The Diagnosis of
    Depressive Syndromes and the Prediction of ECT Response. *British Journal
    of Psychiatry 111*: 659–74.
Cartwright, A. and Jeffreys, M. (1958) Married Women Who Work: Their Own
    and Their Children's Health. *British Journal of Preventive Medicine 12*: 159–72.
Cassel, J. (1974) Psychosocial Processes and 'Stress': Theoretical Formulation.
    International Journal of Health and Services 4: 471–82.
Cioffi, F. (1970) Freud and the Idea of a Pseudo-Science. In R. Borger and F.
    Cioffi (eds.), *Explanation in the Behavioural Sciences*. London: Cambridge
    University Press.
Clayton, P., Desmarais, L. and Winokur, G. (1968) A Study of Normal
    Bereavement. *American Journal of Psychiatry 125*: 168–78.
Clayton, P. J., Halikas, J. A., and Maurice, W. L. (1972) The Depression of
    Widowhood. *British Journal of Psychiatry 120*: 71–7.
Clayton, P. J., Herjanic, M., Murphy, G. E., and Woodruff, R. Jr. (1974)
    Mourning and Depression: Their Similarities and Differences. *Canadian
    Psychiatric Association Journal 19*: 309–12.
Coates, D., Moyer, S., and Wellman, B. (1969) The Yorklea Study of Urban
    Mental Health: Symptoms, Problems and Life Events. *Canadian Journal of
    Public Health 60*: 471–81.
Cobb, S. (1976) Social Support as a Moderator of Life Stress. *Psychosomatic
    Medicine 38*: 300–14.
Cobb, S. and Rose, R. M. (1973) Hypertension/Peptic Ulcer and Diabetes in Air
    Traffic Controllers. *Journal of the American Medical Association 224*: 489–92.
Cobb, S., Schull, W. J., Harburg, E., and Kasl, S. V. (1969) Prologue – The
    Intra-familial Transmission of Rheumatoid Arthritis: An Unusual Study.
    Journal of Chronic Diseases 22: 193–4.
Comstock, G. W. and Helsing, K. J. (1976) Symptoms of Depression in Two
    Communities. *Psychological Medicine 6*: 551–63.
Connolly, J. (1976) Life Events Before Myocardial Infraction. *Journal of Human
    Stress 2*: 3–17.
Cooper, B. (1972) Clinical and Social Aspects of Chronic Neurosis. *Proceedings
    of the Royal Society of Medicine 65*: 509–12.
—— (1976) Psychische Storungen als Reaktion: die Geschichte eines

Psychiatrischen Konzepts. To be published in J. Katschnig (ed.), *Lebens —
Veranderungen und psychische Krankheit.* Munich: Urban & Schwarzgnberg.
Cooper, B. and Sylph, J. (1973) Life Events and the Onset of Neurotic Illness:
An Investigation in General Practice. *Psychological Medicine 3*: 421–35.
Cooper, B., Fry, J., and Kalton, G. (1969) A Longitudinal Study of Psychiatric
Morbidity in a General Practice Population. *British Journal of Preventive and
Social Medicine 23*: 210–17.
Cooper, J. E., Copeland, J. R. M., Brown, G. W., Harris, T., and Gourley, A. J.
(1977) Further Studies on Interviewer Training and Inter-rater Reliability of
the Present State Examination (P.S.E.). *Psychological Medicine 7*: 517–23.
Cooper, J. E., Kendall, R. E., Gurland, B. J., Sharpe, L., Copeland, J. R. M.,
and Simon, R. (1972) *Psychiatric Diagnosis in New York and London. Institute of
Psychiatry, Maudsley Monograph 20.* London: Oxford University Press.
Cosin, B. R., Freeman, C. F., and Freeman, N. H. (1971) Critical Empiricism
Criticized: The Case of Freud. *Journal of Theory of Social Behaviour 1*: 121–51.
Costello, C. G. (1976) *Anxiety and Depression: The Adaptive Emotions.* Montreal:
McGill-Queen's University Press.
Courant, R. and Hilbert, D. (1953) *Methods of Mathematical Physics, Vol. 1.* New
York: Interscience Publishers.

David, M. and Appell, G. (1969) Mother-Child Relations. In J. G. Howells
(ed.), *Modern Perspectives in International Child Psychiatry.* Edinburgh: Oliver
& Boyd.
Davis, F. (1963) *Passage Through Crisis.* Indianapolis: Bobbs-Merril.
Dohrenwend, B. P. (1973) Life Events as Stressors: A Methodological Inquiry.
Journal of Health and Social Behaviour 14: 167–75.
—— (1975) Sociocultural and Social-Psychological Factors in the Genesis of
Mental Disorders. *Journal of Health and Social Behaviour 16*: 365–92.
Dohrenwend, B. P. and Dohrenwend, B. S. (1969) *Social Status and Psychological
Disorder: A Causal Inquiry.* New York: John Wiley.
—— (eds.) (1974a) *Stressful Life Events: Their Nature and Effects.* New York: John
Wiley.
—— (1974b) Psychiatric Disorders in Urban Settings. In G. Caplan (ed.),
*American Handbook of Psychiatry, Vol. II. Child and Adolescent Psychiatry,
Sociocultural and Community Psychiatry.* New York: Basic Books.
Douglas, J. D. (1967) *The Social Meanings of Suicide.* Princeton, N. J.: Princeton
University Press.
Durkheim, E. (1952) *Suicide.* London: Routledge and Kegan Paul.
Dyos, H. J. (1961) *Victorian Suburb: A Study of the Growth of Camberwell.* Leicester
University Press.

Eastwood, M. R. (1972) Psychosomatic Disorders in the Community. *Journal of
Psychosomatic Research 16*: 381–6.
—— (1975) *The Relation Between Physical and Mental Illness.* Toron.): University
Press.
Eastwood, M. R., and Trevelyan, H. (1971) Stress and Coronary Heart
Diseases. *Journal of Psychosomatic Research 15*: 289–92.
Edelston, H. (1943) Separation Anxiety in Young Children: A Study of
Hospital Cases. *Genetic Psychology Monograph 28*: 3–95.
Elinson, J., Padilla, Elena, and Perkins, M. E. (1967) *Public Image of Mental
Health Services.* New York: Mental Health Materials Center, Inc.

Engel, G. L. (1967) A Psychological Setting of Somatic Disease: The 'Giving Up-Given Up Complex'. *Proceedings of the Royal Society of Medicine 60*: 553–5.

Erikson, E. H. (1950) *Childhood and Society*. New York: Norton.

Eversley, D. (1977) Comment. In F. Field (ed.), *Education and the Urban Crisis*. London: Routledge and Kegan Paul.

Eversley, D. and Donnison, D. (1973) *London: Urban Patterns, Problems and Politics*. London: Heinemann.

Eyer, J. (1977) Prosperity as a Cause of Death. *International Journal of Health Services 7*: 125–51.

Fairbairn, W. R. D. (1941) A Revised Psychopathology of the Psychoses and Psychoneuroses. *International Journal of Psycho-Analysis 22*. Reprinted in Fairbairn, W. R. D. (1952) *Psychoanalytic Studies of Personality*. London: Tavistock/Routledge.

—— (1952) *Psychoanalytic Studies of Personality*. London: Tavistock/Routledge.

Farr, W. (1859) *Influence of Marriage on the Mortality of the French People*. London: Savill and Edwards.

Feighner, J. P., Robins, E., Guze, S. B., Woodruff, R. A. Jr., Winokur, G., and Munoz, R. (1972) Diagnostic Criteria for Use in Psychiatric Research. *Archives of General Psychiatry 26*: 56–73.

Fenichel, O. (1945) *The Psychoanalytic Theory of Neurosis*. New York: W. W. Norton.

Field, F. (ed.) (1977) *Education and the Urban Crisis*. London: Routledge and Kegan Paul.

Forrest, A. D., Fraser, R. H., and Priest, R. G. (1965) Environmental Factors in Depressive Illness. *British Journal of Psychiatry 111*: 243–53.

Foulds, G. A. (1973) The Relationship Between the Depressive Illnesses. *British Journal of Psychiatry 122*: 531–33.

Freud, S. (1971) Mourning and Melancholia. In *Collected Papers* Vol. IV. London: Hogarth.

—— (1971) *Introductory Lectures on Psychoanalysis*. London: George Allen and Unwin.

Fried, M. A. (1965) Transitional Functions of Working-Class Communities: Implications for Forced Relocation. In Mildred B. Kantor (ed.), *Mobility and Mental Health*. Springfield, Illinois: Charles C. Thomas.

Frommer, E. A. and O'Shea, G. (1973a) Antenatal Identification of Women Liable to have Problems in Managing their Infants. *British Journal of Psychiatry 123*: 149–56.

—— (1973b) The Importance of Childhood Experience in Relation to Problems of Marriage and Family-Building. *British Journal of Psychiatry 123*: 157–60.

Furman, E. (1974) *A Child's Parent Dies: Studies in Childhood Bereavement*. New Haven: Yale University Press.

Galtung, J. (1967) *Theory and Methods of Social Research*. London: Allen and Unwin.

Garmany, G. (1958) Depressive States: Their Aetiology and Treatment. *British Medical Journal 2*: 341–4.

Garside, R. F., Kay, D. W. K., Wilson, I. C., Deaton, I. D., and Roth, M. (1971) Depressive Syndromes and the Classification of Patients. *Psychological Medicine 1*: 333–8.

Gavron, H. (1966) *The Captive Wife*. Harmondsworth: Penguin Books.

Gaylin, W. (1968) *The Meaning of Despair: Psychoanalytic Contributions to the Understanding of Depression*. New York: Science House, Inc.

Geismer, L. L., Lagay, B., Wolock, I., Gerhart, U. C., and Fink, H. (1972) *Early Supports for Family Life: A Social Work Experiment*. Metuchen, N. J.: The Scarecrow Press.

Ginsberg, S. (1976) Women, Work and Conflict. In N. Fonda and P. Moss (eds.), *Mothers in Employment*. Brunel University.

Goffman, E. (1972) Insanity of Place. In *Relations in Public*. Harmondsworth: Penguin Books.

Goldberg, D. P. (1972) *The Detection of Psychiatric Illness by Questionnaire*. London: Oxford University Press.

Goldberg, D. P. and Blackwell, B. (1970) Psychiatric Illness in General Practice. A Detailed Study Using a New Method of Case Identification. *British Medical Journal ii*: 439–43.

Goldberg, D. P., Cooper, B., Eastwood, R. R., Kedward, H. B., and Shepherd, M. (1970). A Standardized Psychiatric Interview for Use in Community Surveys. *British Journal of Preventive and Social Medicine 24*: 18–23.

Goldberg, D. P., Cooper, B., Eastwood, R. R., Kedward, H. B., and Shepherd, M. (1970). A Standardized Psychiatric Interview for Use in Community Surveys. *British Journal of Preventic and Social Medicine 24*: 18–23.

Goldthorpe, J. H. and Hope, K. (1974) *The Social Grading of Occupations: A New Approach and Scale*. London: Oxford University Press.

Gove, W. R. (1973) Sex, Marital Status and Morality. *American Journal of Sociology 79*: 45–67.

Graham, D. T., Lundry, R. M. and Benjamin, L. S. (1962) Specific Attitudes in Initial Interviews with Patients Having Different 'Psychosomatic' Diseases. *Psychosomatic Medicine 24*: 257–66.

Granville-Grossman, K. L. (1968) the Early Environment of Affective Disorder. In A. Coppen and A. Walk (eds.), *Recent Developments in Affective Disorders*. London: Headley Brothers.

Greer, S. (1964) The Relationship Between Parental Loss and Attempted Suicide: A Control Study. *British Journal of Psychiatry 110*: 698–705.

Greer, S. and Gunn, J. C. (1966) Attempted Suicides from Intact and Broken Parental Homes. *British Medical Journal ii*: 1355–7.

Gruber, H. (1974) *Darwin on Man: A Psychological Study of Scientific Creativity*. London: Wildwood House.

Gruenberg, E. M. A. (1963) A Population Study of Disability from Mental Disorders. *Annals New York Academy of Science 107*: 587–95.

Hagnell, O. (1966) *A Prospective Study of the Incidence of Mental Disorder*. Stockholm: Svenska Bokforlaget Norstedts-Bonniers.

Halbwachs, M. (1930) *Les Causes du Suicide*. Paris: Librairie Felix Alcan.

Hamilton, M. (1960) A Rating Scale for Depression. *Journal of Neurology, Neurosurgery and Psychiatry 23*: 56–61.

Hare, E. H. (1974) The Changing Content of Psychiatric Illness. *Journal of Psychosomatic Research 18*: 283–89.

Hare, E. H. and Shaw, G. K.(1965a) A Study in Family Health: (1) Health in Relation to Family Size. *British Journal of Psychiatry 111*: 461–6.

—— (1965b) *Mental Health on a New Housing Estate. Institute of Psychiatry, Maudsley Monograph 12*. London: Oxford University Press.

Hare, E. H. and Wing, J. K. (1970) (eds.) *An International Symposium: Psychiatric Epidemiology*. London: Oxford University Press.

Harris, T. O. (1976) Social Factors in Neurosis, With Special Reference to Depression. In H. N. van Praag (ed.), *Research in Neurosis*. Amsterdam: Bohn, Scheltema.

Havens, E. M. and Corden Tulley, J. (1972) Female Intergenerational Occupational Mobility: Comparisons of Patterns. *American Sociological Review* 37: 774–7.

Hinde, R. A. (1966) *Animal Behaviour: A Synthesis of Ethology and Comparative Psychology*. Second Edition, 1970. New York: McGraw Hill.

Hinkle, L. E. Jr. (1973) The Concept of 'Stress' in the Biological and Social Sciences. *Science, Medicine, and Man* 1: 31–48.

Hollingshead, A. G. and Redlich, F. C. (1958) *Social Class and Mental Illness*. New York: John Wiley.

Holmes, T. H. and Rahe, R. H. (1967) The Social Readjustment Rating Scale. *Journal of Psychosomatic Research* 11: 213–18.

Hudgens, R. W., Morrison, H. R., and Barchaa, R. G. (1967) Life Events and Onset of Primary Affective Disorders. *Archives of General Psychiatry* 16: 134–45.

Hudgens, R. W., Robins, E., and Delong, W. B. (1970) The Reporting of Recent Stress in the Lives of Psychiatric Patients. *British Journal of Psychiatry* 117: 635–43.

Hughes, C., Tremblay, M. A., Rapoport, R. N., and Leighton, A. H. (1960) *People of Cove and Woodlot*. New York: Basic Books.

Ingham, J. G. and Miller, P. McC. (1976) The Concept of Prevalence Applied to Psychiatric Disorders and Symptoms. *Psychological Medicine* 6: 217–25.

Jacobs, S. C., Prusoff, B. A., and Paykel, E. S. (1974) Recent Life Events in Schizophrenia and Depression. *Psychological Medicine* 4: 444–53.

Jaspers, K. (1962) *General Psychopathology*. Translated by J. Hoenig and M. W. Hamilton. Manchester: Manchester University Press.

Johnstone, A. and Goldberg, D. (1976) Psychiatric Screening in General Practice. *Lancet* i: 605–8.

Kamaroff, A. L., Masuda, M., and Holmes, T. H. (1968) The Social Readjustment Rating Scale: A Comparative Study of Negro, Mexican, and White Americans. *Journal of Psychosomatic Research* 12: 121–8.

Kay, D. W., Garside, R. F., Beamish, P., and Roy, J. R. (1969) Endogenous and Neurotic Syndromes of Depression: A Factor Analytic Study of 104 Cases: Clinical Features. *British Journal of Psychiatry* 115: 377–88.

Kendell, R. E. (1968) *The Classification of Depressive Illnesses. Institute of Psychiatry, Maudsley Monograph 18*. London: Oxford University Press.

—— (1976) The Classification of Depressions: A Review of Contemporary Confusion. *British Journal of Psychiatry* 129: 15–28.

Kendell, R. E., Wainwright, S., Hailey, A., and Shannon, B. (1976) The Influence of Childbirth on Psychiatric Morbidity. *Psychological Medicine* 6: 297–302.

Kessel, W. I. N. (1960) Psychiatric Morbidity in a London General Practice. *British Journal of Preventive and Social Medicine* 14: 16–22.

Kiloh, L. G., and Garside, R. F. (1963) The Independence of Neurotic

Depression and Enodgenous Depression. *British Journal of Psychiatry 109*: 451–63.

Klein, M. (1948) *Contributions to Psychoanalysis 1921–1945*. London: Hogarth.

Komarovsky, M. (1962) *Blue Collar Marriage*. New York: Random House Inc.

Langner, T. S. and Michael, S. T. (1963) *Life Stress and Mental Health*. London: Collier-MacMillan.

Lazarus, R. S. (1966) *Psychological Stress and the Coping Process*. New York: McGraw-Hill.

Lazarsfeld, P. F. and Barton, A. H. (1951) Qualitative Measurement in the Social Sciences: Classification, Typologies, and Indices. In D. Lerner, and H. D. Lasswell, (eds.), *The Policy Sciences*. California: Stanford University Press.

Leff, M. J., Roatch, J. F., and Bunney, W. E. (1970) Environmental Factors Preceding the Onset of Severe Depressions. *Psychiatry 33*: 293–311.

Leighton, A. H. (1959) *My Name is Legion*. New York: Basic Books.

—— (1965) Poverty and Social Change. *Scientific American 212*: 21–27.

Leighton, D. C., Harding, J. S. Macklin, D. B., MacMillan, A. M., and Leighton, A. H. (1963) *The Character of Danger*. New York: Basic Books.

Leighton, D. C., Hagnell, O., Leighton, A. H., Harding, J. S., Kellert, S. R., and Danley, R. A. (1971) Psychiatric Disorder in a Swedish and a Canadian Community: An Exploratory Study. *Social Science and Medicine 5*: 189–209.

Lewis, A. J. (1934) Melancholia: A Clinical Survey of Depressive States. *Journal of Mental Science 80*: 277–378.

—— (1938) States of Depression: Their Clinical and Aetiological Differentiation. *British Medical Journal ii*: 875–8.

—— (1953) Health as a Social Concept. *British Journal of Sociology 4*: 109–124.

Lewis, C. S. (1961) *A Grief Observed*. London: Faber.

Levi, P. (1959) *If This Is a Man*. London: The New English Library.

Lichtenberg, P. (1957) A Definition and Analysis of Depression. *A.M.A. Archives of Neurology and Psychiatry 77*: 519–27.

Lindemann, E. (1944) The Symptomatology and Management of Acute Grief. *American Journal of Psychiatry 101*: 141–8.

Lomas, G. (1975) *The Inner City*. London: London Council of Social Services.

Lorenz, K. (1971) *Studies in Animal and Human Behaviour*, Vol. II. London: Methuen.

Lowenthal, M. F. and Haven, C. (1968) Interaction and Adaptation: Intimacy as a Critical Variable. *American Sociological Review 33*: 20–30.

Lukes, S. (1973) *Emile Durkheim and his Work*. London: Allen Lane.

MacMahon, B. and Pugh, T. F. (1970) *Epidemiology: Principles and Methods*. Boston: Little, Brown & Co.

McCall, G. J. and Simmons, J. L. (1966) *Identities and Interactions*. New York: Free Press.

McHugh, P. (1968) *Defining the Situation. The Organization of Meaning in Social Interaction*. Indianapolis and New York: The Bobbs-Merrill Co.

McKeown, T. (1971) A Historical Appraisal of the Medical Task. In G. McLachlan and T. McKeown (eds.), *Medical History and Medical Care*. Oxford: Oxford University for the Nuffield Provincial Hospitals Trust.

Marris, P. (1958) *Widows and Their Families*. London: Routledge and Kegan Paul.

—— (1974) *Loss and Change*. London: Routledge and Kegan Paul.

Mason, J. W. (1975) A Historical View of the Stress Field. *Journal of Human Stress* 1: 6–12.

Masuda, M. and Holmes, T. H. (1967) The Social Readjustment Rating Scale: A Cross-Cultural Study of Japanese and Americans. *Journal of Psychosomatic Research* 11: 227–37.

Mechanic, D. (1962) *Students Under Stress: A Study in the Social Psychology of Adaptation*. New York: Free Press.

—— (1968) *Medical Sociology: A Selective View*. New York: Free Press.

Mechanic, D. and Newton, M. (1965) Some Problems in the Analysis of Morbidity Data. *Journal of Chronic Diseases* 18: 569–80.

Melges, F. T. and Bowlby, J. (1969) Types of Hopelessness in Psychopathological Process. *Archives of General Psychiatry* 20: 690–9.

Mendels, J. and Weinstein, N. (1972) The Schedule of Recent Experiences: A Reliability Study. *Psychosomatic Medicine* 34: 527–31

Merton, R.K. (1957) *Social Theory and Social Structures*. Revised and enlarged. Glencoe, Illinois: Free Press.

Meyer, R.J. and Haggerty, R.J. (1962) Streptoccocal Infections in Families. *Pediatrics* 29: 539–49.

Mills, C.W. (1959) *The Sociological Imagination*. New York: Oxford University Press.

Moody, R.L. (1946) Bodily Changes During Abreaction. *Lancet* ii: 934–35.

Moore, B. Jr (1972) *Reflections on the Causes of Human Misery*. London: Penguin Press.

Morris, J.N., Chave, S.P.W., Adam, M.B., Sirey, C., Epstein, L., and Sheeham, D.J. (1973) Vigorous Exercise in Leisure Time and the Incidence of Coronary Heart Disease. *Lancet* i: 333–39.

Munro, A. (1966) Parental Deprivation in Depressive Patients. *British Journal of Psychiatry* 122: 443–57.

Navran, L. (1954) A Rationally Derived MMPI Scale to Measure Dependence. *Journal of Consulting Psychology* 18: 192–94.

Ní Bhrolcháin, M. (1977) Psychotic and Neurotic Depression: 1. Some Points of Method (unpublished).

Ní Bhrolcháin, M., Brown, G.W., and Harris, T.O. (1977) Psychotic and Neurotic Depression: II. Clinical Characteristics (unpublished).

Nuckolls, C.B., Cassel, J., and Kaplan, G.H. (1972) Psycho-social Assets, Life Crises and the Prognosis of Pregnancy. *American Journal of Epidemiology* 95: 431–44.

Oakley, A. (1974) *The Sociology of Housework*. Martin Robinson.

Office of Population Censuses and Surveys (OPCS) (1970) *Classification of Occupations*. London: HMSO.

Overall, J.E., Hollister, L.E., Johnson, M., and Pennington, V. (1966) Nosology of Depression and Differential Response to Drugs. *Journal of the American Medical Association* 195: 946–50.

Paffenbarger, R.S. (1964) Epidemiological Aspects of Parapartum Mental Illness. *British Journal of Preventive and Social Medicine* 18 (4): 189–95.

Parad, H.J. and Caplan, G. (1965) A Framework for Studying Families in

Crisis. In J. Parad (ed.), *Crisis Intervention: Selected Readings*. New York: Family Service Association of America.

Parker, J.B., Spielberger, C.D., Wallace, D.K., and Becker, J. (1959) Factors in Manic-Depressive Reactions. *Diseases of the Nervous System 20*: 505–11.

Parkes, C.M. (1964) Recent Bereavement as a Cause of Mental Illness. *British Journal of Psychiatry 110*: 198–204.

—— (1970) 'Seeking' and 'Finding' a Lost Object: Evidence from Recent Studies of the Reaction to Bereavement. *Social Science and Medicine 4*: 187–201.

—— (1971) Psycho-social Transitions: A Field for Study. *Social Science and Medicine 5*: 101–15.

—— (1972) *Bereavement: Studies of Grief in Adult Life*. London: Tavistock.

—— (1973) Factors Determining the Persistence of Phantom Pain in the Amputee. *Journal of Psychosomatic Research 17*: 97–108.

—— (1975) Psycho-social Transitions: Comparison between Reactions to Loss of a Limb and Loss of a Spouse. *British Journal of Psychiatry 127*: 204–10.

Parkes, C.M. and Brown, R.J. (1972) Health after Bereavement. *Psychosomatic Medicine 24*: 449–61.

Parkes, C.M., Benjamin, B., and Fitzgerald, R.G. (1969) Broken Heart: A Statistical Survey of Increased Mortality among Widowers. *British Medical Journal 1*: 740–3.

Parsons, T. (1949) *The Structure of Social Action*. Glencoe: Free Press.

—— (1951) Social Structure and Dynamic Process: The Case of Modern Medical Practice. In *The Social System*. Glencoe: Free Press.

Paykel, E.S. (1971) Classification of Depressed Patients: A Cluster Analysis Derived Grouping. *British Journal of Psychiatry 118*: 278–88.

—— (1973) Life Events and Acute Depression. In J.P. Scott and E.C. Senay (eds.), *Separation and Depression*, Publication 94, American Association for the Advancement of Science, Washington, D.C.

—— (1974) Recent Life Events and Clinical Depression. In E.K.E. Gunderson and R.D. Rahe (eds.), *Life Stress and Illness*. Illinois: Charles C. Thomas.

—— (1977) Contribution of Life Events to Causation of Psychiatric Illness (manuscript).

Paykel, E.S. and Prusoff, B.A. (1973) Response Set and Observer Set in the Assessment of Depressed Patients. *Psychological Medicine 3*: 209–16.

Paykel, E.S. and Uhlenhuth, E.H. (1972) Rating the Magnitude of Life Stress. *Canadian Psychiatric Association Journal* Vol. SS-II: 93–100.

Paykel, E.S., Klerman, G.L., and Prusoff, B.A. (1970) Treatment Setting and Clinical Depression. *Archives of General Psychiatry 22*: 11–21.

Paykel, E.S., Prusoff, B.A., and Klerman, G.L. (1971) The Endogenous-Neurotic Continuum in Depression, Rater Independence and Factor Distributions. *Journal of Psychiatric Research 8*: 73–90.

Paykel, E.S., Prusoff, B.A. and Uhlenhuth, E.H. (1971) Scaling of Life Events. *Archives of General Psychiatry 25*: 340–47.

Paykel, E.S., Myers, J.K., Diendelt, M.N., Klerman, G.L., Lindenthal, J.J., and Pepper, M.P. (1969) Life Events and Depression: A Controlled Study. *Archives of General Psychiatry 21*: 753–60.

Perris, C.A. (1966) A Study of Bipolar (Manic-Depressive) and Unipolar Recurrent Depressive Psychoses. *Acta Psychiatrica Scandinavica 42*: 1–189.

Polani, P.E., Briggs, N.N., Ford, C.E., Clarke, C.M., and Berg, J.M. (1960) A Mongol Girl with 46 Chromosomes. *Lancet i*: 721–24.

Pollitt, J. (1965) *Depression and its Treatment*. London: Heinemann Medical Books.
Popper, K. (1976) *Unended Quest: An Intellectual Autobiography*. London: Fontana/Collins.

Rahe, R.H. (1969) Life Crisis and Health Change. In P.R.A. May and J.R. Winterborn (eds.), *Psychotropic Drug Response: Advances in Prediction*. Springfield, Illinois: C.C. Thomas
Rahe, R.H., Gunderson, E.K.E., and Pugh, W.M. (1972) Illness Prediction Studies. *Archives of Environmental Health 25*: 192–97.
Rees, W.D. and Lutkin, S.G. (1967) Mortality of Bereavement. *British Medical Journal 4*: 1–11.
Reid, I. (1977) *Social Class Differences in Britain*. London: Open Books.
Reiss, E. (1910) Konstitutionelle Verstimmung und Manisch-Depressives. *Irresein, Z. ges. Neurol. Psychiat. Orig. II*: 347.
Richman, N. (1974) The Effects of Housing on Pre-School Children and Their Mothers. *Developmental Medicine and Child Neurology 16*: 53–58.
—— (1976) Depression in Mothers of Pre-School Children *Journal of Child Psychology and Psychiatry 17*: 75–78.
Ritter, K.V. and Hargens, L.L. (1975) Occupational Positions and Class Identifications of Married Working Women: A Test of the Asymmetry Hypothesis. *American Journal of Sociology 80* (4): 934–48.
Robins, L.N. (1966) *Deviant Children Grown Up*. Baltimore: Williams and Wilkins.
Roman, P.M., and Trier, M. (eds.) (1974) *Explorations in Psychiatric Sociology*. Philadelphia: F.A. Davis.
Rosenberg, M. (1968) *The Logic of Survey Analysis*. London: Basic Books.
Rosenstock, I.M. (1966) Why People Use Health Services. *Milbank Memorial Fund Quarterly 3*, Part 2: 94–127.
Roth, M., Gurney, C., Garside, R.F., and Kerr, T.A. (1972) Studies in the Classification of an Affective Disorder. The Relationship of Anxiety and Depressive Illnesses. *British Journal of Psychiatry 121*: 147–61.
Rutter, M.R. (1971) Parent-Child Separation: Psychological Effects on the Children. *Journal of Child Psychology and Psychiatry 12*: 233–60
—— (1972) *Maternal Deprivation Reassessed*. Harmondsworth: Penguin Books.
Rutter, M. and Brown, G.W. (1966) The Reliability of Family Life and Relationships in Families Containing a Psychiatric Patient. *Social Psychiatry 1*: 38–53.
Rutter, M. and Madge, N. (1976) *Cycles of Disadvantage*. London: Heineman.
Rutter, M. and Quinton, D. (1977) Psychiatric Disorder – Ecological Factors and Concepts of Causation. In H. McGurk (ed.), *Ecological Factors in Human Development*. Amsterdam: North Holland.
Rutter, M., Yule, B., Quinton, D., Rowlands, O., Yule, W., and Berger, M. (1975) Attainment and Adjustment in Two Geographical Areas: III. Some Factors Accounting for Area Differences. *British Journal of Psychiatry 126*: 520–33.

Sachar, E.J., MacKenzie, J.M., Binstock, W.A., and Mack, J.E. (1968) Corticosteroid Response to the Psychotherapy of Reactive Depressions. *Psychosomatic Medicine 30*: 23–44.

Sander, L.W. (1962) Issues in Early Mother-Child Interaction. *Journal of the American Academy of Child Psychiatry* 1: 141–66.
—— (1964) Adaptive Relationships in Early Mother-Child Interaction. *Journal of the American Academy of Child Psychiatry* 3: 231–64.
Sargant, W. and Dally, P. (1962) Treatment of Anxiety States by Antidepressant Drugs. *British Medical Journal* i: 6–8.
Scheff, T.J. (1966) *On Being Mentally Ill: A Sociological Theory*. London: Weidenfield and Nicholson.
Schneider, K. (1927) Die abnormen seelischen Reaktionen. In *Handbuch der psychiatrie, Spez. Teil, 7. Abt.* (Hrg. Aschaffenburg, G.). Leipzig and Wien: Deuticke.
Schutz, A. (1954) Concept and Theory Formation in the Social Sciences. *Journal of Philosophy* 51: 257–73. Reprinted in M. Natanson (ed.), *Alfred Schutz: Collected Papers* 1. The Problem of Social Reality, Martin Nijoff, 1962: 48–66. Reprinted in K. Thompson and J. Turnstall (eds.), (1971) *Sociological Perspectives* (1971) Baltimore, Md.: Penguin Books, Part 5, p. 38.
Sedgwick, P. (1973) Illness – Mental and Otherwise. *The Hastings Center* 1: 19–40. Hastings-on-Hudson, New York: Institute of Society, Ethics and the Life Sciences.
Seligman, M.E.P. (1975) *Helplessness: On Depression, Development and Death*. San Francisco: W.H. Freeman.
Selye, H. (1936) *The Stress of Life*. London: Longmans, Green & Co.
Sethi, B.B. (1964) Relationship of Separation to Depression. *Archives of General Psychiatry* 10: 486–95.
Shepherd, M., Cooper, B., Brown, A.C., and Kalton, G. (1966) *Psychiatric Illness in General Practice*. London: Oxford University Press.
Shils, E. (1970) Tradition, Ecology and Institution in the History of Sociology. *Daedalus: Journal of the American Academy of Arts and Sciences* 99: 760–825. The Making of Modern Science: Biographical Studies.
Silverman, C. (1968) *The Epidemiology of Depression*. Baltimore: The Johns Hopkins Press.
Smith, M. Brewster (1974) *Humanizing Social Psychology*. San Francisco: Jossey-Bass.
Sommer, R. (1894) *Diagnostik der Geisteskrankheiten*. Wien & Leipzig: Urban & Schwarzenberg.
Spicer, C.C., Hare, E.H., and Slater, E. (1973) Neurotic and Psychotic Forms of Depressive Illness: Evidence from Age-Incidence in a National Sample. *British Journal of Psychiatry* 123: 535–41.
Srole, L., Langer, T.S., Michael, S.T., Opler, M.K., and Rennie, T.A.C. (1962) *Mental health in the Metropolis*. New York: McGraw Hill.
Stengel, E. (1959) Classification of Mental Disorders. *Bulletin of the World Health Organization* 21: 601–21.
Stott, D.H. (1958) Some Psychosomatic Aspects of Causality in Reproduction. *Journal of Psychosomatic Research* 3: 42–55.
Stromgren, E. (1968) Reactive Psychoses. *Contributions to Psychiatric Epidemiology and Genetics*. Copenhagen: Munksgaard.
Suchman, E. (1967) Appraisal and Implications for Theoretical Development. In S.L. Syme and L.G. Reeder (eds.), Social Stress and Cardiovascular Disease. *Milbank Memorial Fund Quarterly* 45, Part 2: 109–113.
Susser, M. (1973) *Causal Thinking in the Health Sciences*. London: Oxford University Press.

388   Social Origins of Depression

Svendsen, B.B. (1952) Psychiatric Morbidity Among Civilians in Wartime. *Acta Jutlandica 24*, Supplement A. Medical Services 8.
Syme, S.L. (1967) Implications and Future Prospects. *Milbank Memorial Fund Quarterly 16*, No. 2, Part 2.
Szasz, T.S. (1962) *The Myth of Mental Illness*. London: Secker & Warburg.

Taylor, Lord and Chave, S. (1964) *Mental Health and Environment*. London: Longmans.
Thomas, K. (1973) *Religion and the Decline of Magic*. Harmondsworth: Penguin University Books.
Thomson, K. C., and Hendrie, H. C. (1972) Environmental Stress in Primary Depressive Illness. *Archives of General Psychiatry 26*: 130–32.
Tibblin, G. (1971) Risk Factors for Developing Myocardial Infarction and Other Diseases. The 'Men Born in 1913' Study. In G. Tibblin, A. Keys and L. Werkö (eds.), *Preventive Cardiology*. New York: John Wiley.
Tomkins, S.S. (1962) *Affect, Imagery, Consciousness* Vol. I: *The Positive Affects*. London: Tavistock.
—— (1963) *Affect, Imagery, Consciousness* Vol II: *The Negative Affects*. London: Tavistock.
Tuckett, D. (1976) (ed.) *An Introduction to Medical Sociology*. London: Tavistock.

Uhlenhuth, E.H. and Paykel, E.S. (1973) Symptom Configuration and Life Events. *Archives of General Psychiatry 28*: 743–48.

Vaughn, C.E. and Leff, J.P. (1976a) The Influence of Family and Social Factors on the Course of Psychiatric Illness: A Comparison of Schizophrenic and Depressed Neurotic Patients. *British Journal of Psychiatry 129*: 125–37.
—— (1976b) The Measurement of Expressed Emotion in the Families of Psychiatric Patients. *British Journal of Social and Clinical Psychology 15*: 157–65.
Veevers, J.E. (1973) Parenthood and Suicide: An Examination of a Neglected Variable. *Sociology of Science and Medicine 7*: 135–44.

Warheit, G., Holzer, C. III, and Schwab, J. (1973) An Analysis of Social Class and Racial Differences in Depressive Symptom-Aetiology: A Community Study. *Journal of Health and Social Behaviour 4*: 921–99.
Watts, C.A.H. (1966) *Depressive Disorders in the Community*. Bristol: John Wright and Sons.
Webb, E. J., Campbell, D. T., Schwartz, R. D., and Sechrest, L. (1966) *Unobtrusive Measures: Nonreactive Research in the Social Sciences*. Chicago: Rnad McNally.
Weiss, R. (1969) The Fund of Sociability. *Transaction 7*: 36–43.
Weissman, M.M. and Paykel, E.S. (1974) *The Depressed Woman: A Study of Social Relationships*. Chicago: University of Chicago Press.
Westergaard, J., Resler, H. (1976) *Class in a Capitalist Society: A Study of Contemporary Britain*. Hammondsworth: Penguin Books.
Whittet, M.M. (1963) Problems of Psychiatry in the Highlands and Islands. *Scottish Medical Journal 8*: 293–302.
Wilson, I.C., Alltop, L., and Buffaloe, W.J. (1967) Parental Bereavement in Childhood: MMPI Profiles in a Depressed Population. *British Journal of Psychiatry 113*: 761–64.

Wing, J.K. (1973) Social and Familial Factors in the Causation and Treatment of Schizophrenia. *Biochemical Society Specialist Publications I*: 153–63.

Wing, J.K., and Brown, G.W. (1970) *Institutionalism and Schizophrenia*. Cambridge: Cambridge University Press.

Wing, J.K. and Hailey, A.M. (1972) (eds.) *Evaluating a Community Psychiatric Service*. London: Oxford University Press.

Wing, J.K., Cooper, J.E., and Satorius, N. (1974) *The Measurement and Classification of Psychiatric Symptoms: An Instruction Manual for the Present State Examination and CATEGO Programme*. London: Cambridge University Press.

Wing, J.K., Nixon, J.M., Mann, S.A., and Leff, J.P. (1977) Reliability of the PSE (ninth edition) Used in a Population Study (1977). *Psychological Medicine 7*: 505–16.

Winnicott, D.W. (1958) The Capacity To Be Alone. *International Journal of Psycho-Analysis 39*: 416–20. Reprinted in Winnicott, D.W. (1965) *The Maturisational Processes and the Facilitating Environment*. London: Hogarth.

Winokur, G. (1972) Types of Depressive Illness. *British Journal of Psychiatry 120*: 265–66.

Winokur, G., Clayton, P. J., and Keich, T. (1969) *Manic Depressive Illness*. C.V. Mosby

Woodruff, R.A., Guze, S., and Clayton, P. (1971) Unipolar and Bipolar Affective Disorder. *British Journal of Psychiatry 119*: 33–38.

Young, M., Benjamin, L., and Wallis, C. (1963) The Mortality of Widowers. *Lancet ii*: 454–56.

Ziehen, T. (1894) *Psychiatrie fur Arzte und Studirende*. Berlin: Wreden.

Zigler, E. and Phillips, L. (1961) Psychiatric Diagnosis: A Critique. *Journal of Abnormal and Social Psychology 63*: 607–18.

Zung, W.W.K. (1965) A Self-rating Depression Scale. *Archives of General Psychiatry 12*: 63–70.

Index